Intuitive Biostatistics

Intuitive Biostatistics

A Nonmathematical Guide to Statistical Thinking

HARVEY MOTULSKY, M.D.

GraphPad Software, Inc.
hmotulsky@graphpad.com

COMPLETELY REVISED

SECOND EDITION

New York   Oxford

OXFORD UNIVERSITY PRESS

2010

Oxford University Press, Inc., publishes works that further Oxford University's
objective of excellence in research, scholarship, and education.

Oxford   New York
Auckland   Cape Town   Dar es Salaam   Hong Kong   Karachi
Kuala Lumpur   Madrid   Melbourne   Mexico City   Nairobi
New Delhi   Shanghai   Taipei   Toronto

With offices in
Argentina   Austria   Brazil   Chile   Czech Republic   France   Greece
Guatemala   Hungary   Italy   Japan   Poland   Portugal   Singapore
South Korea   Switzerland   Thailand   Turkey   Ukraine   Vietnam

Published by Oxford University Press, Inc.
198 Madison Avenue, New York, New York 10016
http://www.oup.com

ISBN: 978-0-19-973006-3

Printing number: 9 8 7 6 5 4 3 2 1

Printed in the United States of America
on acid-free paper

BRIEF CONTENTS

CONTENTS

PREFACE

My approach in this book is informal and brisk (at least I hope
it is), not ceremonious and plodding (at least I hope it isn't).

JOHN ALLEN PAULOS (2008)

Intuitive Biostatistics provides a comprehensive overview of statistics without
getting bogged down in the mathematical details. In the fourteen years since the
first edition was published, many readers have contacted me. I've been gratified
to learn that people found my approach refreshing and useful. Some scientists
have told me that statistics had always been baffling until they read *Intuitive
Biostatistics*. This enthusiasm encouraged me to (finally!) write a second edition.

Who is this book for?

I wrote *Intuitive Biostatistics* for three audiences:

- Medical (and other) professionals who want to understand the statistical
  portions of journals they read. These readers don't need to analyze any data,
  but they do need to understand analyses published by others. I've tried to
  explain the big picture, without getting bogged down in too many details.
- Undergraduate and graduate students, post-docs, and researchers who
  will analyze data. This book explains general principles of data analysis,
  but it won't teach you how to do statistical calculations, or how to use any
  particular statistical program. It makes a great companion to the more
  traditional statistics texts and to the documentation of statistical software.
- Scientists who consult with statisticians. Statistics often seems like a
  foreign language, and this text can serve as a phrase book to bridge the gap
  between scientists and statisticians. Sprinkled throughout the book are
  "Lingo" sections that explain statistical terminology and point out when
  ordinary words are given very specialized meanings (the source of much
  confusion).

I wrote *Intuitive Biostatistics* to be a guidebook, not a cookbook. The focus
is on how to interpret statistical results, rather than how to analyze data. This
book presents few details of statistical methods and only a few tables required to
complete the calculations.

If you like to think with equations and prefer to learn by following mathematical logic, you have plenty of statistics texts to choose from. This book is for the many students and scientists who find math confusing and prefer verbal explanations. This book does not provide any mathematical proofs or derivations and only includes a few equations to help make concepts clear.

What makes the book unique?

I included many topics often omitted from short introductory texts, including:

- The need for statistical rigor. Chapter 1 shows how often our intuitions can lead us to make incorrect conclusions. This fun chapter explains how common sense can lead you astray and explains the need for statistical thinking.
- Multiple comparisons. It is simply impossible to understand statistical results without a deep understanding of how to think about multiple comparisons. This isn't just a practical issue, but almost a philosophical issue in analyzing data. Chapters 22, 23, and 40 are devoted to this topic. I explain several approaches used to deal with multiple comparisons, including the False Discovery Rate (FDR).
- Nonlinear regression. In many fields of science, nonlinear regression is used more often than linear regression, but most introductory statistics books ignore nonlinear regression completely. This book gives them equal weight. Chapters 34 and 35 set the stage by explaining the concept of fitting models to data and comparing alternative models. Chapter 36 then discusses nonlinear regression.
- Bayesian logic. Bayesian thinking is briefly explained in Chapter 18 as a way to interpret a P value (or a conclusion of statistical significance) in context. This topic returns in Chapter 42, which compares interpreting statistical significance to interpreting the results of clinical laboratory tests.
- Lognormal distributions. These are commonly found in scientific data, but not in statistics books. They are explained in Chapter 11 and are touched upon again in several examples that occur in later chapters. Logarithms and antilogarithms are reviewed in Appendix E.
- Testing for equivalence. Sometimes the goal is not to prove that two groups differ, but rather to prove they are the same. This requires a different mindset, as explained in Chapter 21.
- Normality tests. Many statistical tests assume data are sampled from a Gaussian (also called 'Normal') distribution, and normality tests are used to test this assumption. Chapter 24 explains why these are less useful than many hope.
- Outliers. Values far from the other values are called outliers. Chapter 25 explains how to think about outliers.

- Modern statistical methods. Computer-intensive methods, including resampling and bootstrap, are becoming more popular and this book provides a very brief introduction.
- Model comparison. Statistical hypothesis testing is usually viewed as a way to test a null hypothesis. Chapter 35 explains an alternative way to view statistical hypothesis testing, as a way to compare the fits of alternative models.
- Multiple regression traps. An overview of the many ways that multivariable analyses can be misleading is presented in Chapter 38.
- Detailed review of assumptions and common mistakes. All analyses are based on a set of assumptions, and many chapters discuss these assumptions in depth. This book also provides an in-depth discussion of common mistakes and misunderstandings.

To make space for those topics, I have left out many topics that are traditionally included in introductory texts:

- Probability. I assume that you have at least a vague familiarity with the ideas of probability, and this book does not explain these principles.
- Equations needed to compute statistical tests. I assume that you will either be interpreting data analyzed by others, or using statistical software to run statistical tests. In only a few places do I give enough details to compute the tests by hand.
- Statistical tables. If you aren't going to be analyzing data by hand, there is very little need for statistical tables. I include only a few tables in places where it might be useful to do simple calculations by hand.
- Statistical distributions. You can choose statistical tests and interpret the results without knowing much about z, t and F distributions. This book mentions them, but with very little depth.

How is the second edition different than the first?

Though the spirit of the first edition remains, very few of its words do. It is hard to explain what is new in this edition, since I essentially rewrote the entire book. If you own the first edition and wonder whether this edition is different enough to justify buying it, the answer is yes! I have added new chapters, expanded coverage of some topics that were only touched upon in the first edition, and reorganized everything.

New and expanded topics include:

- Chapter 1 explains how our intuitions can lead us astray in issues of probability and statistics.
- Chapter 11 (and later examples) highlights the fact that lognormal distributions are common.
- Chapter 21 explains the idea of testing for equivalence vs. testing for differences.

- Chapters 22, 23, and 40 discuss the pervasive problem of multiple comparisons.
- Chapters 24 and 25 discuss testing for normality and for outliers.
- Chapter 35 shows how to think about statistical hypothesis testing as comparing the fits of alternative models.
- Chapters 37 and 38 give expanded coverage of the usefulness—and traps—of multiple, logistic, and proportional hazards regression.

The first edition had problems at the end of each chapter. This second edition does not. Instead, it offers three new ways to review concepts and put them into practice:

- New "Q and A" sections review important concepts in a question-and-answer format.
- Chapter 46 is a new review chapter (inspired by, and written with, Bill Greco, SUNY Buffalo). It discusses a single example in great length—with many detours—as a way to review many statistical concepts, identify commonly made mistakes, and examine frequent sources of confusion and doubt that arise in analysis and interpretation of results.
- Chapter 47 is a new chapter that presents 49 multipart problems, with answers in Chapter 48. These problems require little calculation and emphasize statistical concepts.

Which chapters are essential?

If you don't have time to read this entire book, read these 18 chapters to learn the essential concepts of statistics:

1. Statistics and Probability Are Not Intuitive
3. From Sample to Population
4. Confidence Interval of a Proportion
9. Quantifying Scatter
10. The Gaussian Distribution
12. Confidence Interval of a Mean
14. Error Bars
15. Introducing P Values
16. Statistical Significance and Hypothesis Testing
17. Relationship Between Confidence Intervals and Statistical Significance
18. Interpreting a Result That Is Statistically Significant
19. Interpreting a Result That Is Not Statistically Significant
20. Statistical Power
22. Multiple Comparisons Concepts
23. Multiple Comparison Traps
34. Fitting Models to Data
44. Statistical Advice
46. Capstone Example

Who helped?

A huge thanks to the many people who reviewed draft chapters of the second edition:

David Airey, Vanderbilt University
William (Matt) Briggs, New York Methodist Hospital
Peter Chen, University of California, San Diego
Cynthia J Coffman, Duke University
Vincent DeBari, Seton Hall University
Jacek Dmochowski, University of North Carolina, Charlotte
Jim Ebersole, Colorado College
Gregory Fant, George Mason Law School
Joe Felsenstein, University of Washington
Joshua French, Colorado State University
Phillip Ganter, Tennessee State University
Steven Grambow, Duke University
William Greco, SUNY, Buffalo
John Hayes, Pacific University
Laurence Kamin, Benedictine University
Eliot Krause, Seton Hall University
James Leeper, University of Alabama
Yulan Liang, University of Maryland
Longjian Liu, Drexel University
Lloyd Mancl, University of Washington
Sheniz Moonie, University of Nevada
Lawrence "Doc" Muhlbaier, Duke University
Pamela Ohman-Strickland, Rutgers University
Lynn Price, Quinnipac University
Soma Roychowdhury, University of California, Davis
Andrew Schaffner, Cali Polytech State University, San Luis Obispo
Arti Shankar, Tulane University
Patricia A Shewokis, Drexel University
Jennifer Shook, Pennsylvania State University
Sumihiro Suzuki, University of North Texas Health Science Center
Jimmy Walker, Star Training
Paul Weiss, Emory College
Dustin White, Colorado State University
Bill Wimley, Tulane University
Gary Yellen, Harvard University

And a special thanks to the first-edition reviewers: Jan Agosti, Cedric Garland, Ed Jackson, Arno Motulsky, Paige Searle, Christopher Sempos, and Harry Frank, as well as Jeanette Ruby, M.D., who provided extensive help with last minute editing.

I would also like to express appreciation to everyone at Oxford Press: Jason Noe, Senior Editor; Melissa Rubes, Editorial Assistant; Patrick Lynch, Editorial Director; John Challice, Publisher and Vice President; Adam Glazer, Director of Marketing; Preeti Parasharami, Product Manager; Steven Cestaro, Production Director; Miriam Sicilia, Production Editor; Paula Schlosser, Art Director; and Dan Niver and Binbin Li, Designers.

Who am I?

After graduating from medical school and completing an internship in internal medicine, I switched to research in receptor pharmacology (and published over 50 peer-reviewed articles). While I was on the faculty of the Department of Pharmacology at the University of California, San Diego, I was given the job of teaching statistics to first year medical students and to graduate students. The syllabus for those courses grew into the first edition of this book.

I hated creating graphs by hand, so I created some programs to do it for me! I also created some simple statistics programs after realizing that the existing statistical software, while great for statisticians, was overkill for most scientists. These efforts constituted the beginnings of GraphPad Software, Inc., which has been my full-time endeavor for many years (Appendix A). In this role I email with students and scientists almost daily, making me acutely aware of the many ways that statistical concepts can be confusing or misunderstood.

I have organized this book in a unique way, but none of the ideas are particularly original. All of the statistical methods are standard and have been discussed in many texts. I include references for some concepts that are not widely known, but don't provide citations for methods that are in common usage.

Please email me with your comments, corrections, and suggestions for the next edition. I'll post errata and chapter notes at www.intuitivebiostatistics.com.

Harvey Motulsky
hmotulsky@graphpad.com
November 2009

ABBREVIATIONS

Abbreviation	Definition	Chapter where defined
α (alpha)	Significance level	4
CI	Confidence interval	16
df	Degrees of freedom	9
n	Sample size	4
SD or s	Standard deviation	9
SE	Standard error	14
SEM	Standard error of the mean	14
P	P value	15
r	Correlation coefficient	32
W	Margin of error	12

Intuitive Biostatistics

PART A

Introducing Statistics

CHAPTER 1

Statistics and Probability Are Not Intuitive

> If something has a 50% chance of happening, then 9 times out of 10 it will.
>
> YOGI BERRA

The word intuitive *has two meanings. One meaning is "easy to use and understand." That is my goal for this book, hence its title. The other meaning is "instinctive, or acting on what one feels to be true even without reason." Using this definition, statistical reasoning is far from intuitive. This fun (really!) chapter demonstrates how our instincts often lead us astray when dealing with probabilities.*

WE TEND TO JUMP TO CONCLUSIONS

A 3-year-old girl told her male buddy, "You can't become a doctor; only girls can become doctors." To her this made sense, because the three doctors she knew were all women.

When my oldest daughter was 4, she "understood" that she was adopted from China, whereas her brother "came from Mommy's tummy." When we read her a book about a woman becoming pregnant and giving birth to a baby girl, her reaction was, "That's silly. Girls don't come from Mommy's tummy. Girls come from China." With n = 1 in each group, she made a general conclusion. When new data contradicted that conclusion, she questioned the accuracy of the new data rather than the validity of her conclusion.

The ability to generalize from a sample to a population is hard wired into our brains and has even been observed in 8-month-old babies (Xu & Garcia, 2008).

Scientists need statistical rigor to avoid giving in to the impulse to make overly strong conclusions from limited data.

WE TEND TO BE OVERCONFIDENT

Sometimes the phrase "90% confident" is not a result of a statistical calculation, but rather a way to quantify a subjective feeling of uncertainty. How good are people at judging how confident they are? You can test your own ability to quantify uncertainty using a test devised by Russo and Schoemaker (1989). Answer each of these questions with a range that you are 90% confident contains the correct answer. Don't use Google to find the answer. Don't give up and say you don't know. Of course you don't know the answers precisely! The goal is not to provide correct answers, but rather to correctly quantify your uncertainty and come up with ranges of answers that you think are 90% likely to include the true answer. If you have no idea, answer with a superwide interval. For example, if you truly have no idea at all about the answer to the first question, answer with the range 0 to 120 years old, which you can be 100% sure includes the true answer. But try to narrow your responses to each of these questions to a range that you are 90% sure contains the right answer:

- Martin Luther King Jr.'s age at death
- Length of the Nile river, in miles or kilometers
- Number of countries in OPEC
- Number of books in the Old Testament
- Diameter of the moon, in miles or kilometers
- Weight of an empty Boeing 747, in pounds or kilograms
- Year Mozart was born
- Gestation period of an Asian elephant, in days
- Distance from London to Tokyo, in miles or kilometers
- Deepest known point in the ocean, in miles or kilometers

Compare your answers with the correct answers listed at the end of this chapter. If you meet the goal of being 90% confident, you will have created nine intervals that include the correct answer and one that excludes it.

Russo and Schoemaker (1989) tested more than 1,000 people and reported that 99% of them were overconfident. Almost everyone was too confident and answered with narrow ranges that miss the correct answer far more than 10% of the time. The goal was to create ranges that were correct 90% of the time, but most people created ranges that were too narrow and included only 30 to 60% of the correct answers. Similar studies have been done with experts estimating facts in their areas of expertise, and the results are similar.

These results emphasize that you must distinguish computed confidence from informal confidence intervals that are informal guesstimates (even from an expert).

WE SEE PATTERNS IN RANDOM DATA

Most basketball fans believe in "hot hands"—that players occasionally have streaks of successful shots. People think that once a player has successfully made a shot, he is more likely to make the next shot, and that clusters of successful shots will happen more often than predicted by chance.

Gilovich (1985) analyzed data from the Philadelphia 76ers during the 1980–1981 basketball season. Players and fans both strongly agreed that a player

```
– – X – X – X X X – – – – X X X – X X – X X – – – X X – – – X X
X – – X – X X – – X X – – X – X – X – – – X X X X – – X X – – –
X X X X – X X – X – X – X X X – – – – – X – X – X X X – – – – X
– X – X – – X X – X X – X X – – X X X X – – – – X X – X – X – –
– X – X – X X – – – X X – – – – – X – X – X – – X – – X – X X
– – X X X – X – X – – – X X X X – X X X X – – – – – – X X – X X X
X – – X X – – X X X X – X X X – – X – – X X X X X – X X X – – –
X – X – – – X X X X X – – X X – X X – X X X – X X – X – – X – X
X X X – – X X X X X – X – X – X X – X – X X X X – X X – X X X X
– – – X X X – – X X X – X X X – – X – – X – – X – X X X X X – – – X –
```

Table 1.1. Random patterns don't seem random.

Table 1.1 represents 10 basketball players (1 per row) shooting 30 baskets each. An "X" represents a successful shot, and a "–" represents a miss. Is this pattern random? Or does it show signs of nonrandom streaks? Most people tend to see patterns, but in fact the arrangement is entirely random. Each spot in the table had a 50% chance of having an "X."

was more likely to make a shot after making the last one than after missing it, and more likely to miss a shot after missing the prior shot. The data clearly show this is not the case. Additionally, the number of streaks of four, five, or six successful shots in a row was no larger than predicted by chance. The sequence of successes and failures was entirely random, yet almost everyone saw patterns.

Table 1.1 demonstrates the problem. Table 1.1 presents simulated data from 10 basketball players (1 per row) shooting 30 baskets each. An "X" represents a successful shot and a "–" represents a miss. Is this pattern random? Or does it show signs of nonrandom streaks? Look at Table 1.1 before continuing.

Most people see patterns. It just doesn't seem random.

In fact, Table 1.1 was generated randomly. Each spot had a 50% chance of being "X" (successful shot) and 50% chance of being "–" (not successful), without taking into consideration previous shots. The pattern is entirely random, as if it were the result of flipping a coin.

Although I know that the arrangement is entirely random, I can't help but see patterns. The X's *seem* to cluster together more than expected by chance alone, although they really don't. Our brains evolved to find patterns and do so very well. Too well! Statistical rigor is needed to avoid being fooled by apparent patterns among random data.

It is important that we recognize this built-in handicap. Our brains tend to find patterns among random data, so statistical methods are needed to make correct conclusions. Conversely, this makes it impossible to informally generate random numbers or assign subjects randomly to treatments. Attempts at informal randomization never have long enough runs of the same value. If you want random numbers, don't make them up. Flip a coin, throw dice, or use a computer program.

WE DON'T REALIZE THAT COINCIDENCES ARE COMMON

In November 2008, I attended a dinner for the group Conservation International. The actor Harrison Ford is on their board, and I happened to notice that he wore an ear stud. The next day, I watched an episode of the TV show *Private Practice*, and one character pointed out that another character had an ear stud that looked just like Harrison Ford's. The day after that, I happened to read (in a book on serendipity!) that the Nobel prize-winning scientist Baruch Blumberg looks like Indiana Jones, a movie character played by Harrison Ford (Meyers, 2007).

What is the chance that this set of coincidences would happen? Tiny. But that doesn't mean much. It is very unlikely that any particular coincidence will occur. But it is very likely that some astonishing set of unspecified events will occur. That is why remarkable coincidences are always noted in hindsight and never predicted with foresight.

WE HAVE INCORRECT INTUITIVE FEELINGS ABOUT PROBABILITY

Imagine that you can choose between two bowls of jelly beans. The small bowl has 9 white and 1 red jelly bean. The large bowl has 93 white beans and 7 red beans. Both bowls are well mixed, and you can't see the beans. Your job is to pick 1 bean. You win a prize if your bean is red. Should you pick from the small bowl or the large one?

When you choose from the small bowl, you have a 10% chance of picking a red jelly bean. When you pick from the large bowl, the chance of picking a red one is only 7%. So clearly, your chances of winning are higher if you choose from the small bowl. Yet, about two-thirds of people prefer to pick from the larger bowl (Denes-Raj & Epstein, 1994). Many of these people do the math and know that the chance of winning is higher with the small bowl, but they feel better about choosing from the large bowl, because it has more red beans, and offers more chances to win. Of course, it also has more white beans and more chances to lose. Our brains simply are not evolved to deal with probability sensibly, and most people make the illogical choice.

Another example: Many people rated cancer as riskier when it was described as killing 1,286 of 10,000 people than when it was described as killing 24.14 of 100 people, although the latter is double the risk (Yamagishi, 1997).

WE AVOID THINKING ABOUT AMBIGUOUS SITUATIONS

Imagine that you have to choose between two urns. The first urn contains exactly 50 red jelly beans and 50 black jelly beans, randomly mixed together. The second urn also contains 100 jelly beans. Some are red and some are black, but you don't know how many of each. You can reach in and pick a jelly bean at random, but can't see a bean until you choose it. You will win a prize if you happen to pick a red jelly bean, and can choose which urn to select from. Which urn should you choose from?

Now the rules change, and you will win a prize if you happen to pick a black bean. Which urn should you choose from?

Almost everyone chooses the first urn in both cases (Ellsberg, 1961). There is nothing in the problem that tells you whether there are more red jelly beans or more black ones in the second urn, so you are equally likely to pick either. Yet almost everyone prefers to choose from the first urn.

Choosing from the first urn requires that you think about probability—the chance of randomly picking from a 50:50 mixture of red and black jelly beans. Choosing from the second urn is more complicated because it combines ambiguity (you simply don't know whether it contains more red jelly beans, more black ones, or an equal number of each) and probability. Thinking about the second urn makes us feel uncomfortable. Use of functional magnetic-resonance imaging to map blood flow in the brain demonstrates that different parts of the brain deal with risk (probability) and ambiguity. When one thinks about an ambiguous situation (analogous to the second urn above), activity in the fear center in the amygdala increases and activity in the reward center in the caudate decreases (Hsu, Bhatt, Adolphs, Tranel, & Camerer, 2005). Our brains don't like thinking about ambiguous situations, and this prevents us from logically comparing the two situations.

WE FIND IT HARD TO COMBINE PROBABILITIES

Here is a classic brain teaser called the Monty Hall problem, named after the host of a game show. You are a contestant on a game show and are presented with three doors. Behind one is a fancy new car. Behind the others are worthless prizes. You must choose one door and you get to keep whatever is behind it. You pick a door. At this point, the host chooses one of the other two doors to open and shows you that there is no car behind it. He now offers you the chance to change your mind and choose the other door (the one he has not opened).

Should you switch?

Before reading on, you should think about the problem and decide whether you should switch. There are no tricks or traps. Exactly one door has the prize; all doors appear identical; the host (who knows which door leads to the new car) has a perfect poker face and gives you no clues. There is never a car behind the door the moderator chooses to open. Don't cheat. Think it through before continuing.

When you first choose, there are three doors and each is equally likely to have the car behind it. So your chance of picking the winning door is one third. Let's separately think through the two cases—originally picking a winning door or originally picking a losing door.

If you originally picked the winning door, then neither of the other doors has a car behind it, and the host opens one of these. If you switch, you'll switch to the other losing door.

What happens if you originally picked a losing door? In this case, one of the remaining doors has a car behind it and one doesn't. The host knows which door the car is behind and opens the other one. This means that the remaining closed door must be the winning door. If you originally picked one of the two wrong doors, then switching will certainly lead you to win.

Let's recap. If you originally chose the correct door (which has a one-third chance), then switching will make you lose. If you originally picked either of the two losing doors (which has a two-thirds chance), then switching will definitely make you win. Switching from one losing door to the other losing door is impossible, because the host will have opened the other losing door.

Your best choice is to switch! Of course, you can't be absolutely sure that switching doors will help. One-third of the time you will be switching away from the prize. But the other two-thirds of the time you will be switching to the prize. If you repeat the game many times, you will win twice as often by switching doors every time. If you only get to play once, you have twice the chance of winning by switching doors.

Almost everyone (including mathematicians and statisticians) intuitively reaches the wrong conclusion and thinks that switching won't be helpful (Vos Savant, 1997). It is very hard to simultaneously think through two (or more) parallel tracks.

WE DON'T DO BAYESIAN CALCULATIONS INTUITIVELY

Imagine this scenario. You are screening blood samples for the presence of human immunodeficiency virus (HIV). The prevalence of HIV is quite low (0.1%) among the selected donors. The antibody test is quite accurate, but not quite perfect. It correctly identifies 99% of infected blood samples, but also incorrectly concludes that 1% of noninfected samples have HIV. When this test identifies a blood sample as having HIV present, what is the chance that the donor does, in fact, have HIV, and what is the chance the test result is an error (false positive)?

Try to come up with the answer before reading on.

Let's imagine that 100,000 people are tested. Of these, 100 (0.1%) will have HIV, and the test will be positive in 99 (99%) of them. The other 99,900 people do not have HIV, but the test will incorrectly return a positive result in 1% of cases. So there will be 999 false-positive tests. Altogether there will be 99 + 999 = 1,098 positive tests and only 99/1,098 = 9% will be true positives. The other 91% of the positive tests will be false positives. So if a test is positive, there is only a 9% chance that there is HIV in that sample.

Most people, including most physicians, intuitively think that a positive test almost certainly means that HIV is present. Our brains are not wired to combine what we already know (the prevalence of HIV) with the new knowledge (the test is positive).

If the same test is used in a different situation, the results would be different. Imagine the same test is used in a population of IV-drug users in which you expect the prevalence of HIV to be 10%. Again, let's imagine that 100,000 people are tested. Of these, 10,000 (10%) will have HIV, and the test will be positive in 9,900 (99%) of them. The other 90,000 people do not have HIV, but the test will incorrectly return a positive result in 1% of cases. So there will be 900 false-positive tests. Altogether there will be 9,900 + 900 = 10,800 positive tests and 9,900/10,800 = 92% will be true positives. The other 8% of the positive tests will be false positives. So if a test is positive, there is a 92% chance that there is HIV in that sample.

The interpretation of the test result depends greatly on the prevalence of the disease. To reach the correct conclusion, one must combine a baseline frequency with new data. This example gives you a taste of what is called Bayesian logic (which will be discussed more thoroughly in Chapter 18).

WE ARE FOOLED BY MULTIPLE COMPARISON

Austin, Mamdani, Juurlink, and Hux (2006) "mined" a database of health statistics of 10 million residents of Ontario, Canada. They examined 223 different reasons for hospital admission and tested each to see whether it occurred more often in people born under each astrological sign. Seventy-two diseases (reasons for hospital admission) occurred statistically significantly more frequently in one astrological sign than in all the others put together. This means that in each of those 72 cases, the results would occur by chance alone less than 5% of the time (you'll learn more about what "statistical significance" means later in this book).

Sounds impressive, doesn't it? Makes you think that there really is some relationship between astrology and health. But the study wasn't really done to investigate any association between astrological sign and disease; rather, it was done as a warning about the difficulties of interpreting statistical results when many comparisons are performed.

It is misleading to focus on the strong associations between one disease and one astrological sign without considering the others. Austin et al. (2006) examined 223 different reasons for hospital admissions and asked whether each occurred more often in each of 12 astrological signs. Therefore, they made 223 × 12 = 2,676 distinct comparisons. If there truly is no association between astrological sign and disease (and there is no reason to think there is), you'd expect that just by chance, 5% of these comparisons would have P values less than 0.05. Because 5% of 2,676 = 134, one would expect to find about 134 significant associations just by chance. So it is hardly impressive that they found 72 significant associations. That's fewer significant results than you'd expect to find purely by chance.

One of the comparisons was truly striking. People born under the sign of Taurus had 27% more admissions for diverticulitis of the colon. The chance of observing this large a difference in incidence rates by chance alone is 0.0006. This means that if there truly were no association between diverticulitis and being born under the sign of Taurus, the chance of seeing such a striking difference in hospital admissions rates, by chance alone, is 0.06%.

This sounds impressive. Could it be real?

By chance alone, you'd expect to see a P value less than 0.0006 in 1 of 1,667 comparisons (1/0.0006). Since these investigators made nearly 3,000 comparisons of different diseases with different astrological signs, a P value less than 0.0006 is not surprising. You expect such a small P value purely based on chance.

Our brains evolved to spot patterns and are good at it. So we notice when a particular disease is more frequent among those born under a particular astrological sign. It doesn't seem natural to correct for multiple comparisons, but this is essential if you don't want to be fooled by chance associations.

Chapters 22 and 23 explore multiple comparisons in more depth.

WE TEND TO IGNORE ALTERNATIVE EXPLANATIONS

Imagine this scenario (adapted from Bausell, 2007). You are doing a study of acupuncture for osteoarthritis. Patients who come in with severe arthritis pain are treated with acupuncture. They are asked to rate their arthritis pain before and after the treatment. The pain decreases in most patients, but statistical calculations show that such consistent findings are exceedingly unlikely to happen by chance. Therefore, the acupuncture must have worked. Right?

Not really. The decrease in recorded pain may not be caused by the acupuncture. Here are five alternative explanations:

- Placebos reduce pain considerably. If the patients believe in the therapist and treatment, that belief may reduce the pain considerably. The pain relief may be a placebo effect and have nothing to do with the acupuncture.
- The patients want to be polite and may tell the experimenter what he or she wants to hear (that the pain decreased). Thus, the decrease in reported pain may be because the patients are not accurately reporting pain after therapy.
- Before, during, and after the acupuncture treatment, the therapist talks with the patients. Perhaps he recommends a change in aspirin dose, a change in exercise, or nutritional supplements. The decrease in reported pain might be due to these aspects of the treatment, rather than the acupuncture.
- What if three patients experience worse pain with acupuncture, whereas the others get better? The experimenter reviews the records of those three patients carefully and decides to remove them from the study because one of those people actually has a different kind of arthritis than the others, and two had to climb stairs to get to the appointment because the elevator didn't work that day. These kinds of manipulations of the data, although well intentioned, are fraudulent and may explain all the pain relief observed in the study.

- The pain from osteoarthritis varies significantly from day to day. People tend to seek therapy when pain is at its worst. If you start keeping track of pain on the day when it is the worst, it is quite likely to get better, even with no treatment. The next section explores this *regression to the mean*.

WE ARE FOOLED BY REGRESSION TO THE MEAN

Figure 1.1 illustrates simulated pressures. All values were randomly chosen in the same manner. The graph is divided into two columns (before treatment and after treatment) but the values were randomly chosen without regard to the labels. Figure 1.1A illustrates 24 pairs of values. The "before" and "after" groups are about the same. In some cases the value goes up and in others it goes down. If these were real data, you'd conclude that there is no evidence at all that the treatment had any effect on the outcome (blood pressure).

Now imagine the study were designed differently. You've made the before measurements and want to test a treatment for high blood pressure. There is no point in treating individuals whose blood pressure is not high, so you select the people with the highest pressures to study. Figure 1.1B illustrates data for only the 12 individuals with the highest before values. In every case but 1, the after values are lower. If you performed a statistical test (paired t test; see Chapter 31), the results would seem to be extremely convincing. The graph on the bottom-right illustrates the other 12 pairs, those with low values when measured before. In all but 2 pairs, the values go up. Again, these values alone would seem to be convincing evidence that the treatment brings down the value measured (blood pressure).

But these are random data! The before and after values came from the same distribution. What happened?

Variation in blood pressure (and almost any other variable) has two components. Some of the variability is biological. However, this example was constructed to have no systematic (biological) difference between the before and after values. The rest of the variation is random. All the variation in this example is random. For Figure 1.1C, we selected subjects who happened to have the highest blood pressures. When blood pressure is assessed again, there is no reason to expect that the random factor will again lead to a high pressure. So, on average, the after measurements are lower. This is not because of any effect of the treatment, but is purely a matter of chance. When we selected only the people who happened to have low blood pressure, the treatment appeared to cause a substantial increase.

When you select individuals because some measurement is particularly high, a later measurement is likely to be lower. This effect is called *regression to the mean*. People who are especially lucky at picking stocks one year are likely to be less lucky then next year. People who get extremely high scores on one exam are likely to get lower scores on a repeat exam. An athletes that does extremely well in one season is likely to perform more poorly the next season. Athletic

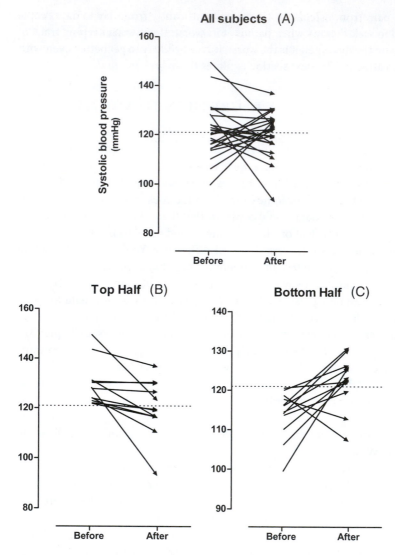

Figure 1.1. Regression to the mean.

All data in (A) were drawn from random distributions (Gaussian, mean = 120, SD = 15) without regard to the designations "before" and "after" and without regard to any pairing. (A) includes 48 random values, divided arbitrarily into 24 before–after pairs (which overlap enough that you can't count them all). (B) includes only the 12 pairs with the highest before values. In all but 1 case, the after values are lower than the before values. (C) shows the pairs with the lowest before measurements. In 10 of the 12 pairs, the after value is "higher" than the before value. If you only saw the graph in (B) or (C), you'd probably conclude that whatever treatment came between before and after had a large impact on blood pressure. In fact, these graphs simply illustrate random values, with no change between before and after. The apparent change is called *regression to the mean*.

performance certainly requires great skill, but random factors also play a major role and will cause regression to the mean. This probably explains much of the *Sports Illustrated* cover jinx—many believe that appearing on the cover of *Sports Illustrated* will bring an athlete bad luck (Wolff, 2002).

Answers to the ten questions in the overconfident section:
Martin Luther King Jr.'s age at death: 39
Length of the Nile river: 4,187 miles or 6,738 kilometers
Number of countries in OPEC: 13
Number of books in the Old Testament: 39
Diameter of the moon: 2,160 miles or 3,476 kilometers
Weight of an empty Boeing 747: 390,000 pounds or 176,901 kilograms
Year Mozart was born: 1756
Gestation period of an Asian elephant: 645 days
Distance from London to Tokyo: 5,989 miles or 9,638 kilometers
Deepest known point in the ocean: 6.9 miles or 11.0 kilometers

CHAPTER 2

Why Statistics
Can Be Hard to Learn

Statistical thinking will one day be as necessary for efficient
citizenship as the ability to read and write.

H. G. WELLS

*F*ear, confusion, and boredom. That is how many react to the idea of
learning statistics. This very short chapter explains why statistics can
be so hard to learn.

REASON 1: FEAR OF MATH

Statistics is a branch of mathematics, so you can't truly understand statistics
without studying many equations. Some fields of statistics simply cannot be fully
understood without first mastering calculus and matrix algebra.

Don't despair. You *can* learn to use statistical tests and interpret the results
without fully understanding how they work. You can learn a lot about statistics
without delving into math, and that is the approach this book uses.

This situation is common in science, because it is impossible for scientists to
truly understand every tool they use. You can interpret results from a pH meter
(which measures acidity) or a scintillation counter (which measures radioactiv-
ity), even if you don't understand exactly how they work. You can effectively use a
radioactively labeled compound in an experiment without really understanding
the nuclear physics of radioactive decay. You can use chemical reagents without
knowing how to synthesize them.

This book has very few equations. In a few places, I show equations as a
way to understand an idea (but never to prove a theorem). And in a few "how
to" sections, I use equations as a way to explain how to do some simple calculations by hand. Compared with most statistics book, this one uses very little
math.

REASON 2: CONFUSING TERMINOLOGY

In Lewis Carroll's *Through the Looking Glass*, Humpty Dumpty says, "When I
use a word, it means exactly what I say it means—neither more nor less." Lewis

Carroll (Charles Dodgson) was a mathematician, and I suspect he was thinking of statisticians when he wrote that line.

All fields use special terminology, and part of mastering any subject is learning its unique vocabulary. One factor that makes statistics particularly difficult to learn is that it endows ordinary words with specialized meanings. This makes it is quite possible to read statistical results and totally misunderstand what they mean.

You will need to learn which words and phrases have technical meanings in statistics that are distinct from their ordinary use. As you read this book, pay special attention to the statistical terms that sound like words you already know. Here is a partial list of such terms:

- Significant
- Error
- Hypothesis
- Model
- Power
- Variance
- Residual
- Normal
- Independent
- Sample
- Population
- Fit
- Confidence
- Distribution
- Control

The first term on the list leads to the most confusion. The phrase *statistically significant* is especially seductive and is often misinterpreted. Chapter 16 will explain what it means and what it doesn't mean.

As much as possible, this book uses plain language rather than statistical jargon. Sprinkled throughout the book are sections labeled "Lingo," which explain statistical terminology.

REASON 3: ABSTRACT THINKING

The goal of statistics is very concrete, to analyze data and make conclusions. But the logic of statistics is quite abstract, even slippery. You can't understand statistical reasoning without mastering concepts such as populations, probability distributions, and null hypotheses. You can't understand the analysis of a set of data without imagining the distribution of other data you didn't actually collect.

When you first encounter statistical thinking, it can seem very weird. In fact, the logic of statistics actually does make sense. Convincing you of that is one goal of this book.

REASON 4: PROBABILITY, NOT CERTAINTY

Many people want statistical calculations to yield definite conclusions. But all that statistics can do is report probabilities. Statistics can be very difficult to learn if you keep looking for certain conclusions. Remember this phrase, popularized by T-shirts, but written by Myles Hollander (according to Welch, 1998): "Statistics means never having to say you're certain!"

CHAPTER 3

From Sample to Population

There is something fascinating about science. One gets such
a wholesale return of conjecture out of a trifling investment
of fact.

MARK TWAIN (*Life on the Mississippi*, 1850)

*T*he goal of data analysis is simple—to make the strongest possible
conclusions from limited amounts of data. Statistics help you extrapolate from a particular set of data (your sample) to make a more general
conclusion (about the population).

STATISTICAL CALCULATIONS GENERALIZE
FROM SAMPLE TO POPULATION

Statisticians say that you extrapolate from a *sample* to a *population*. The distinction between sample and population is key to understanding much of statistics.

Note that the terms *sample* and *population* have a specialized meanings in
statistics that differ from the ordinary uses of those words. As you learn statistics,
you need to know which terms have specialized meanings.

Here are four different contexts in which the terms are used:

- *Quality control.* The terms *sample* and *population* make the most sense in
  the context of quality control. A factory makes lots of items (the population), but randomly selects a few items to test (the sample). The results
  obtained from the sample are used to make inferences about the entire
  population.
- *Political polls.* A random sample of voters (the sample) is polled, and
  the results are used to make conclusions about the entire population of
  voters.
- *Clinical studies.* The sample of patients studied is rarely a random sample
  of the larger population. However, patients included in a study are representative of other similar patients, and the extrapolation from sample to
  population is still useful. But there is often room for disagreement about
  the precise definition of the population. Is the population all such patients
  who come to that particular medical center, all who come to a big city
  teaching hospital, all such patients in the country, or all such patients in

the world? Although the population may be defined rather vaguely, it still is clear that we wish to use the sample data to make conclusions about a larger group.

- *Laboratory experiments.* Extending the terms sample and population to laboratory experiments is a bit awkward. The data you collect are the sample. If you were to repeat the experiment, you'd have a different sample. The population can only be defined abstractly, assuming you would repeat the experiment an infinite number of times. From the sample data you want to make inferences about the ideal, true, underlying situation.

In quality control and in political and marketing polls, the population is usually much larger than the sample, but it is finite and known (at least approximately). In biomedical research, we usually *assume* that the population is infinite or at least very large compared with our sample (and usually not known). All methods in this book are based on this latter assumption. If the population has a defined size and you have sampled a substantial fraction of the population (>10% or so), then you must use special methods that are not presented in this book.

WHAT STATISTICAL CALCULATIONS CANNOT DO

In theory, this is how you should apply statistical analysis to a simple experiment:

1. Define a population you are interested in.
2. Randomly select a sample of subjects to study.
3. Randomly select half the subjects to receive one treatment and give the other half another treatment.
4. Measure a single variable in each subject.
5. From the data you have measured in the samples, use statistical techniques to make inferences about the likely distribution of the variable in the population, and about the effect of the treatment.

When applying statistical analysis to real data, scientists frequently confront several problems that limit the validity of statistical reasoning. For example, consider how you would design a study to test whether a new drug is effective in treating patients infected with HIV.

The population you really care about is all patients in the world, now and in the future, who are or will be infected with HIV. Because you can't access that population, you choose to study a more limited population: for example, HIV patients aged 20 to 40 living in San Francisco who come to a university clinic. You may also exclude from the population patients who are too sick, who are taking other experimental drugs, who have taken experimental vaccines, or who are unable to cooperate with the experimental protocol. Although the population you are working with is defined narrowly, you hope to extrapolate your findings to the wider population of HIV-infected patients.

You want to know whether the drug increases life span. Accumulating survival data will take many years. As an alternative (or first step), you choose to measure the number of helper (CD4) lymphocytes. Patients infected with HIV have low numbers of CD4 lymphocytes, so you can ask whether patients taking the drug have more CD4 cells. To save time and expense, you have switched from an important variable (survival) to an indirect or proxy variable (number of CD4 cells).

Statistical calculations are based on the assumption that measurements are made correctly. In our HIV example, statistical calculations would not be helpful if the antibody used to identify CD4 cells was not really selective for those cells.

Statistical calculations are most often used to analyze one variable measured in a single experiment or a series of similar experiments. But scientists usually draw general conclusions by combining evidence generated by different kinds of experiments. To assess the effectiveness of a drug in combating HIV, you might want to look at several measures of effectiveness: delayed reduction in CD4 cell count, prolongation of life, increased quality of life, and reduction in medical costs. It is also essential to quantify any drug side effects.

In summary, statistical calculations provide limited help in overcoming the following common problems:

- The population you really care about is more diverse than the population from which your data were sampled.
- The subjects in the study were not randomly sampled from a larger population.
- The measured variable is a proxy for another variable you really care about.
- The measurements may be made or recorded incorrectly, and assays may not always measure exactly the right thing.
- Scientific (or clinical) conclusions require your looking at multiple outcomes, not just one.

You must use scientific and clinical judgment, common sense, and sometimes a leap of faith to overcome these problems. Statistical calculations are an important part of data analysis, but interpreting data also requires a great deal of judgment. That's what makes research challenging. This is a book about statistics, so we will focus on the statistical analysis of data. Understanding the statistical calculations is only a small part of evaluating scientific research.

STATISTICAL CONCLUSIONS ARE ALWAYS VAGUE

The whole idea of statistics is to make general conclusions from limited amounts of data. All that statistical calculations can do is quantify probabilities, so every conclusion must include words like "probably," "most likely," or "almost certainly."

Be wary if you ever encounter statistical conclusions that seem 100% definitive. The analysis, or your understanding of it, is probably wrong. Be especially wary of the conclusion that a result is statistically significant, because that phrase is often misunderstood.

LINGO: MODELS AND PARAMETERS

The concept of sampling from a population is an easy way to understand the idea of making generalizations from limited data, but it doesn't always perfectly describe what statistics and science are all about. Another way to think about statistics is in terms of models and parameters.

A *model* is a mathematical description of a simplified view of the world. A model consists of both a general description and *parameters* that have particular values. For example, the model might describe temperature values that follow a Gaussian bell-shape distribution. The parameters of that distribution are its mean and standard deviation. Another example: After ingesting a drug, its concentration in blood decays according to an exponential decay with consistent half-life. The parameter is the half-life (or a rate constant, which can be computed from the half-life).

One goal of statistics is to fit models to data to determine the most likely values of the parameters. Another goal is to compare models to see which best explain the data. Chapters 34 and 35 discuss this idea in more depth.

LINGO: PROBABILITY VERSUS STATISTICS

The words *probability* and *statistics* are often linked together in course and book titles, but they are distinct.

Probability starts with the general case (the population or model) and then predicts what would happen in many samples. These equations can get messy, so it is easy to apply probability theory incorrectly. But the logic is clear. The logic goes from general to specific, from population to sample, from model to data.

Statistics works in the opposite direction (Table 3.1). You start with one set of data (the sample) and make inferences about the overall population or model. The logic goes from a sample to make inferences about the population and from data to make inferences about the model.

n-OF-1 TRIALS

Beware of extrapolating statistical conclusions too far.

Roberts (2004) published 10 different self-experiments that he performed to test ideas about sleep, mood, health, and weight. He was the only subject in his studies, which led to some interesting conclusions. Here is one example: When Roberts looked at faces on television in the morning, his mood was lower that evening (>10 hours later) but elevated the next day (>24 hours later). In another example from that same paper, Roberts found that when he drank unflavored

PROBABILITY

General	→	Specific
Population	→	Sample
Model	→	Data

STATISTICS

General	←	Specific
Population	←	Sample
Model	←	Data

Table 3.1. The logic of probability and statistics.

Probability theory goes from general to specific, from population to sample, from model to data. Statistics theory works in the opposite direction.

fructose water between meals, he lost weight and maintained the lower weight for more than 1 year. These are intriguing ideas, but the analysis of the data he collected on himself may not apply to others.

Therapy of chronic diseases has been improved by performing double-blind trials using single subjects, called *n-of-1 trials*. One therapy is used for 1 week (or month) and then another. The patient doesn't know which therapy he is getting at any particular time. Analysis of many weeks' data can help in choosing optimum treatment (Guyatt et al., 1990; Nikles, Yelland, Glasziou, & Del Mar, 2005). Because all the data (the sample) came from one person (at various times), the conclusions only apply to that one person. You can generalize from limited data collected on one person to the more general situation with that *same* person. This can help optimize the management of chronic diseases and can generate ideas for larger studies. But, the conclusions should not be extrapolated or generalized beyond the one person who was tested.

Most statistical analyses are based on the number of data points collected and usually use the variable "n" to denote this number. Although these single-subject trials are called n-of-1, the value of n within the statistical analysis is the number of values analyzed.

PART B

Confidence Intervals

CHAPTER 4

Confidence Interval
of a Proportion

Confidence intervals can merely indicate how great our
ignorance might be, even if we had strictly random samples
of an adequately defined population.

D. MAINLAND

*A fundamental concept in statistics is the use of a confidence inter-
val to generalize. You compute something from a sample of data,
and the confidence interval allows you to make a more general conclusion. This chapter explains the use of confidence intervals when results
have two possible outcomes summarized as a proportion or fraction. If
you assume the data are sampled from a larger population, a confidence
interval quantifies how precisely you know the population proportion.*

EXAMPLE: DEATHS OF PREMATURE BABIES

To better counsel the parents of premature babies, Allen, Donohue, and Dusman
(1993) investigated the survival of premature infants. They retrospectively studied all premature babies born at 22 to 25 weeks of gestation at the Johns Hopkins
Hospital during a 3-year period. The investigators tabulated infant deaths by
gestational age. Of 29 infants born at 22 weeks of gestation, none survived
6 months. Of 39 infants born at 25 weeks of gestation, 31 survived for at least
6 months.

The investigators presented these data without any confidence intervals
(CI). But, it would only make sense to calculate a CI when the sample is representative of a larger population about which you wish to make inferences. In this
example, it seems reasonable to assume that these data from several years at one
hospital are representative of data from other years at other hospitals, at least at
big-city university hospitals in the United States. If you aren't willing to make
that assumption, you shouldn't calculate or interpret a CI. But the data wouldn't
be worth collecting if the investigators didn't think that the results would be
similar in other hospitals in later years.

Before reading on, write down what you think the CIs (margins of error) are
for the two examples (0/29 and 31/39).

For the infants born at 25 weeks of gestation, the 95% CI of 31/39 ranges from 64 to 91% (calculated by a computer program using a complicated formula). For the infants born at 22 weeks of gestation, the 95% CI of 0/29 extends from 0 to 11.9%. We can be 95% sure that this range includes the overall proportion of surviving infants.

You may get different results depending on which program and options you choose. Computing a CI of a proportion turns out to be tricky and there is no consensus among statisticians as to the best way to calculate the interval (Brown, Cai, & DasGupta, 2001).

These CIs only account for sampling variability. When you try to extrapolate these infant-survival results to results you would expect to see in your hospital, you also must account for the different populations served by different hospitals and the different methods used to care for premature infants. The true CIs, which are impossible to calculate, are almost certainly wider than the ones you calculate.

EXAMPLE: POLLING VOTERS

You polled 100 randomly selected voters just before an election and 33 said they would vote for your candidate. What can you say about the proportion of *all* voters who will vote for your candidate?

Again, there are two issues to deal with. First, you must think about whether your sample is really representative of the population of voters *and* whether people tell the pollsters the truth about how they will vote. Statistical calculations cannot help you grapple with those issues! We'll assume that the sample is perfectly representative of the population of voters and that every person will vote as they said they would when polled. Second, you must think about sampling error. Just by chance, your 100-voter sample will almost certainly contain a smaller or larger fraction of people voting for your candidate than does the overall population.

Because we only know the proportion of favorably inclined voters in one sample, there is no way to be sure about the proportion in the population. The best we can do is to calculate a range of values that bracket the true population proportion. How wide does this range of values have to be? In the overall population, the fraction of voters who will vote for your candidate could be almost anything. So, to create a 95% CI, we accept a 5% chance that the range will not include the true population value.

Before reading on, make your best guess for the 95% CI when your sample proportion equals 33/100.

For the election example, the 95% CI extends from 0.24 to 0.42. Again, you might get slightly different results depending on which program you use.

How good was your guess? Many people assume that the interval is narrower than it is.

Note that there is no uncertainty about what we observed in the voter sample. We are absolutely sure that 33.0% of the people polled said they would vote for our candidate. If we weren't sure of that count, calculation of a CI could not overcome any mistakes that were made in tabulating those numbers or any ambiguity in defining "vote." What we don't know is the proportion of favorable voters in the entire population. However, we can be 95% confident that somewhere between 24 and 42% of population you polled expressed a preference for your candidate on the day the poll was conducted. The phrase "95% confident" is explained in more detail below.

ASSUMPTIONS: CONFIDENCE INTERVAL OF A PROPORTION

The whole idea of a confidence interval is to make a general conclusion from some specific data. Of course, this generalization only makes sense if certain assumptions are true. A huge part of the task of learning statistics is to learn the assumptions upon which statistical inferences are based.

Assumption: Random (or representative) sample

All statistical conclusions are based on the assumption that the sample of data you analyze is sampled from a larger population of data about which you want to generalize. This assumption would be violated in the premature-baby example if the infants included in the sample were somehow selected to be sicker (or less sick) than other premature infants of similar age.

The assumption would be violated in the election example if the sample was not randomly selected from the population of voters. In fact, this mistake was made in the 1936 Roosevelt–Landon U.S. Presidential Election. To find potential voters, the pollsters relied heavily on phone books and automobile registration lists. In 1936, Republicans were far more likely than Democrats to own a phone or a car and, therefore, the poll selected too many Republicans. The poll predicted that Landon would win by a large margin, but that didn't happen.

Reputable polling organizations no longer make this type of mistake and ensure that their samples are representative of the entire population. However, many so-called polls are performed by inviting television viewers to call in their opinion. In the United States, this usually is a 1-900 phone number, and the caller pays for the privilege of being polled! Clearly, the self-selected sample tabulated by such "polls" is not representative of any population, so the data mean nothing. For example, in June 1994 football star O. J. Simpson was arrested for allegedly murdering his ex-wife, and the events surrounding the arrest were given a tremendous amount of television coverage. One news show performed a telephone poll of its viewers asking whether the press was giving too much coverage. The results were meaningless, because people who really thought that there was too much coverage probably weren't watching the show.

Assumption: Independent observations

The 95% CI is only valid when all subjects are sampled from the same population and each has been selected independently of the others.

In the premature-infant example, this would mean that the survival of each infant is not related to the survival of other infants in the sample. This assumption would be violated if some of the infants in the sample were twins, because then some of the propensity for survival would be the result of shared genetic or environmental factors. The assumption also would be violated if some of the deaths were caused by hospital infection or malfunctioning equipment that affected several infants in the study.

The assumption would be violated in the election example if the pollsters questioned both the husband and the wife in each family, if some voters were polled more than once, or if half the subjects were sampled from one city and half from another.

Assumption: Accurate data

The 95% CI is only valid when the number of subjects in each category is tabulated correctly.

In the premature-infant example, the outcome is death, which is pretty unambiguous. But even here, it is possible for the data to be distorted. If the treating physicians knew that 6-month survival was being tracked, they may have used heroic measures to keep a 5-month-old infant alive a few days longer until it was older than 6 months of age. Although this won't help the infant, it would improve the 6-month-survival rate and distort the statistics.

The assumption would be violated in the election example if the pollster recorded some of the opinions incorrectly. It would also be violated if the pollster coerced or intimidated the respondent to answer a certain way, or if the survey questions were poorly phrased to encourage a certain response.

WHAT DOES 95% CONFIDENCE REALLY MEAN?

The true population value either lies within the 95% CI you calculated or it doesn't. There is no way for you to know. If you were to calculate a 95% CI from many samples, the 95% CI would include the population proportion in about 95% of the samples, but would not include the population value in the rest of the samples. This is what it means to be 95% certain that the 95% CI calculated from a sample includes the population proportion.

To show this, we must switch to a simulation where you know *exactly* what population the data were selected from. Assume that you have a bowl of 100 balls, 25 red and 75 black. Mix the balls well and choose one randomly. Put it back in, mix again, and choose another one. Do this 15 times, record the fraction of that sample that are red, and compute the 95% CI for that proportion. Figure 4.1 includes the simulation of 19 such samples. Each 95% CI is illustrated as a vertical bar extending from the lower confidence limit to the upper confidence limit. The value of the observed proportion in each sample is shown as a horizontal line in the middle of each CI. The horizontal line shows the

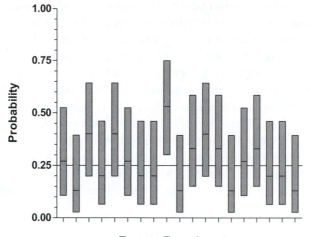

Figure 4.1. What would happen if you collected many samples and computed a 95% CI for each?

Each bar shows one simulated experiment, indicating the proportion of red balls chosen from a mixture of 25% red balls (the rest are black), with n = 15. The percentage success is shown as a line near the middle of the bar, which extends from one 95% confidence limit to the other. In all but one of the simulated samples, the CI includes the true population proportion of red balls (shown as a horizontal line). The 95% CI of Sample 9, however, does not include the true population value. You expect this to happen in 5% of samples. Because Figure 4.1 shows the results of simulations, we know when the CI doesn't include the true population value. When analyzing data, however, the population value is unknown, so you have no way of knowing whether the CI includes the true population value.

true population value (25% of the balls are red). In about half of the samples, the sample proportion is less 25%, and in half the sample proportion is higher. In one of the samples, the population value lies outside the 95% CI. In the long run, assuming no violations of any assumption, 1 of 20 (5%) 95% CIs will not include the population value.

Figure 4.1 helps explain confidence intervals, but you cannot create such a figure when you analyze data. When you analyze data, you don't know the actual population value. You only have results from a single sample. There is no way you can know whether the 95% CI you calculate includes the population value, but it always will contain the value you calculated from your sample. In the long run, 95% of such intervals will contain the population value and 5% will not.

Note that the definition of *confidence interval* specifies the chance that the interval contains the true population value, and not the chance that the population value lies within that interval. The two aren't quite the same. Random chance affects which data you collect, thus affecting the range of the CI. If you repeat the experiment, you'll get a different interval. However, random chance does not affect the true population value, which is fixed and unknowable. It doesn't matter how many times you repeat the experiment; the true population value won't change. That is why it is considered incorrect to say that there is a 95% chance that the population value lies within the CI. That statement implies that the population value is subject to random variation. Instead, it is proper to say the following: "There is a 95% chance that this CI contains the population value." This is a fine distinction that is unlikely to affect your understanding of statistical results.

WHAT IS SPECIAL ABOUT 95%?

Nothing except tradition.

CIs can be computed for any degree of confidence. By convention, 95% CIs are presented most commonly, although 90 and 99% CIs are sometimes published.

If you want to be more confident that your interval contains the population value, the interval will be *wider*. Thus, 99% CIs are wider than 95% CIs. If you are willing to be less confident, then the interval will be *narrower*, so 90% CIs are narrower than 95% CIs.

WHAT IF THE ASSUMPTIONS ARE VIOLATED?

In many situations, the assumptions are not strictly true: The patients in your study may be more homogeneous than the entire population of patients about which you want to make inferences. Measurements made in one lab may not match those made in other labs at other times. The people who take the time to answer the survey may not be representative of the entire population or may have an incentive to lie.

If any assumption is violated, the CI will probably be too optimistic (too narrow). The true CI (taking into account any violation of the assumptions) is likely to be wider than the calculated CI and, perhaps, much wider. This explains why it is possible to see very different CIs when different investigators measure the same thing.

Two different groups used surveys to estimate the number of violent deaths in Iraq between 2002 and 2006 (reviewed in Brownstein & Brownstein, 2008). The two estimates differed by a factor of 5. Each group provided a 95% CI for their estimates, which didn't even come close to overlapping. The upper confidence limit provided by one study was less than half the lower confidence limit of the other study. Computing CIs is easy. Doing science is hard, and doing good science in a war zone is really hard, especially without letting one's political opinions (or those of the people being surveyed) bias data collection.

ARE YOU QUANTIFYING THE EVENT
YOU REALLY CARE ABOUT?

The 95% CI allows you to extrapolate from the sample to the population for the event that you tabulated. For the first example (premature babies), the tabulated event (death in the first month of life) is exactly what you care about. But sometimes you really care about an event that is different from the one you tabulated.

In the voting example, we assessed our sample's responses on a poll on a particular date, so the 95% CI lets us generalize to how the population would respond on that poll on that date. We wish to extrapolate to election results in the future, but can do so only by making an additional assumption—that people will vote as they said they would. This assumption was violated in a classic mistake in the polling prior to the 1948 Dewey versus Truman Presidential Election in the United States. Polls of many-thousand voters indicated that Dewey would win by a large margin. Because the CI was so narrow, the pollsters were very confident. Newspapers were so sure of the results that they prematurely printed the headline "Dewey Beats Truman." In fact, Truman won. Why was the poll wrong? The polls were performed in September and early October, and the election was held in November. Many voters changed their mind in the interim period. The 95% CI computed from data collected in September was inappropriately used to predict voting results 2 months later.

LINGO

CI versus confidence limits

The two ends of the CI are called the *confidence limits*. The CI extends from one confidence limit to the other. The CI is a range, whereas each confidence limit is a value.

Many scientists use the terms confidence interval and confidence limits interchangeably. Fortunately, mixing up these terms does not get in the way of understanding statistical results.

Estimate

The sample proportion is said to be a *point estimate* of the true population proportion. The CI is said to be an *interval estimate*.

Note that "estimate" has a special meaning in statistics. It does not mean an approximate calculation or an informed hunch, but rather is the result of a defined calculation. "Estimate" is used because the value computed from your sample is only an estimate of the true value in the population (which you can't know).

Confidence level

There is nothing special about 95%. The term confidence level is used to describe the desired amount of confidence. If you generate a 99% CI, the confidence level equals 99%.

HOW IT WORKS: CI OF A PROPORTION

Many computer programs and Web calculators calculate the CI of a proportion. This section explains approximate calculations you can easily do yourself.

Why are there several methods?

Several methods have been developed for computing the CI, and there is no consensus about which is best (Brown et al., 2001). Fortunately, the methods all give results that are pretty similar.

Below, we describe the *modified Wald method*, developed by Agresti and Coull (1998). It is quite accurate and is also easy to compute by hand. Simulations with many sets of data demonstrate that the true confidence level calculated by this method depends on the values of the numerator and denominator. On average, the confidence level is 95%, but it will be less than 95% with some combinations of numerator and denominator and higher with others (Brown et al., 2001; Ludbrook & Lew, 2009).

The other commonly used method, the so-called *exact method of Clopper and Pearson* (1934), always has a confidence level of at least 95%, but the confidence level is actually higher than that with some values of the numerator and denominator. Accordingly, the intervals tend to be a bit wider than the modified Wald intervals. The Clopper method cannot be easily computed by hand.

Modified Wald method

1. Define z based on the confidence level you want. For 95% CI, $z = 1.960$. For 90% intervals, $z = 1.645$. For 99% intervals, $z = 2.576$.
2. Calculate p′ from the number of successes (S) and the number of trials (n). Its value will be between the observed proportion (S/n) and 0.5.

$$p = \frac{S+z}{n+z^2}$$

For 95% CIs, this simplifies to

$$p' \approx \frac{S+2}{n+4}.$$

3. Compute W, the margin of error (or half width) of the CI.

$$W = z\sqrt{\frac{p'(1-p')}{n+z^2}}$$

For 95% confidence, this simplifies to

$$W \approx 2\sqrt{\frac{p'(1-p')}{n+4}}.$$

4.   Compute the 95% CI.

From $(p' - W)$ to $(p' + W)$

Note that the variable p' used here is not the same as a *P value* (which we will discuss extensively in later chapters). The use of the letter P for both purposes is potentially confusing. This book uses an upper-case P for P values and a lower-case p for proportions, but not all books follow this convention.

For the survival data for the 25-week infants given at the beginning of this chapter, the sample proportion is 31/39, or 79.5%. The 95% CI, computed with the modified Wald method, ranges from 64 to 89%. The Clopper method generates a wider CI, ranging from 64 to 91%.

Standard Wald method

Many books, including the first edition of this one, present the simpler *standard* Wald equation. It replaces step 2 above by computing p' as S/n and leaves out z^2 from step 3. This method works well when n is large and the proportion is far from 0.0 and 1.0, but it can work very poorly (giving actual confidence levels much lower than 95%) in other cases. The modified Wald method presented above is preferred because it works well with any sample, yet is no harder to compute.

If the proportion is 0 or 100%

In one of the previous examples, none of the 29 babies born at 22 weeks of gestation survived. It still makes sense to compute a CI, because the true proportion in the population may not be zero. Of course, the lower confidence limit must be 0%, because there is no possibility of a proportion being negative. There are two ways to define the upper confidence limit in this situation.

As usually defined, the 95% CI allows for a 2.5% chance that the upper confidence limit doesn't go high enough to include the true population proportion and a 2.5% chance that the lower confidence limit doesn't go low enough to include the true population proportion. This leaves a 95% chance that the interval includes the true population proportion.

If you use this approach when the numerator is zero, there is a 2.5% chance that the upper interval doesn't go high enough. But there is no chance that the lower interval doesn't go low enough, because it is bounded at zero. Because the uncertainty only goes in one direction, this "95%" CI really gives you 97.5% confidence. Calculated in this way, the 95% CI for the percentage of surviving babies extends from 0 to 13.9%.

The alternative approach is to compute the upper confidence limit such that there is a 5% chance it doesn't go high enough to include the true population value. This approach creates a true 95% CI, but is not consistent with other intervals. Calculated this way, the 95% CI for babies surviving extends from 0 to 10.2%.

If the numerator and denominator are equal, the sample proportion is 100%, which is also the upper limit of the CI. As explained above, there are two ways to define the lower limit.

PROPORTION	MARGIN OF ERROR (%)	APPROXIMATE 95% CI
5/10	32	18 to 82
50/100	10	40 to 60
500/1000	3	47 to 53
5000/10000	1	49 to 51

Table 4.1. Approximate CI of a proportion when the observed proportion is 50%.

This table's values should not be used for formal data analysis because they are approximations. Remember these values when you wish to rapidly evaluate published data. The margin of error is approximately equal to the reciprocal of the square root of n.

HOW TO: APPROXIMATE CIs

Shortcut for proportions near 50%
When the proportion is near 50%, the margin of error of the CI is approximately equal to the square root of 1/n. This leads to the rules of thumb listed in Table 4.1. Many political polls use a sample size of about 1,000, and many polls have results very near 50:50. The margin of error is 3%, a value you'll often see reported in newspapers as the margin of error of a poll.

Shortcut when the numerator is zero: The rule of three
Hanley and Lippman-Hand (1983) devised a simple shortcut equation, called the *rule of three*, for determining the 95% CI of a proportion when the numerator is zero. If you observe zero events in n trials, the 95% CI extends from 0.0 to 3.0/n. This defines the interval so that it truly has 95% confidence.

In the preceding example, 0 of 29 infants born at 22 weeks survived. Using the rule of three, the 95% CI for the survival proportion extends from 0.0 (of course) to 3/29, or 10.3%.

Another example follows: You have observed no adverse drug reactions in the first 250 patients treated with a new antibiotic. The CI for the true rate of drug reactions extends from 0.0 to about 3/250, or 1.20%.

Shortcut when the numerator is 1 or 2: The rules of 5 and 7
Similar shortcut equations let you approximate the CI when the numerator is 1 or 2 (Montori et al., 2004).

What is the CI of 1/n? The lower limit will clearly be close to zero and probably won't be of interest. But what is the upper limit? It can be approximated as 5/n. For example, if you observe 1 success in 50 tries, the upper 95% confidence limit is very close to 5/50, or 0.10.

PROPORTION	UPPER 95% CONFIDENCE LIMIT (APPROXIMATE)
0/n	3/n
1/n	5/n
2/n	7/n

Table 4.2. The rules of 3, 5, and 7.

If the proportion is 0, 1, or 2 over n (and n is fairly large), these rules will compute an approximation of the upper 95% confidence limit. The lower limit will be a small value (zero, when the numerator is zero) and usually is not of interest.

Similarly, if the numerator is 2, the upper 95% confidence limit is close to 7/n. So if you observe 2 successes in 50 tries, the upper 95% confidence limit is very close to 7/50, or 0.14.

Table 4.2 summarizes the rules of 3, 5, and 7.

LOOKING FORWARD: PARAMETERS AND MODELS

Let's put these examples into a wider perspective and introduce a few new terms.

To interpret the CI, we had to accept a number of assumptions listed above. More generally, we created a model of the population. In this case the model is quite simple, that each person in the population has one of two possible outcomes. The model is defined by one parameter, the overall proportion in the population with one of those outcomes. For one example, this was the fraction of premature babies who died. For the other example, it was the fraction of voters who say they'd vote for a particular candidate.

We also need a model for how the individuals in the population vary from one another. In this example, that is easy. Each individual has one of two outcomes. Read about this in advanced statistics books by reading about the *binomial* distribution.

The experimental sample is then used to find the most likely value for this parameter. Of course, in these examples, the proportions observed in the sample are the most likely values for the population values. Statisticians say that the sample proportions are the best *estimates* of the population parameters. The CIs quantify the precision of those estimates and are called *interval estimates*.

For understanding proportions and CIs of proportions, the mindset of models and parameters really doesn't add anything. But, as you'll see in the last part of this book, this approach is very useful for more complicated situations.

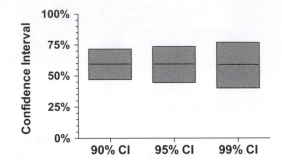

Figure 4.2. Effect of degree of confidence on the width of a CI.
Each bar represents a sample with a 60% success rate and n = 40. The
graph illustrates the 90, 95, and 99% CIs for the percentage success in the
population the data were drawn from. When you choose less confidence,
the CI is narrower.

Q & A

What's the difference between a 95% CI and a 99% CI?	To be more certain that an interval contains the true population value, you must generate a wider interval. A 99% CI is wider than a 95% CI. See Figure 4.2.
Is it possible to generate a 100% CI?	A 100% CI would have to include every possible value, so it would extend from 0.0 to 100.0%. That is always the same, regardless of the data, so it isn't at all useful.
How do CIs change if you increase the sample size?	The width of the CI is approximately proportional to the reciprocal of the square root of the sample size. So, if you increase the sample size by a factor of 4, you can expect to cut the length of the CI in half. Figure 4.3 illustrates how the CI gets narrower if the sample size gets larger.
Why isn't the CI symmetrical around the observed proportion?	Because a proportion cannot go below 0.0 or above 1.0, the CI will be lopsided when the sample proportion is far from 0.50 or the sample size is small. See Figure 4.4.

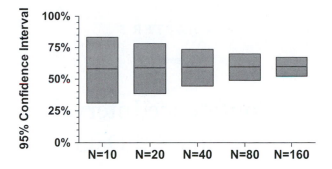

Figure 4.3. **Effect of sample size on the width of a CI.**

Each bar represents a sample with a 60% success rate, and the graph shows the 95% CI for the percentage success in the population the data were drawn from. When the samples are larger, the CI is narrower.

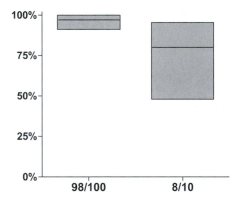

Figure 4.4. **Asymmetrical CI.**

If the proportion is far from 50%; the 95% CI of a proportion is noticeably asymmetrical, especially when the sample size is small.

CHAPTER 5

‒⟍

Confidence Interval
of Survival Data

In the long run, we are all dead.
JOHN MAYNARD KEYNES

*O*utcomes that can only happen once (i.e., death) are often displayed
*as graphs showing percentage survival as a function of time. This
chapter explains how survival curves are created and how to interpret
their confidence intervals.*

SURVIVAL DATA

The term *survival curve* is a bit misleading. In fact, survival curves can plot
time to any well-defined end point or event, such as occlusion of a vascular
graft, date of first metastasis, or rejection of a transplanted kidney. The event
does not have to be dire. The event could be restoration of renal function, dis-
charge from a hospital, resolution of a cold, or graduation. The event must be
a one-time event. Events that can recur should not be analyzed with survival
curves.

The methods described here (and in Chapter 29) apply when you know the
survival time of each subject (or know when the data were censored, as explained
in the next section). These methods are not appropriate for analyzing, for example, the survival of many thousands of cells, because you don't know the survival
time of each individual cell. Instead, you would simply plot the percentage survival versus time and fit a curve or connect with point-to-point lines.

CENSORED SURVIVAL DATA

If each subject's survival time were known, creating a survival curve would be
trivial. But many survival times are not known.

Many studies enroll patients over a period of several years. The patients who
enroll later are not followed for as many years as patients who enrolled early.
Imagine a study of a cancer treatment that enrolled patients between 1995 and

STARTING DATE	ENDING DATE	WHAT HAPPENED
Feb. 7, 1998	Mar. 2, 2002	Died
May 19, 1998	Nov. 30, 2004	Moved; no longer on protocol
Nov. 14, 1998	Apr. 3, 2000	Died
Mar. 4, 1999	May 4, 2005	Study ended
Jun. 15, 1999	May 4, 2005	Died
Dec. 1, 1999	Sep. 4, 2004	Died
Dec. 15, 1999	Aug. 15, 2003	Died in car crash

Table 5.1. Sample survival-data details for the data plotted in Figure 5.1.

2000 and ended in 2008. If a patient enrolled in 2000 and was still alive at the end of the study, his survival time is unknown, but must exceed 8 years. Although the study lasted 13 years, the fate of that patient after Year 8 is unknown.

During the study, some subjects dropped out—perhaps they moved to a different city or wanted to take a medication disallowed on the protocol. If a patient moved after 2 years on the study, his survival time is unknown, but must exceed 2 years. Even if you knew how long he lived, you couldn't use the data because he was no longer taking the experimental drug. However, the analysis must account for the fact that he lived at least 2 years on the protocol.

Information about these patients is said to be *censored*. The word *censor* has a negative connotation. It sounds like the subject has done something bad. Not so. It's the data that have been censored, not the subject! These censored observations should not be removed from the analyses—they must just be accounted for properly. The survival analysis must take into account how long each subject is known to have been alive and following the experimental protocol, and not use any information after that.

Table 5.1 presents data for a survival study. It only has seven patients. That would be a very small study, but it makes the example easy to follow. The data for three patients are censored for three different reasons. One of the censored observations is for someone who is still alive at the end of the study. We don't know how long he will live after that. Another person moved away from the area and thus left the study protocol. Even if we knew how much longer he lived, we couldn't use the information, because he was no longer following the study protocol. One person died in a car crash. Different investigators handle this differently. Some define a death to be a death, no matter what the cause. Here we will define a death from a clearly unrelated cause (such as a car crash) to be a censored observation. We know he lived 3.67 years on the treatment, and don't know how much longer he would have lived, because his life was cut short by a car accident.

Table 5.2 demonstrates how these data are entered into a computer program. The codes for death (1) and censored (0) are commonly used, but are not completely standard.

YEARS	CODE
4.07	1
6.54	0
1.39	1
6.17	0
5.89	1
4.76	1
3.67	0

Table 5.2. How the data of Table 5.1 are entered into a computer program.

GRAPHING PERCENTAGE SURVIVAL VERSUS TIME

There are two slightly different methods for creating a survival table. With the *actuarial* method, the X-axis is divided up into regular intervals, perhaps months or years, and survival is calculated for each interval. With the *Kaplan-Meier* method, survival time is recalculated with each patient death. This method is preferred, unless the number of patients is huge. The term *life-table analysis* is used inconsistently, but usually includes both methods.

The Kaplan-Meier method is logically simple. To calculate the fraction of patients who survived on a particular day, simply divide the number alive at the end of the day by the number alive at the beginning of the day (excluding any who were censored on that day from both the numerator and the denominator). This gives you the fraction of patients who were alive at the beginning of a particular day who were still alive at the beginning of the next day. To calculate the fraction of patients who survive from Day 0 until a particular day, multiply the fraction of patients who survive Day 1 times the fraction of those patients who survive Day 2 times the fraction of those patients who survive Day 3...times the fraction who survive Day k. This method automatically accounts for censored patients, because both the numerator and the denominator are reduced on the day a patient is censored. Because we calculate the product of many survival fractions, this method is also called the *product-limit* method. The method is part of many computer programs, so there is no need to learn the tedious details.

Time zero is not some specified calendar date; rather, it is the time that each patient entered the study. In many clinical studies, time zero spans several calendar years as patients are enrolled. At time zero, by definition, all patients are alive, so survival equals 100%. Whenever a patient dies, the percentage of surviving patients decreases. If the study (and thus the X-axis) were extended far enough, survival would eventually drop to zero.

Table 5.3 includes the computed survival percentages, with 95% CI, at each time a patient dies. Figure 5.1 plots these data four ways. Each time a patient dies, the curve drops down. The censored subjects are shown as circles in the upper panels and as ticks in the lower-left panel.

NO. OF YEARS	LOWER LIMIT	% SURVIVAL	UPPER LIMIT
0.00	100.00	100.00	100.00
1.39	33.39	85.71	97.86
3.67	33.39	85.71	97.86
4.07	21.27	68.57	91.21
4.76	11.77	51.43	81.33
5.89	4.81	34.29	68.56
6.17	4.81	34.29	68.56
6.54	4.81	34.29	68.56

Table 5.3. Kaplan-Meier survival proportions with 95% confidence limits computed by computer (not using the approximate equations presented in this chapter).

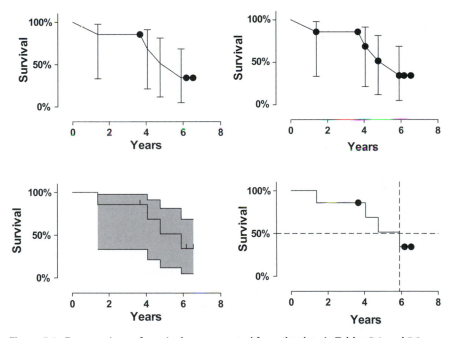
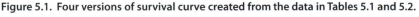

Figure 5.1. Four versions of survival curve created from the data in Tables 5.1 and 5.2.
The X axis plots the number of years after each subject was enrolled. Note that time zero does not have to be any particular day or year. The Y axis plots percentage survival. The three censored patients are shown as symbols in the three of the graphs, and as upward blips in the fourth. Four of the subjects died. You can see each death as a downward step in the curves. The 95% CIs for the populations are shown as error bars in the top two graphs, and as a shaded region (confidence bands) in the bottom-left graph. The bottom right graph shows the median survival time, which is the time at which half of the subjects have died and half are still alive. Read across at 50% to determine median survival, which is 5.89 years in this example. If fewer than half of the subjects have died by the end of the study, you cannot determine median survival.

An essential part of data analysis includes computing and interpreting a CI. Programs that compute survival curves can compute a 95% CI at each time that a death occurs. These can then be joined to plot 95% confidence bands, as shown in the lower-left panel of Figure 5.1. The survival curve shows exactly what happened in the sample we studied. Given certain assumptions (see below), we can be 95% sure that the true population survival at any time lies within the 95% confidence bands.

HOW TO: CALCULATE THE CONFIDENCE INTERVAL OF SURVIVAL

Calculation of confidence intervals is best left to computer programs. But it isn't too hard to compute an approximate CI, so you can interpret a survival curve published without them.

The margin of error of the survival proportion p, at some particular time, is approximately equal to

$$W = 2\sqrt{\frac{p(1-p)}{n}}.$$

In this equation, n is not the number of subjects in the study. Instead, n is that total number of subjects minus the number censored prior to the time for which you are computing the CI. The value of n changes as you progress along the curve. The variable p is the proportion survival at a particular time point and is not a P value.

Subtract W from p to obtain the lower confidence limit. If this value is less than 0, define the lower limit to be 0. Add W plus p to get the upper limit. If this value is greater than 100%, define the upper limit to be 100%.

Let's use the above equation to figure out the approximate CI for survival for the example at 4.07 years. We started with seven patients. Only one subject was censored before 4.07 years. Thus, for this calculation n = 7 – 1 = 6. Reading off the curve, p ≈ 0.686. Plugging p and n into the equation, the 95% CI extends in each direction by approximately 0.371, so it extends from about 31.4 to 100%. The graph illustrates CIs computed by a more exact method.

MEDIAN SURVIVAL

It can be convenient to summarize an entire survival curve by one value, the median survival. The median is the middle value (the 50th percentile) of a set of numbers, so median survival is how long it takes until half the subjects have died.

It is easy to derive the median survival time from a survival curve: Draw a horizontal line at 50% survival and note where it crosses the survival curve.

Then look down at the X axis to read the median survival time. The lower-right panel of Figure 5.1 indicates that the median survival in this example is 5.89 years.

Calculations of median survival are ambiguous in two situations. Median survival is undefined when more than half the subjects are still alive at the end of the study. In this case, the survival curve never crosses the 50% survival line. The median survival is greater than the last duration of time plotted on the survival curve, but there is no way to know how much greater. The other ambiguous situation is when the survival curve is horizontal at 50% survival. One way to define median survival in this case is to average the first and last times when survival is 50%.

FIVE-YEAR SURVIVAL

Survival with cancer is often quantified as 5-year survival. A vertical line is drawn at $X = 5$ years, and the Y value that line intersects is the 5-year percentage survival. Of course, there is nothing special about 5 years (rather than 2 or 4 or 6 or...) except tradition.

ASSUMPTIONS: SURVIVAL ANALYSIS

When evaluating any statistical analysis, it is critical to review all assumptions. Analyses of survival curves depend on these assumptions.

Assumption: Random (or representative) sample

The whole idea of all statistical analyses is to generalize the data from your sample to a more general situation. If your sample is not randomly selected from a defined population, then you must *assume* that your sample is representative of that population.

Assumption: Independent subjects

The results of any statistical analyses can only be interpreted if the data from each subject offer independent information. If the study pools data from two hospitals, the subjects are not independent. It is possible that subjects from one hospital have different average survival times than subjects from another hospital, and you could alter the survival curve by choosing more subjects from one hospital and fewer from the other hospital. Because most diseases have a genetic component, another way to violate the assumption of independence would be to include two (or more) people from one family (in one treatment group).

Assumption: Entry criteria are consistent

Typically, subjects are enrolled over a period of months or years. In these studies, it is important that the entry criteria do not change during the enrollment period.

Imagine a cancer-survival curve starting from the date that the first metastasis was detected. What would happen if improved diagnostic technology detected metastases earlier? Patients would die at the same age they otherwise would, but now they are diagnosed at a younger age and, therefore, live longer with the diagnosis. Even with no change in therapy or in the natural history of the disease, survival time will apparently increase simply because the entry criteria changed.

Airlines use this trick to improve their "on-time departure" rates. Instead of planning to close the doors at the scheduled departure time, they now plan to close the airplane's door 10 minutes before the "scheduled departure time." This means that the doors can close 10 minutes later than actually planned, yet the flight will still be defined to be "on time."

Assumption: End point defined consistently

If the curve is plotting duration of time until death, there can be ambiguity about which deaths to count. In a cancer trial, for example, what happens to subjects who die in car crashes? Some investigators count these as deaths; others count them as censored subjects. Both approaches can be justified, but the approach should be decided before the study begins. If there is any ambiguity about which deaths to count, the decision should be made by someone who doesn't know which patient is in which treatment group.

If the curve plots duration of time until an event other than death, it is crucial that the event be assessed consistently throughout the study.

Assumption: Starting time clearly defined

The starting point should be an objective date—perhaps the date of first diagnosis, or first hospital admission. You may be tempted to use an earlier starting criterion instead, such as the time when a patient remembers first observing symptoms. Don't do it. Such data are invalid because a patient's recollection of early symptoms may be altered by later events.

What happens when subjects die before they receive the treatment they were supposed to get? It is tempting to remove these subjects from the study. But this can lead to biases, especially if one treatment (such as a medication) is started immediately, but another (surgery) requires preparation or scheduling. If you remove the patients who die early from the surgical group but not from the medication group, the two groups will have different survival times, even if the treatments are equivalent. To avoid such biases, most studies follow a policy of *intention to treat*. Each subject's survival is analyzed as if he or she received the assigned treatment, even if the treatment was not actually given.

Assumption: Censoring unrelated to survival

The survival analysis is only valid when the reasons for censoring are unrelated to survival. If data from a large fraction of subjects are censored, the validity of this assumption is critical to the integrity of the results.

Data for some patients are censored because they are alive at the end of the study. With these patients, there is no reason to doubt the assumption that censoring is unrelated to survival.

The data for other patients are censored because they drop out of the study. If the reason these patients dropped out could be related to survival, then the analysis won't be valid. Examples include patients who quit the study because they were too sick to come to the clinic, patients who felt well and stopped treatment, and patients who quit because they didn't think the treatment was working. These reasons all relate to disease progression or response to therapy, and it is quite possible that the survival of these patients is related to their reason for dropping out. Including these subjects (and censoring their data) violates the assumption that censoring is unrelated to survival. But excluding these subjects entirely can also lead to biased results. The best plan is to analyze the data both ways. If the conclusions of the two analyses are similar, then the results are straightforward to interpret. If the conclusions of the two analyses differ substantially, then the study results are simply ambiguous.

Assumption: Average survival doesn't change during the study

Many survival studies enroll subjects over a period of several years. The analysis is only meaningful if you assume that the first few patients are sampled from the same population as the last few subjects.

If the nature of the disease changes during the time the study accrues patients, the results will be difficult to interpret. This is quite possible when studying rapidly evolving infectious diseases. It is also important that the treatment (including supportive care) does not change over the course of the study.

Q & A: Survival Curves	
Why is percentage survival graphed as staircases, rather than point to point?	The tradition is to plot the actual experience in the sample. So, when a subject dies, the curve drops down in a staircase fashion. Connecting the points diagonally might do a better job of demonstrating your best estimate for survival in the overall population, but this is not standard.
What if subjects enter the study on different dates?	That's OK. The X-axis shows time from entry in the study, so it does not correspond to calendar dates.
Why is the confidence band asymmetrical?	Because the percentage survival cannot go below 0.0 or above 100, the CI will be lopsided. This asymmetry is very noticeable when the sample survival percentage is far from 50 or the sample size is small.
Why is no CI plotted at time zero?	At time zero, 100% survival is a given. Subjects who are not alive at time zero are not included in the study! So the survival at time zero is not a value subject to sampling error. It is 100% for sure.

Continued

Q&A Continued

My confidence band is too wide to be useful. How can I make it narrower?	Collect more data, a lot more data. The width of the CI is approximately proportional to the reciprocal of the square root of the sample size. So, if you increase the sample size by a factor of 4, you can expect the CI to be half as wide.
Why report median survival time rather than the mean (average) survival time?	This is because the mean survival time can only be computed when there are no censored observations and the study continues long enough for all subjects to have died. In contrast, median survival can be computed when some observations are censored and when the study ends before all subjects have died. Once half of the subjects have died, the median survival is unambiguous even without knowing how long the others will live.
In the example, two of seven subjects survived. Why doesn't the curve end at Y = 2/7 or 29%?	Survival curve calculations properly account for censored data. After data are censored, that subject doesn't contribute to computing the percentage survival. Data for two subjects were censored prior to the last time point, so the simple computation (2/7 = 29% still survive) is not correct. In fact, the curve ends with 34.9% survival.
Can the data be plotted as percentage death rather than percentage survival?	Yes! See Figure 5.2.

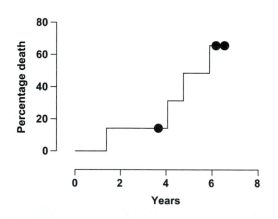

Figure 5.2. A graph of percentage death, rather than percentage survival, illustrates the same information.

When only a small percentage of subjects have died by the end of the study, this kind of graph can be more informative (because the Y-axis doesn't have to extend all the way to 100).

CHAPTER 6

———

Confidence Interval
of Counted Data

> Not everything that can be counted counts; and not every-
> thing that counts can be counted.
>
> ALBERT EINSTEIN

*W*hen events occur randomly, independently of one another, and
*with an average rate that doesn't change over time, the number of
events counted in a certain time interval (or the number of objects counted
in a certain volume) follow a Poisson distribution. From the number of
events actually observed (or the number of objects actually counted), a
confidence interval (CI) can be computed for the average number of events
per unit of time (or objects per unit volume).*

THE POISSON DISTRIBUTION

Some outcomes are expressed as the number of objects in some volume or the
number of events in some time interval. Examples include the number of babies
born in an obstetrics ward each day, the number of eosinophils seen in one microscope field, or the number of radioactive disintegrations detected by a scintillation counter in one minute.

As you'd expect, if you repeatedly sample time intervals (or volume), the
number of events (or objects) will vary. This random distribution is called a
Poisson distribution. Given the population's average number of occurrences in
one unit of time (or space), the Poisson distribution predicts how often you'll
observe any particular number of events or objects.

Figure 6.1 presents examples of the Poisson distribution. Background radiation depends on which types of radiation you measure and how sensitive (and
large) the detector is, but ranges from a few to a few dozen counts per minute.
Figure 6.1 illustrates the predictions of the Poisson distribution with an average
population rate of 1.6 counts/minute (left) and 7.5 counts/minute (right). In any
particular minute, the number of detected radiation counts may be higher or
lower than the average. The number of disintegrations counted will always be an
integer and will follow a Poisson distribution. The right half of Figure 6.1 shows

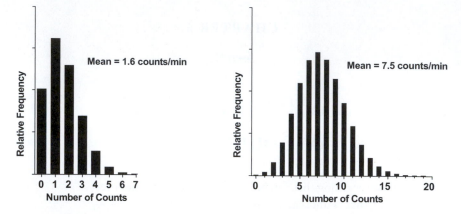

Figure 6.1. The Poisson distribution.

Assume that the average number of radiation counts is 1.6 counts/minute (left) or 7.5 counts/minute (right). In any particular minute, the count may be higher or lower than the average, as illustrated by these Poisson distributions. The horizontal axis lists the number of radioactive disintegrations actually counted (not normalized to counts per minute), and the vertical axis plots the frequency.

the predictions of a Poisson distribution when the average number of counts is 7.5 counts/minute. This Poisson distribution is nearly symmetrical and looks like a Gaussian distribution (see Chapter 10). The left half of Figure 6.1 shows the predictions of a Poisson distribution with an average of 1.6 counts per minute. This Poisson distribution is notably asymmetrical.

Because the number of objects or events cannot be less than zero, but has no upper limit, the Poisson distribution is skewed (asymmetrical), especially if the counts are very low. With larger population mean counts, this asymmetry is unnoticeable, and the Poisson distribution approximates a Gaussian distribution (to be explained in Chapter 10).

ASSUMPTIONS: POISSON DISTRIBUTION

Calculations based on the Poisson distribution can be used for number of events per unit time or number of objects in a certain volume.

Assumptions for number of events

Calculations about events assume the following:

- The event is clearly defined.
- Each event occurs randomly, independent of other events. This assumption might be violated if you tracked the number of babies born each day, because of the occurrence twins and triplets. Instead, count the number of deliveries (counting twins and triplets as one delivery).

- The average rate doesn't change over time.
- Each event is counted only once. This assumption was violated in a study conducted to find out how often airplanes nearly collide. They surveyed pilots and copilots, but the initial analysis overestimated the number of near misses. The problem is that this study design allowed for a single near miss to be reported four times—by both pilots in both planes ("NASA Blows Millions," 2007).

Assumptions for number of objects
Calculations about objects assume the following:

- Objects are randomly dispersed, with no clumps.
- Each object is only counted once.
- Objects are well-defined, with no ambiguity about what to count (or not count). If you are counting cells in a microscope field, you must be able to accurately differentiate cells from debris, and the cells must not be clumped.

CIs BASED ON POISSON DISTRIBUTIONS

The Poisson distribution can be used to compute a CI. All you need to know is the actual number of objects counted in a volume, or the number of events that occurred in one time interval, and it is possible to compute a CI for the average number of objects in that volume, or counts in that time interval. The calculations are explained later in this chapter. These examples are meant to explain the concept, not the calculations.

Raisins in bagels
You carefully dissect a bagel and find 10 raisins. If you assume that raisins are randomly distributed among bagels, with no clumping of raisins (perhaps a dubious assumption), and that the average number of raisins per bagel isn't changing over time (the recipe is constant), then the Poisson distribution applies. The 95% CI ranges from 4.8 to 18.4 (Table 6.1). You are 95% certain that the average number of raisins per bagel lies in that range.

Radioactive counts
You have counted 120 radioactive counts in 1 minute. Radioactive counts occur randomly and independently, and the average rate doesn't change (within a reasonable time frame much shorter than its half-life). Thus, the Poisson distribution is a reasonable model. The 95% CI for the average number of counts per minute is 99.5 to 143.5.

Note that you must base this calculation on the actual number of radioactive disintegrations counted. If you counted the tubes for 10 minutes, the calculation must be based on the counts in 10 minutes and not on the calculated number of counts in 1 minute. This is explained below.

C	LOWER	UPPER	C	LOWER	UPPER	C	LOWER	UPPER
0	0.00	3.69	41	29.42	55.62	82	65.21	101.78
1	0.03	5.57	42	30.27	56.77	83	66.11	102.89
2	0.24	7.22	43	31.12	57.92	84	67.00	104.00
3	0.62	8.77	44	31.97	59.07	85	67.89	105.10
4	1.09	10.24	45	32.82	60.21	86	68.79	106.21
5	1.62	11.67	46	33.68	61.36	87	69.68	107.31
6	2.20	13.06	47	34.53	62.50	88	70.58	108.42
7	2.81	14.42	48	35.39	63.64	89	71.47	109.52
8	3.45	15.76	49	36.25	64.78	90	72.37	110.63
9	4.12	17.08	50	37.11	65.92	91	73.27	111.73
10	4.80	18.39	51	37.97	67.06	92	74.16	112.83
11	5.49	19.68	52	38.84	68.19	93	75.06	113.93
12	6.20	20.96	53	39.70	69.33	94	75.96	115.03
13	6.92	22.23	54	40.57	70.46	95	76.86	116.13
14	7.65	23.49	55	41.43	71.59	96	77.76	117.23
15	8.40	24.74	56	42.30	72.72	97	78.66	118.33
16	9.15	25.98	57	43.17	73.85	98	79.56	119.43
17	9.90	27.22	58	44.04	74.98	99	80.46	120.53
18	10.67	28.45	59	44.91	76.11	100	81.36	121.63
19	11.44	29.67	60	45.79	77.23	101	82.27	122.72
20	12.22	30.89	61	46.66	78.36	102	83.17	123.82
21	13.00	32.10	62	47.54	79.48	103	84.07	124.92
22	13.79	33.31	63	48.41	80.60	104	84.98	126.01
23	14.58	34.51	64	49.29	81.73	105	85.88	127.11
24	15.38	35.71	65	50.17	82.85	106	86.78	128.20
25	16.18	36.90	66	51.04	83.97	107	87.69	129.30
26	16.98	38.10	67	51.92	85.09	108	88.59	130.39
27	17.79	39.28	68	52.80	86.21	109	89.50	131.49
28	18.61	40.47	69	53.69	87.32	110	90.41	132.58
29	19.42	41.65	70	54.57	88.44	111	91.31	133.67
30	20.24	42.83	71	55.45	89.56	112	92.22	134.77
31	21.06	44.00	72	56.34	90.67	113	93.13	135.86
32	21.89	45.17	73	57.22	91.79	114	94.04	136.95
33	22.72	46.34	74	58.11	92.90	115	94.94	138.04
34	23.55	47.51	75	58.99	94.01	116	95.85	139.13
35	24.38	48.68	76	59.88	95.13	117	96.76	140.22
36	25.21	49.84	77	60.77	96.24	118	97.67	141.31
37	26.05	51.00	78	61.66	97.35	119	98.58	142.40
38	26.89	52.16	79	62.55	98.46	120	99.49	143.49
39	27.73	53.31	80	63.44	99.57	121	100.40	144.58
40	28.58	54.47	81	64.33	100.68	122	101.31	145.67

Table 6.1. The 95% CIs of Poisson (counted) data.

C is the number of events or number of objects that you actually counted. The 95% CI for the average number of events per unit time, or number of objects per unit of volume is given. Be sure not to normalize C to some standard unit. C must be the number of events or objects actually counted. For larger C, use the equation:

$$C - 1.96\sqrt{C} \text{ to } C + 1.96\sqrt{C}$$

People-years

Exposure to an environmental toxin caused 1.6 deaths per 1,000 person-years exposure. What is the 95% CI? To calculate the CI, you must know the exact number of deaths that were observed in the study. This study observed 16 deaths in observations of 10,000 person-years (they might have studied 10,000 people for 1 year or 500 people for 20 years). Set $C = 16$, and the 95% CI for the number of deaths ranges from 9.15 to 25.98. Divide by the denominator (10,000 person-years) to express the 95% CI for the death rate, which ranges from 0.92 to 2.6 deaths per 1,000 person-years exposure.

HOW TO: CALCULATE THE POISSON CI

To compute the CI of a count, all you need is the count (C) from one sample. If you have multiple samples, just add the counts from each sample to calculate a total count. It is essential that you base the calculations on the number of events (or objects) actually observed. Don't normalize to a more convenient time scale or volume until after you have calculated the CI. If you attempt to calculate a CI based on the normalized count, the results will be meaningless.

When C is large (greater than 25 or so), here is a useful shortcut approximation for the 95% CI of C:

$$C - 1.96\sqrt{C} \text{ to } C + 1.96\sqrt{C}$$

So if C is 25, the approximate 95% CI extends from 15 to 35, whereas the exact CI ranges from 16.2 to 36.9 (Table 6.1).

If your count combined multiple samples, divide both ends of the interval by the number of samples to calculate the CI of the number of counts per sample.

THE ADVANTAGE OF USING LONGER TIME INTERVALS (OR BIGGER VOLUMES)

Figure 6.2 demonstrates the advantage of using a longer time interval. One tube containing a radioactive sample was counted repeatedly. The left side of Figure 6.2 illustrates radioactive decays counted in 1-minute intervals. The right side of Figure 6.2 illustrates radioactive decays counted in 10-minute intervals. The graph plots counts per minute, so the number of radioactive counts counted in each 10-minute interval was divided by 10.0 before being graphed.

When computing the CIs for Poisson variables, it is essential to do the calculations with the number of objects or events actually counted. If you count 700

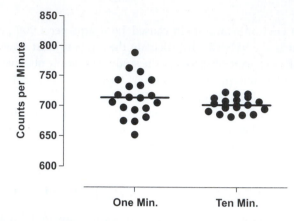

Figure 6.2. The advantages of counting radioactive samples for a longer time interval.

One radioactive sample was repeatedly measured for 1-minute intervals (left) and 10-minute intervals (right). The number of radioactive counts detected in the 10-minute samples was divided by 10, so both parts of the graph show counts per minute. By counting longer, there is less Poisson error. Thanks to Arthur Christopoulos for providing the data.

radioactive disintegrations in 1 minute, the 95% CI for the average number of disintegrations per minute ranges from about 650 to 754. If you count 7,000 disintegrations in 10 minutes, the 95% CI for the average number of disintegrations per 10 minutes ranges from 6,836 to 7,164. Divide those values by 10 to obtain the 95% CI for the average number of decays per minute, which ranges from 684 to 716. Counting for a longer period of time gives you a more precise assessment of the average number of counts per interval.

Let's revisit the example of raisins in bagels. Instead of counting raisins in one bagel, imagine that you had dissected seven individual bagels and found counts of 9, 7, 13, 12, 10, 9, and 10 raisins. In total, there were 70 raisins in seven bagels, so an average of 10 raisins per bagel. The CI should be computed on the total counted. Given 70 objects counted in a certain volume the 95% CI for the average number ranges from 54.57 to 88.44. This is the number of raisins per seven bagels. Divide by 7 to express these results in more useful units. The 95% CI ranges from 7.8 to 12.6 raisins per bagel.

It is essential that you normalize time (or volume) units only *after* computing the CI from the actual number of events or objects that were counted. If you first normalized to counts per minute, you would get the wrong result when computing the CI.

Q & A: Poisson Distribution

What is the difference between the binomial and Poisson distributions?	Both the binomial and Poisson distributions are used for outcomes that are counted, but the two are very different. The binomial distribution describes the distribution of two possible outcomes. The Poisson distribution describes the possible number of objects you'll find in a certain volume, or the number of events you'll observe in a particular time span.
Why use 1.96 in the equation in the previous section?	You'll learn about this in Chapter 10. In a Gaussian distribution, 95% of the values lie within 1.96 standard deviations of the mean. With large values of C, the Poisson distribution approximates a Gaussian distribution, with a standard deviation equal to the square root of C.
Is it possible to compute a CI when the observed number of counts is zero?	Yes. When you observe zero objects in a certain volume or zero events in a certain time, the 95% CI for the average number of objects in that volume (or events in that time interval) ranges from 0.0 to 3.69.

Continuous Variables

PART 4

Continuous Variables

CHAPTER 7

Graphing Continuous Data

When you can measure what you are speaking about and
express it in numbers, you know something about it; but when
you cannot measure it, when you cannot express it in numbers,
your knowledge is of the meager and unsatisfactory kind.

LORD KELVIN

*When results are continuous (blood pressure, enzyme activity, IQ
score, blood hemoglobin, oxygen saturation, temperature, etc.),
the first step (too often neglected) is to visualize the data. This chapter
shows how the actual distribution of values can be graphed, without any
statistical calculations.*

CONTINUOUS DATA

When analyzing data, it is essential to choose methods appropriate for the kind
of data you are working with. To highlight this point, this book began with dis-
cussions of three kinds of data. Chapter 4 discussed data expressed as two possible outcomes, summarized as a proportion; Chapter 5 explained survival data
and how to account for censored observations; and Chapter 6 discussed data
expressed as the actual number of events counted in a certain time, or as objects
counted in a certain volume.

This chapter begins a discussion of continuous data, such as blood pressures,
enzyme activity, weights, and temperature. Continuous data are more common
than other kinds of data.

THE MEAN AND MEDIAN

Mackowiak and colleagues (1992) measured body temperature from hundreds
of healthy individuals to see what the normal temperature range really is. A
subset of 12 of these values is shown in Table 7.1. These values, and the sugges-
tion to use them to explain basic statistical principles, come (with permission)
from Schoemaker (1996).

Calculating an *arithmetic mean* or average is easy: Add up all the values and
divide by the number of observations. The mean of the smaller (n = 12) subset
is 36.77°C. If the data are contaminated with an outlier (a value far from the

37.0
36.0
37.1
37.1
36.2
37.3
36.8
37.0
36.3
36.9
36.7
36.8

Table 7.1. The body temperature of 12 individuals in degrees centigrade.

These values are used as sample data.

others), the mean won't be very representative. For example, if the largest value (37.1) were mistakenly entered into the computer as 371 (that is, without the decimal point), the mean would increase to 64.6°C, which is larger than all the other values.

The mean is one way to quantify the middle or central tendency of the data, but it is not the only way. Here are some others:

- The *median* is the middle value. Rank the values from lowest to highest and identify the middle one. This definition ensures that the median is not influenced by an outlier, or even a bunch of outliers. If there are an even number of values, average the two middle ones. For the n = 130 data set, the median is the average of the 65th and 66th ranked values, 36.85°C.

- The *geometric mean* is calculated by transforming all values to their logarithms, computing the mean of each logarithm, and then taking the antilog of that mean (logarithms and antilogarithms are reviewed in Appendix E). Because a logarithm is only defined for values greater than zero, the geometric mean cannot be calculated if any values are zero or negative. None of the temperature values is zero or negative, so the geometric mean could be computed. But it would not be useful with the sample temperature data, because 0.0 does not mean "no temperature." Temperature in degrees centigrade is not a ratio variable (defined in Chapter 8). Read more about the geometric mean in Chapter 11.

- The *harmonic mean* is calculated by first transforming each value to its reciprocal and then computing the (arithmetic) mean of those reciprocals. The harmonic mean is the reciprocal of that mean. If the values are all positive, larger numbers effectively get less weight than lower numbers.

The harmonic mean is not commonly used in the biological sciences. It can't be computed if any values are zero or negative.

- The *trimmed mean* is the mean of most of the values, ignoring the highest and lowest values. Olympic ice skating used to be scored this way, with the largest and smallest score eliminated before averaging the scores from all other judges. Sometimes several of the highest and lowest values are ignored.

- The *mode* is the value that occurs most commonly in the data set. It is not useful with continuous variables assessed with at least several digits of accuracy, because each value will be unique. The mode can be useful with variables that can only be expressed as integers. Note that the mode doesn't always assess the center of a distribution. Imagine, for example, a medical survey where one of the questions is "How many times have you had surgery?" In many populations, the most common answer will be zero, so that is the mode. In this case, some values will be higher than the mode, but none will be lower.

Q & A: Mean and Median

Can the mean or median equal zero? Can it be negative?	Yes. The mean (or median) can have any value, including negative values and zero.
Which is larger, the mean or median?	It depends on the data. If the distribution of values is symmetrical, the mean and median will be similar. If the distribution is skewed to the right, with an excess of large values, then the mean will be larger than the median.
Are "mean" and "average" synonyms?	Yes, they are interchangeable.
What units are the mean and median expressed in?	The mean and median are expressed in the same units as the data.
Can the mean and median be computed when $n=1$? When $n=2$?	Computing a mean or median from two values is no problem. The whole idea of a mean or median makes no sense when there is only one value, but you could say that the mean and the median both equal that value.
Can the mean and median be calculated when some values are negative?	Yes. But the geometric and harmonic means can only be calculated when all values are positive.
Is the 50th percentile the same as the median?	Yes.

LINGO: ERROR AND BIAS

In Figure 7.1 the temperatures range from 35.7 to 38.2°C (Figure 7.1). Most of this variation is probably the result of biological variability. People (and animals, and

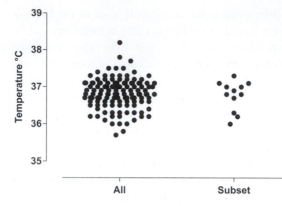

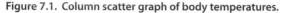

Figure 7.1. Column scatter graph of body temperatures.
(Left) The entire dataset, with n = 130. (Right) A randomly selected subset (n = 12). In a column scatter graph, the vertical position of each symbol denotes its value. The horizontal position (within each lane) is adjusted (jittered) to prevent points from overlapping (too much).

even cells) are different from one another, and these differences are important! Moreover, people (and animals) vary over time because of circadian variations, aging, and alterations in activity, mood, and diet. In biological and clinical studies, much or most of the scatter is often caused by biological variation.

It is possible that some of the variation in the temperature values comes from imprecision or experimental error. Reading a thermometer takes a bit of judgment and can be prone to error. Many statistics books (especially those designed for engineers) implicitly assume that most variability is the result of imprecision. In medical studies, biological variation can often contribute more variation than experimental imprecision.

Mistakes and glitches could also contribute to variability. It is possible that a value was written down incorrectly or that the thermometer wasn't positioned properly.

The word *error* is often used to refer to all three of these sources of variability. Note that this statistical use of "error" is quite different from the everyday use of the word to mean *mistake*. The terms *scatter* or *variability* are more understandable than the term error, but statistics books tend to use *error* when referring to any kind of variation.

Another term you should know is *bias*. Biased measurements result from systematic errors. Bias can be caused by any factor that consistently alters the results: the proverbial thumb on the scale, defective thermometers, bugs in computer programs (maybe the temperature was measured in centigrade and the program that converted the values to Fahrenheit was buggy), the placebo effect, and so on. As used in statistics, the word bias refers to anything that leads to systematic errors, not only the preconceived notions of the experimenter.

GRAPHING DATA TO SHOW SCATTER
OR DISTRIBUTION

Scatter plots indicate every value

Figure 7.1 plots the temperature data as a column scatter plot. The left side of the graph shows all 130 values. The right side of the graph shows the randomly selected subset of 12 values (Table 7.1), which we will analyze separately. Each value is plotted as a symbol. Within each half of the graph, symbols are moved to the right or left to prevent too much overlap; the horizontal position is arbitrary, but the vertical position, of course, denotes the measured value.

This kind of column scatter graph, or dot plot, demonstrates exactly how the data are distributed. You can see the lowest and highest value and the distribution. There is no need to plot a mean and error bar, because each value is visible. A horizontal line is commonly drawn at the mean or median.

With huge numbers of values, column scatter graphs get unwieldy with so many overlapping points. The left side of Figure 7.1, with 130 circles, is pushing the limits of this kind of graph. But the right side, with 12 circles, is quite clear and takes the same amount of space as a graph with mean and error bars, while showing more information.

Box-and-whiskers plots

A box-and-whiskers plot gives you a good sense of the distribution of data, without showing every value (Figure 7.2). Box-and-whisker plots work great when you have too many data points to show clearly on a column scatter graph, but you don't want to take the space to show a full frequency distribution.

A horizontal line marks the median of each group. The median is the 50th percentile. Half of the values are larger than the median and half are lower. If there is an even number of values, then the median is the average of the middle two values.

The boxes extend from the 25th to the 75th percentiles and, therefore, contain half the values. A quarter (25%) of the values are higher than the top of the box and 25% of the values are below the bottom of the box. If you try to calculate the quartiles yourself, note that calculating the percentiles is trickier than you'd guess. Eight different equations can be used to compute percentiles (Harter, 1984). All methods compute the same result for the median (50th percentile), but not for other percentiles. With large data sets, however, the results are all similar.

The whiskers can be graphed in various ways. The first box-and-whiskers plot in Figure 7.2 plots the whiskers down to the 5th and up to the 95th percentiles, and plots individual dots for values lower than the 5th and higher than the 95th percentile. The other box-and-whisker plot in Figure 7.2 plots whiskers down to the smallest value and up to the largest, and so it doesn't plot any individual points. Whiskers can be defined in other ways as well.

Frequency distribution histograms

A frequency distribution lets you see the distribution of many values. Divide the range of values into a set of smaller ranges (bins), and graph how many

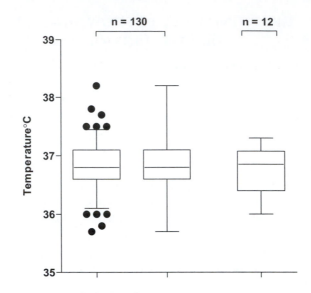

Figure 7.2. Box-and-whisker plots.
(Left) Box-and-whisker plots of the entire dataset. The whiskers extend down to the 5th percentile and up to the 95th, with individual values showing beyond that. (Middle) The whiskers show the range of the data. (Right) The box-and-whiskers plot of the subset of 12 values.

values are in each bin. Figure 7.3 illustrates frequency-distribution histograms for the temperature data. If you add the height of all the bars, you'll get the total number of values.

The trick in constructing frequency distributions is deciding how wide to make each bin. The three graphs in Figure 7.3 use different bin widths. The graph on the left has too few bins (each bin covers too wide a range of values), so it doesn't really show you enough detail about how the data are distributed. The graph on the right has too many bins (each bin covers too narrow a range of values), so it shows you too much detail. The graph in the middle is the most informative.

The term *histogram* is usually defined as a frequency distribution plotted as a bar graph, as illustrated in Figure 7.3. Sometimes, however, the term histogram is used more generally to refer to any bar graph, even one that is not a frequency distribution.

Cumulative frequency distribution
One way to avoid choosing a bin width is to plot a cumulative frequency distribution, where each Y value is the number of values less than X. The cumulative distribution begins at Y = 0 and ends at Y = n, the number of values in the data set. This kind of graph can be made without choosing a bin width. Figure 7.4 illustrates a cumulative frequency distribution of the temperature data.

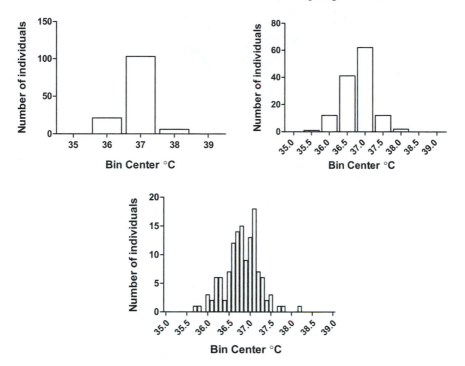

Figure 7.3. Frequency distribution histograms of the temperature data with various bin widths.

With too few bins (top-left), you don't get a sense of how the values vary. With too many bins (bottom), the graphs shows too much detail. Each bar plots the number of individuals whose body temperature is in a defined range (bin). The centers of each range, the bin centers, are labeled.

Figure 7.5 shows the same graph, but the Y-axis plots the percentage (rather than number) of values greater than each X value. The right side of Figure 7.5 illustrates the same distribution plotted with the Y-axis transformed in such a way that a cumulative distribution from a *Gaussian distribution* (see Chapter 10) becomes a straight line.

BEWARE OF DATA MASSAGE

Published graphs sometimes don't plot the data that were actually collected, but instead plot the result of computations. Pay attention to the decisions and calculations done between data collection and graphing.

Removing impossible values

Data sets are often screened to remove impossible values. Weights can't be negative. The year of death cannot be before the year of birth. The age of a child cannot be greater than the age of the mother. It makes no sense to run statistical

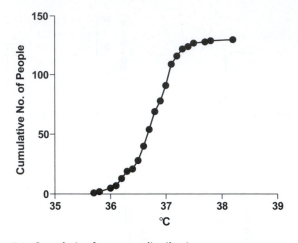
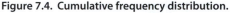

Figure 7.4. Cumulative frequency distribution.

Each circle illustrates the number of people whose temperature was less than (or equal to) the X value. With a cumulative distribution, there is no need to choose a bin width. This graph plots the distribution of 130 values. But since the data were recorded only to within 0.1 degree, there are only 21 unique values. Accordingly, the graph has 21 points.

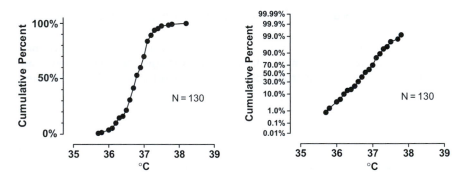
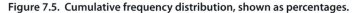

Figure 7.5. Cumulative frequency distribution, shown as percentages.

(Left) The graph is the same as Figure 7.4, except that the Y-axis plots the percentage of values greater than each X value (rather than the actual number). (Right) Plot of the data with the Y-axis transformed in such a way that a cumulative Gaussian distribution (to be explained in Chapter 10) becomes a straight line, as seen here.

analyses on obviously incorrect data. These values must be fixed (if the mistake can be traced) or removed.

But beware! Eliminating "impossible" values can also prevent you from seeing important findings. In 1985, researchers first noticed the drop in ozone levels over Antarctica (which turned out to be caused by chlorofluorocarbons).

But measurements from a satellite demonstrated no such drop. Why the discrepancy? It seems that the satellite had been reporting a drop in ozone levels for years, but these data were automatically removed because they were considered to be impossible values (Sparling, 2001). That story is disputed, but is illuminating, even if false. One must be very careful when automatically filtering out impossible values.

Adjusting data

The values analyzed by statistical tests are often not direct experimental measurements. It is common to adjust the data, so it is important to think about whether these adjustments are correct and whether they introduce errors. If the numbers going into a statistical test are questionable, then so are the statistical conclusions.

In some cases many adjustments are needed, and these adjustments can have a huge impact. As a case in point, NASA provides historical records of temperature. An examination of how temperature has changed over the past century has convinced many people that the world is getting warmer. The temperature record, however, requires many corrections. Corrections are needed to account for the fact that cities are warmer than surrounding areas (because of building heat), that different kinds of thermometers have been used at different historical times, that the time of day that temperatures have been taken is not consistent, etc. (Goddard, 2008). The net result of all these adjustments pushed earlier temperatures down by almost 1°C, which is about half of the observed temperature increase in the past century. These adjustments require judgment, and different scientists may do the adjustments differently. Anyone interpreting the data must understand the contribution of these adjustments to the overall observed effect, and the degree to which these adjustments could possibly be biased by the scientists' desire to make the data come out a certain way.

When interpreting published data, ask about how the data were adjusted before they were graphed or entered into a statistics program.

Smoothing

When plotting data that change over time, it is temping to smooth the data or plot a rolling average. The idea is to remove much of the variability in order to make the overall trend more visible.

Smoothed data should not be entered into statistical calculations. If given smoothed data, the results reported by most statistical tests will be invalid. Smoothing removes information, so most analyses of smoothed data are not useful.

Look ahead to Figure 33.4 to see an example of how analysis of smoothed data can lead to a very misleading conclusion.

Variables that are the ratio of two measurements

Often the value one cares about is the ratio of two values. For example, divide enzyme activity or number of binding sites by the cell count or the protein concentration. Calculating the ratio is necessary to express the variable in a way that can be interpreted and compared, for example as enzyme activity per milligram of protein. The numerator is usually what you are thinking about. The denominator is just housekeeping. But, of course, the accuracy of the ratio depends on the accuracy of both numerator and denominator.

Normalized data

Some scientists normalize data to run from 0 to 100%. When you see these kinds of data, you should wonder about how the values defined to equal 0% and 100% were chosen. Ideally, the definition of 0 and 100% is based on theory, or on control experiments with plenty of data. If 0 and 100% are not clearly defined, or seem to be defined sloppily, then the normalized values won't be very useful.

CHAPTER 8

Types of Variables

Get your facts first, then you can distort them as you please.

MARK TWAIN

The past four chapters have discussed four kinds of data. This chapter reviews the distinction between different kinds of variables. Much of this chapter is simply terminology, but these definitions commonly appear in exam questions.

INTERVAL VARIABLES

Chapter 7 used body temperature in degrees centigrade for its examples. This kind of continuous variable is termed an *interval variable* (but not a ratio variable). It is an interval variable because a difference (interval) of 1°C means the same thing all the way along the scale, no matter where you start.

Computing the difference between two values can make sense with interval variables. The 10°C difference between a temperature of 100 and 90°C has the same meaning as the difference as between 90 and 80°C.

Calculating the ratio of two temperatures is not useful. The problem is that the definition of zero is arbitrary. A temperature of 0.0°C is defined as the temperature where water freezes and certainly does not mean "no temperature." A temperature of 0.0°F is a completely different temperature (–17.8°C). Because the zero point is arbitrary (and doesn't mean no temperature), it would make no sense at all to compute ratios of temperatures. A temperature of 100°C is not twice as hot as 50°C.

Figure 8.1 illustrates average body temperatures of several species (Blumberg, 2004). The platypus has an average temperature of 30.5°C, whereas a canary has an average temperature of 40.5°C. It is incorrect to say that a canary has a temperature 33% higher than a platypus. If you did that same calculation using degrees Fahrenheit, you'd get a different answer.

Figure 8.1A is misleading. The bars start at zero, inviting you to compare their relative heights and to think about the ratio of those heights. But that comparison is not useful. This graph is also not helpful because it is difficult to see the differences between values.

Figure 8.1B uses a different baseline to demonstrate the differences. The bar for canary is about three times as high as the bar for platypus, but this ratio

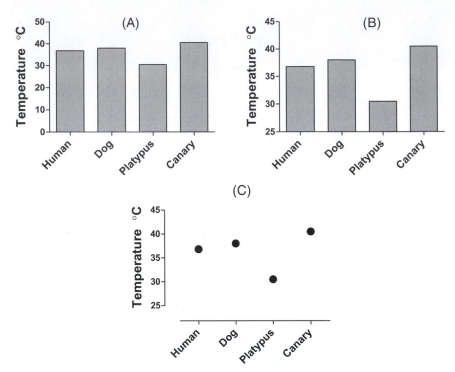

Figure 8.1. Body temperature of four species.

(A) is misleading. It invites you to compare the relative heights of the bars. But because a temperature of 0°C does not mean no temperature, the ratio of bar heights is not a meaningful value. (B) uses a different baseline to emphasize the differences. The bar for canary is about three times as high as the bar for platypus, but this ratio (indeed, any ratio) can be misleading. (C) illustrates the most informative way to graph these values.

(indeed, any ratio) is not useful. Figure 8.1C illustrates the most informative way to graph these values. The use of points, rather than bars, doesn't suggest thinking in terms of a ratio. A simple table might be better than any kind of graph for these values.

RATIO VARIABLES

With a *ratio variable*, zero is not arbitrary. Zero height is no height. Zero weight is no weight. Zero enzyme activity is no enzyme activity. So height, weight, and enzyme activity are ratio variables.

As the name suggests, it can make sense to compute the ratio of two ratio variables. A weight of 4 grams is twice the weight of 2 grams, because weight is a ratio variable. But, a temperature of 100°C is not twice as hot as 50°C, because temperature in °C is not a ratio variable. Note, however, that temperature in

OK TO COMPUTE...	NOMINAL	ORDINAL	INTERVAL	RATIO
Frequency distribution	Yes	Yes	Yes	Yes
Median and percentiles	No	Yes	Yes	Yes
Add or subtract	No	No	Yes	Yes
Ratio	No	No	No	Yes
Mean, standard deviation, standard error of the mean	No	No	Yes	Yes
Coefficient of variation	No	No	No	Yes

Table 8.1. Calculations that are meaningful with various kinds of variables.
The standard deviation and coefficient of variation will be explained in Chapter 9, and the standard error of the mean will be explained in Chapter 14.

degrees Kelvin is a ratio variable, because 0.0 degrees Kelvin really does mean (at least to a physicist) no temperature.

Like interval variables, you can compute the difference between ratio variables, as well as their ratio.

OTHER KINDS OF VARIABLES

The term *continuous variable* is applied to both interval and ratio variables. The next six chapters deal with continuous variables.

An *ordinal variable* expresses rank. The order matters, but not the exact value. For example, pain is expressed on a scale of 1 to 10. A score of 7 means more pain than a score of 5, which is more than a score of 3. But, it doesn't make sense to compute the difference between two values, because the difference between 7 and 5 may not be comparable to the difference between 5 and 3. The values simply express an order. Another example would be movie or restaurant ratings from one to five stars.

To complete the list of terms describing kinds of variables, here are two more. Categorical outcomes with two possibilities are called *binomial variables*. Categorical outcomes with more than two possible outcomes (not in any particular order) are *nominal variables*.

Table 8.1 summarizes which kinds of calculations are meaningful with which kinds of variables. Table 8.1 refers to the standard deviation and coefficient of variation, both of which are explained in Chapter 9, and the standard error of the mean (explained in Chapter 14).

NOT QUITE AS DISTINCT AS THEY SEEM

Note that the categories are nowhere near as distinct as they may sound (Velleman & Wilkinson, 1993). Here are some ambiguous situations:

- Color: In a psychological study of perception, different colors would be regarded as categories, so color is a nominal variable. But color can be quantified by wavelength, and thus be considered a ratio variable. Alternatively, you could rank the wavelengths and consider color an ordinal variable.

- The number of cells actually counted in a certain volume: It has all the properties of a ratio variable, except the number must be an integer. Is that a ratio variable or an ordinal variable?
- EC_{50}: An EC_{50} is a measure of a drug's potency. It is the drug concentration that elicits 50% of the maximum response. An EC_{50} cannot equal zero, but it is very useful to think about ratios of two EC_{50} values. So, it is sort of a ratio variable, but not quite.
- Percentages: Outcomes measured as a ratio or interval variables are often normalized, so they are expressed as percentages. For example, a pulse rate (heartbeats per minute, a ratio variable) could be normalized to a percentage of the maximum possible pulse rate. A discrete outcome with a set of mutually exclusive categories can also be expressed as a percentage. For example, what percentage of transplanted kidneys are rejected within a year of surgery? But these two situations are very different, and different kinds of statistical analyses are needed. The fact that data are expressed as percentages does not tell you what kind of variable it is.

CHAPTER 9

Quantifying Scatter

The average human has one breast and one testicle.
DES MCHALE

Chapter 7 demonstrated various ways to graph data in order to make it easy to see the degree of variability. This chapter explains how variation can be quantified with the standard deviation, variance, coefficient of variation, interquartile range, and median absolute deviation.

INTERPRETING A STANDARD DEVIATION

The variation among values can be quantified as the *standard deviation* (SD), which is expressed in the same units as the data.

You can interpret the SD using the following rule of thumb: About two thirds of the observations in a population usually lie within the range defined by the mean minus 1 SD to the mean plus 1 SD. This definition is unsatisfying because the word *usually* is so vague. Chapter 10 gives a more rigorous interpretation of the SD for data sampled from a Gaussian distribution.

Let's turn to the larger (n = 130) sample in Figure 9.1. The mean temperature is 36.82°C and the SD is 0.41°C. Figure 9.1 plots the mean with error bars extending 1 SD in each direction (error bars can be defined in other ways, as you'll see in Chapter 13).

The range 36.4 to 37.2°C extends below and above the mean by 1 SD. Figure 9.1 (left) is a column scatter graph of the body-temperature data, and you can see that about two thirds of the values are within that range.

Take a good look at Figure 9.1. Often you'll only see the mean and SD, as shown on the right, and you will need to imagine the actual scatter of the data. If you publish graphs, consider showing the actual data, as on the left side of Figure 9.1, rather than just the mean and SD.

HOW IT WORKS: CALCULATE A SD

It would seem that the simplest way to quantify a variability would be to ask how far each value is from the mean (or median) of all values, and then to report

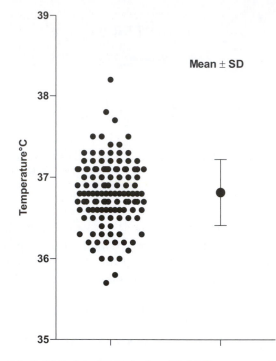

Figure 9.1. (Left) Each individual value. (Right) The mean and SD.

the average or median of those values. That wouldn't work, because the positive deviations would balance out the negative deviations so the average deviation would always equal zero. Another approach might be to take the average, or the median, of the absolute values of the deviations of each value from the mean. Indeed, *median absolute deviation* (MAD) is one way to quantify variability, and it is discussed later in this chapter. However, the most common way to quantify variation is by calculating the SD.

Of course, you'll use computer programs to compute the SD. Even so, the best way to understand the SD is to know how it is calculated.

1. Calculate the mean (average). For the n = 12 body-temperature sample in Figure 7.1, the mean is 36.77°C.
2. Calculate the difference between each value and the mean.
3. Square each of those differences.
4. Add up those squared differences. For the example data, the sum is 1.767.
5. Divide that sum by n–1, where n is the number of values. For the example, n = 12 and the result is 0.161. This value is called the variance.
6. Take the square root of the value you calculated in Step 5. The result is the SD. For this example, the SD = 0.40°C.

That recipe can be shown as an equation, where Y_i stands for one of the n values, and $\overline{Y}$ is the mean.

$$SD = \frac{\Sigma(Y_i - \overline{Y})^2}{n-1}$$

WHY n-1?

When calculating the SD, the sum of squares is divided by n–1. Why n–1 rather than n?

The numerator is the sum of the squares of the difference between each value and the mean of those values. Except for the rare case where the sample mean happens to equal the population mean, the data will be closer to the sample mean than it will be to the true population mean (which you can't know). Therefore, the sum of squares will probably be a bit smaller (and can't be larger) than what it would be if you computed the difference between each value and the true population mean. Because the numerator is a bit "too small," the denominator must be made smaller too.

Why n–1? If you knew the sample mean and all but one of the values, you could calculate what that last value must be. The nth value is absolutely determined from the sample mean and the other n–1 values. Only n–1 of the values are free to assume any value. Therefore, we calculate the average of the squared deviations by dividing by n–1, and say that there are n–1 *degrees of freedom* (df).

Many people find the concept of df to be quite confusing. Fortunately, being confused about df is not a big handicap! You can choose statistical tests and interpret the results with only a vague understanding of df.

The n–1 equation is used in the common situation where you are analyzing a sample of data and wish to make more general conclusions. The SD computed in this way (with n–1 in the denominator) is the most accurate estimate of the value of the SD in the overall population. This value is sometimes called the *sample SD*. It is the best possible estimate of the SD of the entire population, as determined from one particular sample, and so it should be used routinely in clinical and experimental science.

If you simply want to quantify the variation in a particular set of data, and don't plan to extrapolate to make wider conclusions, then you can compute the SD using n in the denominator. The resulting SD is correct for those particular values, but would usually underestimate the SD of the population from which those values were drawn. Use the equation with n in the denominator only when you are not trying to make general conclusions from the data. One example would be when a teacher wants to quantify variation among exam scores. The goal is not to make inferences about a larger population of hypothetical scores but just to quantify the variation among those particular scores.

	ANIMAL A	ANIMAL B	ANIMAL C
	47.7	64.7	39.3
	43.1	65.4	40.0
	52.3	88.3	23.9
	55.2	64.0	36.6
	42.5	71.9	48.9
Mean	48.2	70.9	37.7

Table 9.1. What is n?

Data from three animals (three columns), each with five replicate measurements (rows). Because there are not 15 independent values here, it is not correct to compute a SD and CI using n = 15. Instead, average the values from each animal and then compute the SD and CI from those three means using n = 3.

SITUATIONS WHERE n CAN SEEM AMBIGUOUS

When calculating SD (and various statistical tests), the definition of the sample size "n" can seem ambiguous in some situations.

Replicates

Table 9.1 presents a common situation. Data were collected from three animals (represented by the three columns), each with five replicate measurements (rows). In total, 15 values were collected. But these are not 15 independent samples from one population. There are two sources of variability here: variation between animals, and variation between replicate measurements in one animal. Lumping these together would lead to invalid analyses. It is not correct to compute a SD (and CI; see Chapter 12) using n = 15.

The simplest way to analyze such data is to average the values from each animal. For this example, there are three means (one for each animal). You would then compute the SD (and CI) from those three means using n = 3. The results can then be extrapolated to the population of animals you could have studied.

n-of-1 trials

Another situation where the definition of n is potentially ambiguous is the n-of-1 trial mentioned in Chapter 3. Such trials are conducted with only one patient (serving as his or her own control). But despite n-of-1 name, the n value used in statistical analysis is not 1, but rather is the number of values collected. The results can then be extrapolated to the population of results you could have collected from that one person.

SD AND SAMPLE SIZE

For the full body-temperature dataset (n = 130), as shown in Figure 7.1, SD = 0.41°C. For the smaller sample (n = 12, randomly sampled from the larger sample), SD = 0.40°C. Many find it surprising that the SD is so similar in samples of such different sizes. This is to be expected. The SD quantifies the variation within a population. As you collect larger samples, you'll be able to quantify the variability more accurately, but collecting more data doesn't change the variability among the values. Increasing sample size is equally likely to increase or decrease the SD.

Here is a way to think about this concept mathematically. Both the numerator and denominator of the equation at the top of page 73 grow equally when the sample size gets larger. The ratio, and thus the SD, does not change in a predicable direction.

COEFFICIENT OF VARIATION

For ratio variables, variability can be quantified as the coefficient of variation (CV), which equals the SD divided by the mean. If the CV equals 0.25, you know that the SD is 25% of the mean.

Because the SD and mean are both expressed in the same units, the CV is a fraction with no units. Often the CV is expressed as a percentage.

For the preceding temperature example, the CV would be completely meaningless. Temperature is an interval variable, not a ratio variable, because zero is defined arbitrarily (see Chapter 8). A CV computed from temperatures measured in degrees centigrade would not be the same as a CV computed from temperatures measured in degrees Fahrenheit. Neither CV would be meaningful, because the idea of dividing the mean by a measure of scatter only makes sense for ratio variables, where zero really means zero.

The CV is useful for comparing scatter of variables measured in different units. You could ask, for example, whether the variation in pulse rate is greater than or less than the variation in the concentration of serum sodium. The pulse rate and sodium are measured in completely different units, so comparing their standard deviations would make no sense. Comparing their coefficients of variation might prove useful to a physiological investigation of homeostasis.

VARIANCE

The *variance* equals the SD squared, and so is expressed in the same units as the data—squared. In the body-temperature example, the variance is 0.16°C squared.

Statistical theory is based on variances, rather than SD, because variances can be partitioned into various components. You can ask what fraction of that variance is caused by various factors, but it makes no sense to partition the SD in this way.

If you are not a mathematical statistician, you'll find it easier to avoid the concept of variance with its weird units. Use the SD instead.

Q & A: SD	
Can the SD ever equal zero? Can it be negative?	The SD will equal zero if all the values are identical. The SD can never be a negative number.
In what units do you express the SD?	The SD is expressed in the same units as the data.
Can the SD be computed when n = 1? When n = 2?	The SD quantifies variability, so it cannot be computed from a single value. It can be computed from two values (n = 2).
Is the SD the same as the standard error of the mean (SEM)?	No. They are very different. See Chapter 14.
Can the SD be computed if the data clearly do not come from a Gaussian distribution?	Yes. The SD can be computed from any set of values. The Gaussian distribution is explained in Chapter 10. If the data do not come from a Gaussian population, you cannot necessarily use the rule of thumb that roughly two-thirds of the values are expected to be within 1 SD of the mean.
Is the SD larger or smaller than the CV?	The SD is expressed in the same units as the data. The CV is a unitless ratio, often expressed as a percentage. Because the two are not expressed in the same units, it makes no sense to ask which is larger.
Is the SD larger or smaller than the variance?	The variance is the SD squared, so it is expressed in different units. It makes no sense to ask which is larger.

OTHER WAYS TO QUANTIFY VARIABILITY

The SD is not the only way to quantify variability.

Interquartile Range

Subtract the 25th percentile from the 75th percentile and you have the *interquartile range*. Because both of these percentile values are expressed in the same units as the data, the interquartile range is also expressed in the same units.

For the body-temperature data (n = 12 subset), the 25th percentile is 36.4°C and the 75th percentile is 37.1°C, so the interquartile range is 0.7°C. For the full (n = 130) data set, the 25th percentile is 36.6°C and the 75th percentile is 37.1°C, so the interquartile range is 0.5°C.

MEDIAN ABSOLUTE DEVIATION

The median absolute deviation (MAD) is a simple way to quantify variation. Half of the values are closer to the median than the MAD and half are farther away.

The best way to understand the MAD is to understand the "recipe" for how it is calculated. First, compute the median of all values. The median is the 50th percentile. Then calculate how far each value is from the median of all values. Regardless of whether the value is greater or less than the median, express the distance between it and the median as a positive value (that is, take the absolute value of the difference between the value and the median). Now find the median of that set of differences. The result is the MAD. (Some investigators take the mean of that set of differences and call the result the *mean absolute deviation*, also abbreviated MAD.)

For the body-temperature data (n = 12 subset), the median is 36.85°C, and the MAD is 0.2°C. For the full (n = 130) data set, the median is 36.8°C, and the MAD is 0.3°C.

Note one point of confusion. There are two distinct computations of the median. First, one computes the median (the 50th percentile) of the actual data. Then you compute the median of the absolute values of the distances of the data from the 50th percentile.

Like the interquartile range, but unlike the SD, computation of the MAD is resilient to the presence of outliers (Chapter 25).

Half of the values are within 1 MAD of the median. Therefore, a symmetrical range that extends 1 MAD in each direction from the median will contain about half of the values. The interquartile range also contains half of the values. The distinction is that the interquartile range can be asymmetrical around the median.

CHAPTER 10

The Gaussian Distribution

> Everybody believes in the normal approximation, the experi-
> menters because they think it is a mathematical theorem, the
> mathematicians because they think it is an experimental fact.
> G. LIPPMAN (1845–1921)

*Many statistical methods assume that data follow a Gaussian dis-
tribution. This chapter briefly explains the origin and use of the
Gaussian distribution. Chapter 24 will explain how to test for deviations
from a Gaussian distribution.*

ORIGIN OF THE GAUSSIAN DISTRIBUTION

The Gaussian bell-shape distribution is the basis for much of statistics. It arises when many random factors create variability. This happens because random factors tend to offset each other. Some will push the value higher and others will pull it lower. The effects usually partly cancel one another, so many values end up near the center (the mean). Sometimes many random factors will tend to work in the same direction, pushing a value away from the mean. Rarely, the random factors will nearly all work in the same direction, pushing that value far from the mean. Thus, many values are near the mean, some values are further from the mean, and very few are quite far from the mean. When you plot the data on a frequency distribution, the results is a symmetrical, bell-shape distribution, idealized as the *Gaussian distribution.*

Mathematicians have proven that scatter will approximate a Gaussian distribution when there are many sources of variation, so long as the various contributors to variation are summed to get the final result and the sample size is large. As you have more and more sources of scatter, the predicted result approaches a Gaussian distribution.

Interpreting many statistical tests requires an assumption that pervades much of statistics: The data must be sampled from a population that follows a Gaussian distribution. This is often a reasonable assumption. For example, in a laboratory experiment, variation between experiments might be caused by several factors: imprecise weighing of reagents, imprecise pipetting, the random nature of radioactive decay, nonhomogenous suspensions of cells or membranes, etc. Variation in a clinical value might be caused by many genetic and environmental

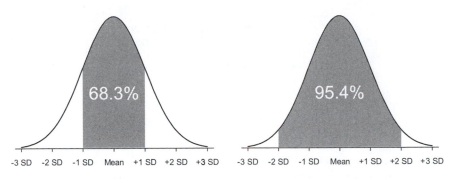

Figure 10.1. Ideal Gaussian distributions.
The horizontal axis plots various values, and the vertical axis plots their relative abundance. The area under the curve represents all values in the population. The fraction of that area within a range of values tells you how common those values are. (Left) About two thirds of the values are within 1 SD of the mean. (Right) Slightly more than 95% of the values are within 2 SD of the mean.

factors. When scatter is the result of many independent causes, the distribution will tend to follow a bell-shape Gaussian distribution.

SD AND THE GAUSSIAN DISTRIBUTION

Figure 10.1 illustrates an ideal Gaussian distribution. The horizontal axis shows various values that can be observed, and the vertical axis quantifies their relative frequency. The mean, of course, is the center of the Gaussian distribution. The Gaussian distribution is high near the mean, because that is where most of the values are. As you move away from the mean, the distribution drops down with its characteristic bell shape. The distribution is symmetrical, so the median and the mean are identical.

The SD is a measure of the spread or width of the distribution. The area under the entire curve represents the entire population. The left side of Figure 10.1 shades the area under the curve within 1 SD of the mean. You can see that the shaded portion is about two-thirds (68.3%) of the entire area, demonstrating that about two thirds of the values in a Gaussian population are within 1 SD of the mean. The right side of Figure 10.1 demonstrates that about 95% of the values in a Gaussian population are within 2 SD of the mean (the actual multiplier is 1.96).

Scientific papers and presentations often show the mean and SD, but not the actual data. If you assume that the distribution is approximately Gaussian, you can recreate the distribution in your head. Going back to the sample body-temperature data in Figure 9.1, what could you infer if you knew only that the mean is 36.82°C and its SD is 0.41°C (n = 130)? If you assume a Gaussian distribution, you could infer that about two thirds of the values lie between 36.4 and 37.2°C and that 95% of the values lie between 36.0 and 37.6°C. If you look back at Figure 9.1, you can see these estimates are not far off.

z	PERCENTAGE OF STANDARD NORMAL DISTRIBUTION BETWEEN −z AND z
0.67	50.00%
0.97	66.66%
1.00	68.27%
1.65	90.00%
1.96	95.00%
2.00	95.45%
2.58	99.00%
3.00	99.73%

Table 10.1. The standard normal distribution.

Table 10.1 is best understood by example. The range between z = −1 and z = +1 contains 68.27% of a standard normal distribution.

THE STANDARD NORMAL DISTRIBUTION

When the mean equals 0 and the SD equals 1.0, the Gaussian distribution is called a *standard normal curve*. Figure 10.1 would be a standard normal distribution if the labels went from −3 to +3, without using the labels SD and mean.

All Gaussian distributions can be converted to a standard normal distribution. To do this, subtract the mean from each value and divide the difference by the SD.

$$z = \frac{\text{Value} - \text{Mean}}{\text{SD}}$$

The variable "z" is the number of SD away from the mean. When z = 1, a value is 1 SD above the mean. When z = −2, a value is 2 SD below the mean. Table 10.1 tabulates the fraction of a normal distribution between −z and +z for various values of z.

If you work in pharmacology, don't confuse this use of the variable z with the specialized Z-factor used to assess the quality of an assay used to screen drugs (Zhang, Chung, & Oldenburg, 1999). The two are not related.

THE "NORMAL" DISTRIBUTION DOES NOT DEFINE NORMAL LIMITS

A Gaussian distribution is also called a *normal* distribution. This is another case where statistics has endowed an ordinary word with a special meaning. Don't mistake this special use of the word "normal" with its more ordinary meaning to describe commonly observed value, or a value of a lab test or clinical measurement that does not indicate disease.

Here is a simple, but flawed, approach that is often used: Assume that the body temperatures (from the examples of the previous chapters) in the population follow a Gaussian distribution and define 5% of the population to be abnormal.

Using the sample mean and SD from our study, the normal range can be (incorrectly) defined as the mean plus or minus 1.96 SD: 36.816 ± (1.96 · 0.405), which ranges from 36.0 to 37.6°C.

There are a number of problems with this approach:

- It really doesn't make sense to define normal and abnormal just in terms of the distribution of values in the general population. We know that high body temperature can be an indication of infection or inflammatory disease. So, the question we really want to answer is: When is a temperature high enough that it needs investigation? The answer to this question requires scientific or clinical context and cannot be answered by statistical calculations.
- Our definition of normal and abnormal really should depend on other factors such as age and sex. What is abnormal for a 25-year old may be normal for an 80-year old.
- In many cases, we don't really want a crisp boundary between normal and abnormal. It often makes sense to label some values as "borderline."
- Even if the population is approximately Gaussian, it is unlikely to follow a Gaussian distribution exactly. The deviations from Gaussian are likely to be most apparent in the tails (extreme values) of the distribution, where the abnormal values lie.
- This approach defines just as many people as having abnormally high values as abnormally low values. Is having a temperature in the lowest 2.5% really an indication that something is wrong and that further medical workup is warranted? There is no reason to define the normal limits symmetrically around the mean or median.

Defining the normal limits of a clinical measurement is not straightforward and requires clinical thinking. Simple statistics rules based on the mean, SD, and the Gaussian distribution should not be used.

WHY THE GAUSSIAN DISTRIBUTION IS SO CENTRAL TO STATISTICAL THEORY

The Gaussian distribution plays a central role in statistics because of a mathematical relationship known as the *central limit theorem*. You'll need to read a more theoretical book to really understand this theorem, but the explanation below gives you the basics.

To understand this theorem, follow this imaginary experiment:

1. Create a population with a known distribution that is not Gaussian.
2. Randomly pick many samples of equal size from that population.
3. Tabulate the means of these samples.
4. Graph the frequency distribution of the means.

The central limit theorem says that if your samples are large enough, the distribution of means will follow a Gaussian distribution, although the population is not Gaussian. Because most statistical tests (such as the t test and analysis of variance) are concerned only with differences between means, the central limit theorem explains why these tests work well even when the populations are not Gaussian.

Q & A: Gaussian Distribution

Who was Gauss?	Karl Gauss was a mathematician (one of the greatest of all time) who used this distribution in 1809 to analyze astronomical data. Although his name is now attached to the distribution, others (Laplace and de Moivre) actually used it earlier.
Is the Gaussian distribution the same as a normal distribution?	Yes, the two terms are used interchangeably.
Are all bell-shape distributions Gaussian?	As you can see in Figure 10.1, the Gaussian distribution is bell-shaped. But not all bell-shape curves are Gaussian.
Will numerous sources of scatter always create a Gaussian distribution?	No. A Gaussian distribution is formed only when each source of variability is independent and additive with the others, and no one source dominates. Chapter 11 discusses what happens when the sources of variation multiply.

CHAPTER 11

The Lognormal Distribution and Geometric Mean

42.7 percent of all statistics are made up on the spot.
STEVEN WRIGHT

*L*ognormal distributions are not an obscure mathematical quirk, but *are very common in many fields of science. This chapter explains how lognormal distributions arise, and how to analyze lognormal data. Read this chapter to prevent making the common mistake of choosing analyses that assume sampling from a Gaussian distribution, when working with data that are actually sampled from a lognormal distribution.*

EXAMPLE: RELAXING BLADDERS

And you thought statistics was never relaxing!

Frazier, Schneider, and Michel (2006) measured the ability of isoprenaline (a drug which acts much like the neurotransmitter norepinephrine) to relax the bladder muscle. The results are expressed as the EC_{50}, which is the concentration required to relax the bladder halfway between its minimum and maximum possible relaxation. The graph on the left side of Figure 11.1 illustrates the data plotted on a linear scale.

The distribution is far from symmetrical and is quite skewed. One value lies distant from the rest and almost looks like a mistake.

THE ORIGIN OF A LOGNORMAL DISTRIBUTION

Chapter 10 explained that a Gaussian distribution arises when variation is caused by many factors that are additive. Some factors push a value higher and some pull it lower, and the cumulative result is a symmetrical bell-shape distribution that approximates a Gaussian distribution.

But some factors act in a multiplicative, rather than additive, manner. If a factor works multiplicatively, it is equally likely to double a value as to cut it in half. If that value starts at 100 and is multiplied by 2, it ends up at 200. If it is divided by 2, it ends up at 50. So that factor is equally likely to increase a value by 100 or decrease it by 50. The effect is not symmetrical.

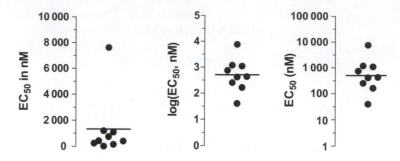

Figure 11.1. Lognormal data.

These data demonstrate the EC_{50} of isoprenaline for relaxing bladder muscle (Frazier et al., 2006). Each dot indicates data from the bladder of a different animal. The EC_{50} is the concentration required to relax the bladder halfway between its minimum and maximum possible relaxation , in nanomoles per liter (nM). The graph on the left plots the original concentration scale. The data are far from symmetrical, and the highest value appears to be an outlier. The middle graph plots the logarithm (base 10) of the EC_{50} and it is symmetrical. The graph on the right plots the raw data on a logarithmic axis. This kind of graph is a bit easier to read.

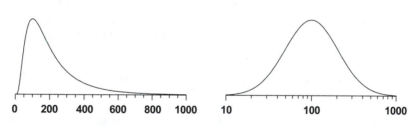

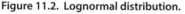

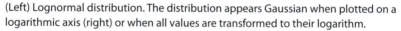

Figure 11.2. Lognormal distribution.

(Left) Lognormal distribution. The distribution appears Gaussian when plotted on a logarithmic axis (right) or when all values are transformed to their logarithm.

If many factors act in a multiplicative manner, the resulting distribution is asymmetrical, as shown in Figure 11.2 (left). This distribution is called a *lognormal distribution*. Logarithms? How did logarithms enter this picture? As the next section will demonstrate: The logarithms of the values follow a Gaussian distribution, but the raw data do not.

HOW TO ANALYZE LOGNORMAL DATA

If you transform all values from a lognormal distribution to their logarithms, the distribution becomes Gaussian. Logarithms (and antilogarithms) are reviewed in Appendix E.

The middle graph in Figure 11.1 plots the logarithm of the EC_{50} values. Note that the distribution is symmetrical.

The graph on the right in Figure 11.1 illustrates an alternative way to plot the data. The axis has a logarithmic scale. Note that every major tick on the axis represents a value 10 times higher than the previous value. The distribution of data points is identical to that in the middle graph, but the graph on the right is easier to comprehend because the Y values are in natural units of the data, rather than logarithms.

GEOMETRIC MEAN

The mean of the data from Figure 11.1 is 1,333 nM. This is illustrated as a horizontal line in the left panel of Figure 11.1. The mean is larger than all but one of the values, so it is not a good measure of the central tendency of the data.

The middle panel plots the logarithms of the values on a linear scale. The horizontal line is at the mean of the logarithms, 2.71. About half of the values are higher and half are smaller.

The right panel in Figure 11.1 uses a logarithmic axis. The values are the same as those of the graph on the left, but the spacing of the values on the axis is logarithmic. The horizontal line is at the antilog of the mean of the logarithms. This graph uses logarithms base 10, so the antilog is computed by calculating $10^{2.71}$, which equals 513. The value 513 nM is called the *geometric mean*.

To compute a geometric mean, first transform all the values to their logarithms. Then calculate the mean of those logarithms. Then transform that mean of the logarithms back to the original units of the data.

Q&A: Lognormal Distributions

Where can I review logarithms and antilogarithms?	In Appendix E.
Lognormal or log-normal?	Both forms are commonly used.
Are values in a lognormal distribution always positive?	Yes. The logarithm of zero and negative numbers is simply not defined. Distributions that contain zero or negative values cannot be treated as lognormal distributions.
Can the geometric mean be computed if any values are zero or negative?	No.
When computing the geometric mean, should I use natural logarithms or logs base 10?	It doesn't matter, as long as you are consistent. More often, scientists use logarithms base 10, so the reverse transform is the power of 10. The geometric mean will have exactly the same value, whichever log base is used, as long as the antilog transform is chosen to match. See Appendix E.

Continued

Q&A Continued

Are lognormal distributions common?	Yes, they occur commonly (Limpert, Stahel, & Abbt, 2001). For example, the potency of a drug (assessed as EC_{50}, IC_{50}, K_m, K_i, etc.) is almost always lognormal. For this reason, it makes sense to compare treatment groups using ratios rather than differences, and to summarize data with a geometric mean. Other examples of lognormal distributions are the blood-serum concentrations of many natural or toxic compounds.
Should I use a logarithmic axis when plotting data from a lognormal distribution?	Yes, this can make it easier to understand. See Figure 11.1 (right).
What happens if you analyze data from a lognormal distribution as if they were sampled from a Gaussian distribution?	It depends on the details of the data and the sample size. It is likely that the results of any statistical analysis that assumes a Gaussian distribution will be misleading. You may also be misled about the presence of outliers (Chapter 25). An easy mistake would be to view the left graph of Figure 11.1 and conclude that these values are sampled from a Gaussian distribution, but contaminated by the presence of a single outlier. Running an outlier test would confirm that conclusion. But that would be misleading. Outlier tests assume that all the values (except for any outliers) are sampled from a Gaussian distribution. When presented with data from a lognormal distribution, outlier tests are likely to incorrectly flag very high values as outliers, when in fact those high values are expected in a lognormal distribution.
What units are used to express the geometric mean?	The same units as used with the values being analyzed. Thus, the mean and geometric mean are expressed in the same units.
Is the geometric mean larger or smaller than the regular mean?	The geometric mean is always smaller.

CHAPTER 12

Confidence Interval of a Mean

It is easy to lie with statistics. It is hard to tell the truth
without it.

ANDREJS DUNKELS

*C*hapters 4 through 6 have explained confidence intervals of proportions, counts, and survival fractions. This chapter extends those concepts to the confidence interval of a mean, a calculation which depends
on the size of the sample and the variability of the values (expressed as
the standard deviation).

INTERPRETING A CI OF A MEAN

For our ongoing n = 130 body-temperature example (Figure 7.1), any statistics program will calculate that the 95% CI of the mean ranges from 36.75 to
36.89°C. For the smaller n = 12 subset, the 95% CI of the mean ranges from 36.51
to 37.02°C.

Note that there is no uncertainty about the sample mean. We are 100% sure
that we have calculated the sample mean correctly. Any errors in recording the
data or computing the mean will not be accounted for in computing the CI of the
mean. By definition, the CI is always centered on the sample mean. The population mean is not known and can't be known. However, we can be 95% sure that
the calculated interval contains it.

What exactly does it mean to be "95% sure"? When you have measured only
one sample, you don't know the value of the population mean. The population
mean either lies within the 95% CI or it doesn't. You don't know, and there is no
way to find out. If you calculate a 95% CI from many independent samples, the
population mean will be included in the CI in 95% of the samples, but will be
outside of the CI in the other 5% of the samples. Using data from one sample,
therefore, you can say that you are 95% confident that the 95% CI includes the
population mean.

The correct syntax is to express the CI as "36.75 to 36.89" or as "[36.75,
36.89]." It is considered bad form to express the CI as "36.75–36.89," because the
hyphen would be confusing when the values are negative. Although it seems sensible to express the CI as "36.82 ± 0.07," that format is rarely used.

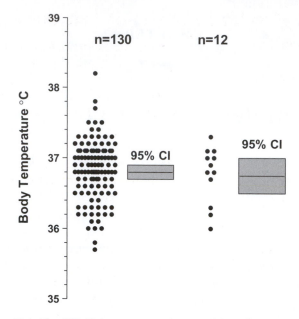

Figure 12.1. The 95% CI does not contain 95% of the values, especially when the sample size is large.

WHAT VALUES DETERMINE THE CI OF A MEAN?

The CI of a mean is computed from four values:

- The sample mean. Our best estimate of the population mean is the sample mean. Accordingly, the CI is centered on the sample mean.
- The SD. If the data are widely scattered (large SD), then the sample mean is likely to be farther from the population mean than if the data are tight (small SD). The width of the CI, therefore, is proportional to the sample SD.
- Sample size. Our sample has 130 values, so the sample mean is likely to be quite close to the population mean, and the CI will be very narrow. With tiny samples, the sample mean is likely to be further from the population mean, so the CI will be wider. The width of the CI is inversely proportional to the square root of the sample size. If the sample were four times larger, the CI would be half as wide (assuming the same SD). Note that the CI from the n = 12 sample is wider than the CI for the n = 130 sample (Figure 12.1).
- Degree of confidence. Although CIs are typically calculated for 95% confidence, any value can be used. If you wish to have more confidence (i.e., 99% confidence), you must generate a wider interval. If you are willing to accept less confidence (i.e., 90% confidence), you can generate a narrower interval.

ASSUMPTIONS: CI OF A MEAN

To interpret a CI of a mean, you must accept the following assumptions:

Assumption: Random (or representative) sample

The 95% CI is based on the assumption that your sample was randomly selected from the population. In many cases, this assumption is not true. You can still interpret the CI as long as you assume that your sample is representative of the population.

In clinical studies, it is not feasible to randomly select patients from the entire population of similar patients. Instead, patients are selected for the study because they happened to be at the right clinic at the right time. This is called a *convenience sample* rather than a *random sample*. For statistical calculations to be meaningful, we must assume that the convenience sample adequately represents the population, and that the results are similar to what would have been observed had we used a true random sample.

This assumption would be violated in the body-temperature example if the people who participated chose to join a study of body temperature because they knew (or suspected) that their own temperature was consistently higher or lower than that of most other people.

Assumption: Independent observations

The 95% CI is only valid when all subjects are sampled from the same population and each has been selected independently of the others. Selecting one member of the population should not change the chance of selecting any other person. This assumption would be violated if some individuals' temperatures were measured twice and both values were included in the sample. The assumption would also be violated if several of the subjects were siblings, because it is likely that genetic factors affect body temperature.

Assumption: Accurate data

The 95% CI is only valid when each value is measured correctly. This assumption would be violated if subjects didn't place the thermometer in their mouths correctly, or if the thermometer was misread.

Assumption: Assessing an event you really care about

The 95% CI allows you to extrapolate from the sample to the population for the event that you tabulated. But sometimes you might really care about a different event. In this example, what you really want to know is the core body temperature. Instead, temperature under the tongue was measured. The difference in this example is trivial, but it is always worth thinking about the distinction between what is measured and what one really wants to know.

Low levels of high-density lipoprotein (HDL, "good cholesterol") are associated with an increased risk of atherosclerosis and heart disease. Pfizer developed torcetrapib, a drug that elevates HDL, with great hope that it would prevent heart disease. Barter and colleagues (2007) gave the drug to thousands of patients with a high risk of cardiovascular disease. "Bad" (low-density lipoprotein, LDL) cholesterol decreased 25% and good (HDL) cholesterol increased 72%. The CIs were narrow, and the P values were tiny (<0.001). If the goal were to improve cholesterol levels, the drug was a huge success. Unfortunately, however, treatment with torcetrapib also increased the number of heart attacks by 21% and increased the number of deaths by 58%. Although the drug had the intended effects on blood lipids, it had the opposite effect on the events you really care about.

Assumption: The population is distributed in a Gaussian manner, at least approximately.

The most common method of computing the CI of a mean is based on the assumption that the data are sampled from a population that follows a Gaussian distribution. This assumption is less important when the sample is large. An alternative resampling method of computing the 95% CI that does not assume sampling from a Gaussian distribution is explained below.

What if the assumptions are violated?

In many situations, these assumptions are not strictly true. The patients in your study may be more homogeneous than the entire population of patients. Measurements made in one lab will have a smaller SD than measurements made in other labs at other times. More generally, the population you really care about may be more diverse than the population that the data were sampled from. Furthermore, the population may not be Gaussian. If any assumption is violated, the CI will probably be too optimistic (too narrow). The true CI (taking into account any violation of the assumptions) is likely to be wider than the calculated CI.

HOW TO: CALCULATE THE CI OF A MEAN

Although computers will do the calculations, it is easier to understand a CI of a mean once you know how it is computed. The CI is centered on the sample mean (m). To calculate the width requires taking account of the SD (s), the number of values in the sample (n), and the degree of confidence you desire (usually 95%).

Use Table 12.1 (reprinted in Appendix D) to determine the value of a constant based on the sample size and the degree of confidence you desire. This value is called a constant from the t distribution, and this book uses the abbreviation t*. For the body-temperature example, n = 12, so df = 11, and t* (for 95% confidence) is 2.201. The next chapter explains the t distribution.

Calculate the margin of error of the CI, w, from t*, the standard deviation (s), and the sample size (n).

$$w = \frac{t^* \cdot s}{\sqrt{n}}$$

DF	DEGREE OF CONFIDENCE				DF	DEGREE OF CONFIDENCE			
	80%	90%	95%	99%		80%	90%	95%	99%
1	3.0777	6.3138	12.7062	63.6567	27	1.3137	1.7033	2.0518	2.7707
2	1.8856	2.9200	4.3027	9.9248	28	1.3125	1.7011	2.0484	2.7633
3	1.6377	2.3534	3.1824	5.8409	29	1.3114	1.6991	2.0452	2.7564
4	1.5332	2.1318	2.7764	4.6041	30	1.3104	1.6973	2.0423	2.7500
5	1.4759	2.0150	2.5706	4.0321	35	1.3062	1.6896	2.0301	2.7238
6	1.4398	1.9432	2.4469	3.7074	40	1.3031	1.6839	2.0211	2.7045
7	1.4149	1.8946	2.3646	3.4995	45	1.3006	1.6794	2.0141	2.6896
8	1.3968	1.8595	2.3060	3.3554	50	1.2987	1.6759	2.0086	2.6778
9	1.3830	1.8331	2.2622	3.2498	55	1.2971	1.6730	2.0040	2.6682
10	1.3722	1.8125	2.2281	3.1693	60	1.2958	1.6706	2.0003	2.6603
11	1.3634	1.7959	2.2010	3.1058	65	1.2947	1.6686	1.9971	2.6536
12	1.3562	1.7823	2.1788	3.0545	70	1.2938	1.6669	1.9944	2.6479
13	1.3502	1.7709	2.1604	3.0123	75	1.2929	1.6654	1.9921	2.6430
14	1.3450	1.7613	2.1448	2.9768	80	1.2922	1.6641	1.9901	2.6387
15	1.3406	1.7531	2.1314	2.9467	85	1.2916	1.6630	1.9883	2.6349
16	1.3368	1.7459	2.1199	2.9208	90	1.2910	1.6620	1.9867	2.6316
17	1.3334	1.7396	2.1098	2.8982	95	1.2905	1.6611	1.9853	2.6286
18	1.3304	1.7341	2.1009	2.8784	100	1.2901	1.6602	1.9840	2.6259
19	1.3277	1.7291	2.0930	2.8609	150	1.2872	1.6551	1.9759	2.6090
20	1.3253	1.7247	2.0860	2.8453	200	1.2858	1.6525	1.9719	2.6006
21	1.3232	1.7207	2.0796	2.8314	250	1.2849	1.6510	1.9695	2.5956
22	1.3212	1.7171	2.0739	2.8188	300	1.2844	1.6499	1.9679	2.5923
23	1.3195	1.7139	2.0687	2.8073	350	1.2840	1.6492	1.9668	2.5899
24	1.3178	1.7109	2.0639	2.7969	400	1.2837	1.6487	1.9659	2.5882
25	1.3163	1.7081	2.0595	2.7874	450	1.2834	1.6482	1.9652	2.5868
26	1.3150	1.7056	2.0555	2.7787	500	1.2832	1.6479	1.9647	2.5857

Table 12.1. Critical values of the t distribution for computing CIs.

When computing a CI of a mean, df equals n−1. More generally, df equals n minus the number of parameters being estimated.

Q&A: CI of a Mean

Why 95% confidence?	CIs can be computed for *any* degree of confidence. By convention, 95% CIs are presented most commonly, although 90 and 99% CIs are sometimes published. To be more confident that your interval contains the population value, the interval must be wider. Thus, 99% CIs are wider than 95% CIs, and 90% CIs are narrower than 95% CIs.
Does a CI quantify variability?	No. It is a common mistake to assume that the CI tells you about the spread of the values. It doesn't. The width of a CI depends partly on the scatter among the values, but also on the sample size. You do not expect 95% of the actual values to lie within the CI of a mean. In fact, with large samples, only a tiny fraction of the values lie within the CI. The CI of the mean tells you how precisely you have determined the population mean. It does not tell you about scatter among values.
When can I use the rule of thumb that a 95% CI equals the mean plus or minus 2 SD?	Never! In a Gaussian distribution, you expect to find about 95% of the individual values within 2 SD of the mean. But the idea of a CI is to define how precisely you know the population mean. For that, you need to take into account sample size.
When can I use the rule of thumb that a 95% CI equals the mean plus or minus 2 SEM?	When n is large. Chapter 13 explains the SEM.
Do 95% of values lie within the CI?	No! The CI quantifies how precisely you know the population mean. With large samples, you can estimate the population mean quite accurately, so the CI is quite narrow and includes only a small fraction of the values (see Figure 12.1).
If I collect more data, should I expect 95% of the new values to lie within this CI?	No! The CI quantifies how precisely you know the population mean. With large samples,
	you can estimate the population mean quite accurately, so the CI is quite narrow and will include only a small fraction of values you sample in the future.
Is the 95% CI of the mean always symmetrical around the mean?	It depends on how it is computed. But with the standard method, explained in the previous section, the CI always extends equally above and below the mean.
Is a 99% CI wider or narrower than a 90% CI?M	Wider (see Figure 12.2).

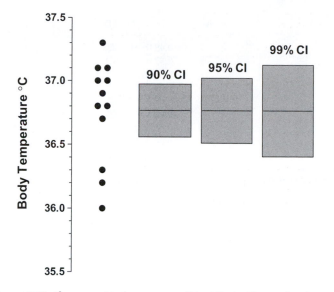

Figure 12.2. If you want to be more confident that a CI contains the population mean, you must make the interval wider.

The 99% interval is wider than the 95% interval, which is wider than the 90% CI.

For the example data, s = 0.40°C, so w = 0.254 (for 95% confidence). The CI covers this range:

m − w to m + w

For the example data, m = 36.77°C, so the 95% CI extends from 36.52 to 37.02°C.

If you want 90% confidence, t* = 1.7959 (n = 12 so df = 11), w = 0.207, and the 90% CI extends from 36.56 to 36.98°C.

ONE-SIDE CIs (ADVANCED TOPIC)

CIs are almost always calculated and presented as described above—an interval defined by two limits. But it is also possible to create one-side confidence limits.

For the example, the 90% CI extends from 36.56 to 36.98°C. Because this is a 90% two-side CI, there is room for 5% error on each end. There is a 5% chance that the upper limit (36.98) is less than the population mean. There is also a 5% chance that the lower limit (36.56) is greater than the population mean. That leaves a 90% (100−5−5%) chance that the interval 36.56 to 36.98°C includes the true population mean.

n	95% CI OF SD
2	0.45 to 31.9·SD
3	0.52 to 6.29·SD
5	0.60 to 2.87·SD
10	0.69 to 1.83·SD
25	0.78 to 1.39·SD
50	0.84 to 1.25·SD
100	0.88 to 1.16·SD
500	0.94 to 1.07·SD
1000	0.96 to 1.05·SD

Table 12.2. The CI of an SD.

Assuming random sampling from a Gaussian population, Table 12.2 gives the 95% CI for the population SD, given the sample SD and sample size (n). These values were computed using equations from page 197 of Sheskin (2007).

But what if we are clinically interested only in fevers, and want to know only the upper confidence limit? Because there is a 5% chance that the population mean is greater than 36.98°C (see previous paragraph), that leaves a 95% chance that the true population mean is less than 36.98°C. This is a one-side 95% CI. More precisely, you could say that the range from minus infinity to 36.98°C is 95% likely to contain the population mean.

CI OF A SD (ADVANCED TOPIC)

A CI can be determined for nearly any value you calculate from a sample of data. With the n = 12 body-temperature data, the SD was 0.40°C. It isn't done often, but it is possible to compute a 95% CI of the SD itself. In this example, the 95% CI of the SD extends from SD = 0.28°C to SD = 0.68°C (calculated using a web-based calculator at http://graphpad.com).

The interpretation is straightforward. Given the same assumptions as those used when interpreting the CI of the mean, we are 95% sure that the calculated interval contains the true population SD. With the n = 130 body-temperature data, the SD is 0.41°C. Because the sample size is so much larger, the sample SD is a more precise estimate of the population SD, and the CI is narrower, ranging from SD = 0.37°C to SD = 0.47°C.

Table 12.2 presents the CI for a standard deviation for various sample sizes.

CI OF A GEOMETRIC MEAN (ADVANCED TOPIC)

Chapter 11 explained how to compute the geometric mean. This is easily extended to computing the 95% CI of the geometric mean. The first step in computing a geometric mean is to transform all the values to their logarithms. Then the mean of the logarithms is computed and reverse transformed to its antilog. The result is the geometric mean.

To create a CI of the geometric mean, compute the CI of the mean of the logarithms and then reverse transform each confidence limit.

For the EC_{50} example in Chapter 11, the mean of the logarithms is 2.71, and the 95% CI of this mean extends from 2.22 to 3.20. Reverse transform each of these values, and the 95% CI of the geometric mean (which equals 512 nM) ranges from 167 to 1,569 nM. Note that the CI of the geometric mean is not symmetrical around the geometric mean.

CHAPTER 13

The Theory of Confidence Intervals

Confidence is what you have before you understand the problem.

WOODY ALLEN

The statistical theory underlying confidence intervals is hard to understand. Probability theory starts with a known population, and then computes the probabilities of obtaining various possible samples. Statistical analysis flips the theory. It starts with data, and then computing the likelihood that the data were sampled from various populations. This chapter tries to give you a general sense of how the theory is flipped. It includes more equations than the rest of the book, but it is OK to skip or skim this chapter. Later chapters do not assume you have mastered this one.

CI OF A MEAN VIA THE t DISTRIBUTION

What is the t distribution?

Chapter 12 demonstrated how to calculate a CI of a mean, a method which required our finding a value from the t distribution. A full understanding of the t distribution requires a mathematical approach beyond this book, but here is an overview.

Let's assume we know a population follows a Gaussian distribution. The mean of this population is designated by the Greek letter μ (mu). Let's assume we also know the standard deviation of this population, designated by the Greek letter σ (sigma).

Using a computer program, one can randomly choose values from this defined population. Pick n values and compute the mean of this sample, which we'll abbreviate m. Also compute the SD of this sample, which we'll abbreviate s. This sample was chosen randomly, so m and s won't equal the population values μ and σ.

Repeat thousands of times. For each random sample, compute the ratio t:

$$t = \frac{\mu - m}{s/\sqrt{n}}$$

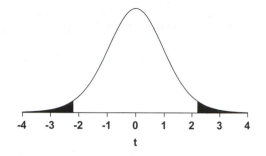

Figure 13.1. The t distribution for 11 df.
The shaded areas in the two tails each represent 2.5% of the area under the curve, which leaves 95% in the unshaded area. Because 95% of the time a value sampled from this t distribution is between –2.201 and 2.201, a 95% CI is computed by setting t* equal to 2.201.

Because these are simulated data from a hypothetical population, the value of μ is known and constant, as is n. For each sample, compute m and s, and then use the equation above to compute t.

For each random sample, the sample mean is equally likely to be larger or smaller than the population mean, so the t ratio is equally likely to be positive or negative. It will usually be fairly close to zero, but can be far away. How far? It depends on sample size (n), variability (s) and chance. Figure 13.1 illustrates the distribution of t computed for a sample size of 12. Of course, there is no need to actually perform these simulations. Mathematical statisticians have derived the distribution of t using calculus.

Sample size, n, is included in the equation that defines t, so you might expect the distribution of t to be the same regardless of sample size. In fact, the t distribution depends on sample size. With small samples, the curve in Figure 13.1 would be wider. With large samples, the curve would be narrower. With huge samples, the curve in Figure 13.1 would become indistinguishable from the Gaussian distribution shown in Figure 10.1.

The critical value of t

The area under the curve in Figure 13.1 represents all possible samples. Chop off the 2.5% tails on each side (shaded) to determine a range of t ratios that includes 95% of the samples. For this example with n = 12 and df = 11, the t ratio has a value between –2.201 and 2.201 in 95% of the samples. Let's define the variable t* to equal 2.201 (this abbreviation is not standard).

The value of t* depends on sample size and on the degree of confidence you want (here we chose the standard, 95%). Note that its value does not depend on the actual data we are analyzing. You can look up this value in Appendix D.

The flip!

Here comes the most important step, where the math is flipped around to compute a CI.

In any one sample, the sample mean (m) and standard deviation (s) are known, as is the sample size (n). What is not known is the population mean. That is why we want to generate a CI.

Rearrange the equation from the previous section to put the unknown value μ on the left:

$$\mu = m \pm t^* \cdot \frac{s}{\sqrt{n}}$$

For the example, n = 12, m = 36.77°C and s = 0.40°C. The t ratio has a 95% probability of being between –2.201 and +2.201, so t* = 2.201. Plug in those values and compute the population mean twice. The first time use the plus sign, and then do the calculations again using the minus sign. The results are the limits of the 95% CI, which ranges from 36.51 to 37.02°C.

How it works

The t distribution is defined by assuming the population is Gaussian, and investigating the variation among the means of many samples. The math is then flipped to make inferences about the population mean from the mean and SD of one sample.

CI OF A MEAN VIA RESAMPLING

The resampling approach

One of the assumptions of the usual (t distribution) method for computing a CI of a mean is that the values were sampled from a Gaussian distribution. What if you can't support that Gaussian assumption?

Resampling, also called *bootstrapping,* is an alternative approach to statistics that does not assume a Gaussian (or any other) distribution.

Create many pseudosamples via resampling

The first step is to generate many more pseudosamples via resampling.

The data set we are analyzing has 12 values, so each of our "resampled samples" will also have 12 values. To find the first value, pick a random integer between 1 and 12. If it is 3, pick the third value from the original sample. To find the second value, pick again a random integer between 1 and 12, and pick the corresponding value. It might be the third value again, but is likely to be one of the other 11 values. Repeat again until you have a new *pseudosample* with 12 values.

Repeat this many times to create, say, 500 pseudosamples. These new samples are created by sampling from the same set of values (12 in this example). Those same 12 values appear over and over, and no other values ever appear. But the samples aren't all identical. In each sample, some values are repeated and others are left out.

For each of the 500 new samples, compute the mean (because we want to know the CI of the population mean). Next, determine the 2.5th and 97.5th percentiles of that list of means. For this example, the 2.5th percentile is 36.55°C and the 97.5th percentile is 36.97°C. Because the difference between 97.5 and 2.5 is 95, we can say that 95% of the means of the pseudosamples are between 36.55 and 36.97°C.

The flip!

Statistical conclusions require flipping the logic from the distribution of multiple samples to the CI of the population mean. With the resampling approach, the flip is simple. The range of values that contains 95% of the resampled means (36.55 to 36.97°C) is the 95% CI of the population mean.

For this example, the resampling CI is nearly identical to the CI computed using the conventional method (which assumes a Gaussian distribution). But the resampling method did not require assuming a Gaussian distribution and is more accurate when that assumption is not justified. The only assumption used in the resampling approach is that the values in our sample vary independently and are representative of the population.

That's it?

This resampling method seems too simple to be useful! It is surprising that randomly resampling from the *same set of values* gives useful information about the population from which that sample was drawn. But it does create useful results. Plenty of theoretical and practical (simulations) work has validated this approach, which some statisticians think should be widely used.

CI OF A PROPORTION VIA RESAMPLING

Let's revisit the voting example from Chapter 4. When polled, 33 of 100 people said they would vote a certain way. Our goal is to find the 95% CI for the true population proportion.

The resampling approach is easier to use for proportions than for means. The sample proportion is 33% with n = 100. To resample, simply assume the population proportion is 0.33, draw numerous random samples, and find the range of proportions that includes 95% of those samples.

Figure 13.2 illustrates the answer. If the entire population of voters has 33% in favor of your candidate, then if you collect many samples of 100 voters, 95% of those samples will have between 24 and 42% in favor of your candidate.

That range tells you about multiple samples from one population. We want to know what can be inferred about the population from one sample. It turns out that that same range is the CI. Given our one sample, we are 95% sure the true population value is somewhere between 24 and 42%.

With continuous data, the resampling approach is more versatile than the t distribution approach, because it doesn't assume a Gaussian (or any other) distribution. With binomial data, there is no real advantage to the resampling

Observed proportion (33/100)

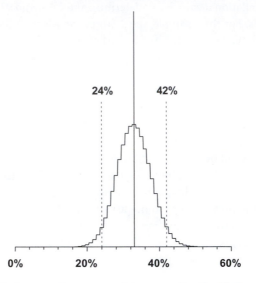

Figure 13.2. A resampling approach to computing the CI of a proportion.

If the true proportion of "success" (voting for your candidate, in this example) were 33%, the graph illustrates the probability distribution of the success rate in many samples of 100 people. After removing the 2.5% tails on each side, you can see that 95% of samples will have success rates between 24 and 42%. Surprisingly, you can flip the logic and use this graph as a way to derive CIs.

approach, except that it is a bit easier to understand than the approach based on the binomial distribution (see the next section).

CI OF A PROPORTION VIA BINOMIAL DISTRIBUTION

When polled, 33 of 100 people said they would vote a certain way. The goal is to find two confidence limits, L (lower) and U (upper), so that the 95% CI of the proportion ranges from L to U. This section demonstrates one approach, summarized in Figure 13.3. As mentioned in Chapter 4, there are several approaches to compute CIs of proportions, and they don't give exactly the same result.

The lower 95% CI (L) is determined by an indirect approach. Probability equations can answer the question: If the population proportion equals L, what is the probability that a sample proportion (n = 100) will equal 0.33 (as we observed in our sample) or more? To compute a 95% CI, each tail of the distribution must be 2.5%, so we want to find the value of L that makes the answer to that question be 2.5%.

Observed proportion (33/100)

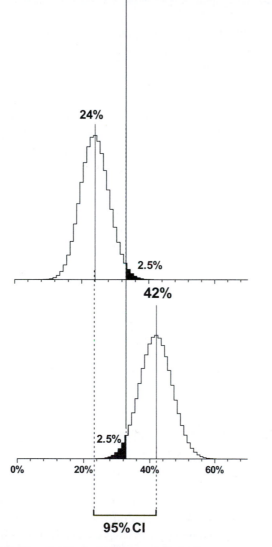

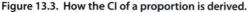

Figure 13.3. How the CI of a proportion is derived.

The solid vertical line is at 33%, which is the sample proportion (33/100). The top probability distribution demonstrates the probability of various outcomes if the true population proportion were 24%. It is centered on 24%, but the right tail of the distribution indicates that there is a 2.5% chance that the observed proportion in one particular sample will be 33% or higher. The bottom distribution indicates the probability of various outcomes if the population proportion were 42%. The left tail demonstrates that there is a 2.5% chance that the observed proportion in one particular sample will be 33% or lower. Subtracting 2.5% from 100% twice, we are left with a 95% interval ranging from 24 to 42%.

The upper 95% confidence limit of a proportion (U) uses a similar approach. If the population proportion equals U, what is the probability that a sample proportion (n = 100) will equal 0.33 or less? We want the answer to be 2.5% and solve for U.

Using the binomial distribution to solve for L and U is not straightforward. A brute force approach is to try lots of possible values of L or U, so as to find values where the cumulative binomial distribution gives a result of 2.5%. Excel's Solver can automate this.

For the example, L equals 0.24, or 24%. If fewer than 24% of voters were truly in favor of your candidate, there would be less than a 2.5% chance of randomly choosing 100 subjects of which 33% (or more) are in favor of your candidate.

For the example, U equals 0.42, or 42%. If more than 42% of voters really were in favor of your candidate, there would be less than a 2.5% chance of randomly choosing 100 subjects of which 33% (or less) were in favor of your candidate.

So far, we have been asking about which sample proportions are likely given known population proportions (L and U). Now we want to make inferences about the population from one sample. That requires a flip in reasoning. Here it comes.

Calculate 100%-2.5%-2.5%, which leaves 95%. Therefore, there is a 95% chance that the true percentage of voters in favor of your candidate is between 24 and 42%.

This method uses probability calculations that are logically simple, and flips them to answer questions about data analysis. Depending on how you look at it, the previous paragraph (the flip) is either really obvious or deeply profound. Thinking about this kind of inverse probability is tricky and has kept statisticians and philosophers busy for centuries.

LEARN MORE

To learn more about the resampling approach—also called the *bootstrapping*, or *computer-intensive*, method—start by reading books by Wilcox (2001) and Manly (2006). The method explained in Chapter 13 is called a *percentile-based resampling confidence interval*. Fancier methods create slightly more accurate CIs.

A huge advantage of the resampling approach is that it is so versatile. It can be used to obtain the CI of the median, of the interquartile range, or of almost any other parameter. Resampling approaches are extensively used in the analysis of genomics data.

CHAPTER 14

Error Bars

The only role of the standard error...is to distort and conceal the data. The reader wants to know the actual span of the data; but the investigator displays an estimated zone for the mean.

A. R. FEINSTEIN

Scientific papers often tabulate or graph results as means ± SD or means ± SEM. This chapter explains the difference. The SEM does not quantify variation. It quantifies the precision of the mean, which a CI does more exactly. Error bars can plot the SD, the SEM, or other values, so graphs with error bars should always contain labels explaining what they mean.

SEM

What is the SEM?
The ratio of the SD (s) divided by the square root of the sample size (n) is called the *standard error of the mean*, abbreviated SEM. It is defined by this equation:

$$SEM = \frac{s}{\sqrt{n}}$$

Often the SEM is referred to as the *standard error*, with the word *mean* missing, but implied. Like many statistical terms, this jargon is confusing. The SEM has nothing to do with standards or errors, and standard errors can be computed for values other than the mean (for example, the standard error of the best-fit value of a slope in linear regression; see Chapter 33).

The SEM does not quantify the variability among values.
Note that the SEM does *not* directly quantify scatter or variability among values in the population. Many scientists misunderstand this point. The SEM can be small even when the SD is large, provided that the sample size is large. With huge samples, the SEM is always tiny. For the n = 130 sample of the body-temperature data, the SEM equals 0.0359°C.

The SEM quantifies how precisely you know the population mean.

Imagine taking many samples of sample size n from your population. These sample means will not be identical, so you could quantify their variation by computing the SD of the set of means. The SEM computed from one sample value is your best estimate of what the SD among sample means would be if, in fact, you collected (infinitely) many samples.

Chapter 12 defined the margin of error (w) of a CI of a mean as follows:

$$w = \frac{t^* \cdot s}{\sqrt{n}}$$

Substituting the definition of the SEM,

$$w = t^* \cdot SEM$$

So the width of a CI of the mean is proportional to the SEM.

HOW TO: COMPUTE THE SD FROM THE SEM

Many scientists present the SEM in papers and presentations. Remember this equation, so you can easily calculate the SD (s):

$$s = SEM \cdot \sqrt{n}$$

For the n = 12 body-temperature sample, the SEM equals 0.1157°C. If that is all you knew, you could compute the SD. Multiply 0.1157 times the square root of 12, and the SD equals 0.4008°C. This is an exact calculation, not an approximation.

Q & A: SEM Versus SD	
What does the SD quantify?	The SD quantifies scatter—how much the values vary from one another.
What does the SEM quantify?	The SEM quantifies how accurately you know the true mean of the population. The value of the SEM depends upon both the SD and the sample size.
Are the SD and SEM expressed in the same units?	Yes. Both are expressed in the same units as the data.
Which is smaller?	The SEM is always smaller than the SD.
If you increase the sample size, is the SD expected to get larger, get smaller, or stay about the same?	The SD does not change predictably as you acquire more data. The SD quantifies the scatter of the data, and increasing the size of the sample does not change the scatter. The SD is equally likely to get larger or smaller as the sample size increases.

Continued

Q&A Continued

	Fine print: For all sample sizes, the *square* of the sample SD is the best possible estimate of the population variance. It is said to be unbiased, regardless of n. In contrast, when n is small, the *sample SD* tends to slightly underestimate the population SD. Increasing n, therefore, is expected to increase the SD a bit. Because all statistical theory is based on the variance rather than the SD, the bias in the sample SD is not worth worrying about or correcting for. Few statistics books even mention it.
If you increase the sample size, is the SEM expected to get larger, get smaller, or stay about the same?	Get smaller. The SEM quantifies how precisely the sample mean has been determined. Larger samples define the sample mean with more precision, so they tend to have smaller SEMs. This makes sense, because the mean of a large sample is likely to be closer to the true population mean than is the mean of a small sample. Of course, in any particular experiment you can't be sure that increasing n will decrease SEM. It is a general rule, but it is also a matter of chance. It is possible, but unlikely, that the SEM might increase if you collect a larger sample size.
When can I use the rule of thumb that the 95% CI of a mean equals the mean plus or minus 2 SEMs?	Calculating a CI requires using a multiplier from the t distribution, abbreviated (in this book) as t*. With large samples, t* has a value close to 2.0. Hence the rule of thumb that a 95% CI of a mean extends about 2 SEM in each direction from the mean. With small sample sizes, this approximate CI will be too narrow because the correct multiplier is greater than 2.0. It isn't enough to double the SEM. You need to multiply by an even larger value (see Appendix D). For example, if n = 3, a 95% CI extends 3.18 SEM in each direction from the mean.
Graphs often show an error bar extending 1 SEM in each direction from the mean. What does that denote?	The range defined by the mean plus or minus 1 SEM has no simple interpretation. With large samples, that range is a 68% CI of the mean. But the degree of confidence depends on sample size. When n = 3, that range is only a 58% CI. You can think of the mean plus or minus 1 SEM as covering about a 60% CI.
Why are SEM error bars used so often?	SEM error bars are popular because they are always smaller than the SD, and because they are a compact way to show how precisely you know the mean.

WHICH KIND OF ERROR BAR SHOULD I PLOT?

Your choice depends on your goals.

Goal: To show the variation among the values

If each value represents a different individual, you probably want to show the variation among values. Even if each value represents a different lab experiment, it often makes sense to show the variation.

With fewer than 100 or so values, you can create a scatter plot that shows every value. What better way to show the variation among values than to show every value? If your data set has more than 100 or so values, a scatter plot becomes messy. Alternatives include a box-and-whiskers plot, a frequency distribution (histogram), or a cumulative frequency distribution (see Chapter 7).

What about plotting mean and SD? The SD does quantify scatter, so this is indeed one way to graph variability. But, since a SD is only one value, it is a pretty limited way to show variation. A graph showing mean and SD error bars is less informative than any of the other alternatives. I see no advantage to plotting a mean with SD error bars as opposed to a column scatter graph, a box-and-whiskers plot, or a frequency distribution.

Of course, if you do decide to show SD error bars, be sure to say so in the figure legend, so it won't be confused with an SEM.

If you are creating a table, rather than a graph, there are several ways to show the data, depending on how much detail you want to show. One choice is to show the mean as well as the smallest and largest values. A more compact choice is to tabulate the mean ± SD.

Goal: To show how precisely you have determined the mean

If your goal is to compare means with a t test (Chapter 30) or ANOVA (Chapter 39), or to show how closely your data come to the predictions of a model, the goal may be to show how precisely the data define the mean, rather than to show variability among values. In this case, the best approach is to plot the 95% CI of the mean (or perhaps a 90 or 99% CI).

What about the SEM? Graphing the mean with SEM error bars is a method commonly used to show how well you know the mean. The only advantage of SEM error bars is that they are shorter, but it is harder to interpret SEM error bars than it is to interpret a CI.

Whatever error bars you choose to show, be sure to state your choice.

Goal: To create persuasive propaganda

Simon (2005) "advocated" the following approach in his excellent Weblog. Of course he meant it as a joke!

- If your goal is to emphasize small and unimportant differences in your data, show your error bars as SEM and hope that your readers think they show the SD.
- If your goal is to cover up large differences, show SD error bars, and hope that your readers think they show the SEM.

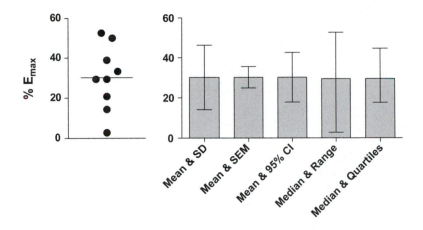

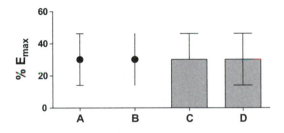

Figure 14.1. (Left) The actual data. (Right) Five kinds of error bars, each representing a different way to portray variation.

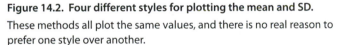

Figure 14.2. Four different styles for plotting the mean and SD.

These methods all plot the same values, and there is no real reason to prefer one style over another.

THE APPEARANCE OF ERROR BARS

Frazier et al. (2006) measured how well the neurotransmitter norepinephrine relaxes bladder muscle. Chapter 11 examined the concentrations required to get half-maximal bladder relaxation (EC_{50}), as an example of lognormal data. Now let's look at the maximal relaxation (abbreviated % E_{max}) that can be achieved with large doses of norepinephrine in old rats. Figure 14.1 (left) illustrates the raw data plotted as a column scatter plot.

Figure 14.1 (right) shows how error bars can represent several different quantities. Here, error bars represent the SD, SEM, 95% CI, range, and interquartile range. When you create graphs with error bars, be sure to state clearly how they were computed.

Figure 14.2 illustrates four different ways to plot the mean and error bar (in this case, representing the SD). There is no reason to prefer one style over another. It is a matter of preference and style.

P Values and Significance

CHAPTER 15

Introducing P Values

Imperfectly understood CIs are more useful and less dangerous than incorrectly understood P values.

HOENIG AND HEISEY (2001)

Many statistical analyses are reported with P values, which are explained in this essential chapter. P values are often misunderstood, because they answer a question you probably never thought to ask.

EXAMPLE 1: COIN FLIPPING

You flip a coin 20 times and find that 16 of the flips lead to heads and 4 to tails. How unlikely is that?

Defining the P value

Because the probability of heads is 50%, you'd expect about 10 heads in 20 flips. The probability of getting 16 heads will be small, but how small?

First we need to make an assumption—that each coin flip has a 50:50 chance of heads or tails, and that the results are accurately recorded and tabulated. This is an example of a *null hypothesis*. In this example, we expect the coin toss to be fair, and so we expect the null hypothesis to be true. In many (probably most) examples, the null hypothesis is something the scientist hopes to prove false.

If the null hypothesis were true, what would we expect to see? Since each coin toss has two possible outcomes, and the results would follow what is called a *binomial distribution*. The equation that describes the binomial distribution is a bit messy and won't be shown here. But, the equation is built in to Excel, R, and Web calculators, so you can use it to answer any question you pose.

We observed 16 heads, but are not really interested in knowing the chance of obtaining exactly 16 heads of 20 tosses. If we had observed 17 heads, it would have been even more unusual. So we want to know the chance of obtaining 16 or more heads. But wait, we aren't done. If there had been 16 or more tails and thus 4 or fewer heads, that would have also been unusual.

The relevant question is: If the coin tosses were random and the answers were recorded correctly, what is the chance that when you flip the coin 20 times

111

you'll observe either 16 or more heads or 4 or fewer heads (which means there were 16 or more tails)? The answer is 1.19%.

The probability, 1.19%, is called a *P value*. It is usually reported as a fraction (0.0119) rather than a percentage. The P value answers this generic question: If the null hypothesis were true, what would be the chance of observing results as extreme, or even more extreme, as the results observed in this particular experiment?

Putting the P value in context

How should the P value be interpreted? It depends on the context.

If you are 100% certain that the coin is fair, the tosses are random, and the results are recorded fairly, then you can be 100% sure this streak of many heads is just a chance event. You can be 100% sure that the null hypothesis is true, despite the small P value.

If this is part of a magic show, you can be pretty sure that trickery invalidates the assumptions that the coin is fair, the tosses are random, and the results are recorded fairly. You can be almost 100% certain the null hypothesis is false.

Those two extremes point out that interpretation of a small P value depends on the scientific context. This is a really important, often overlooked point that we'll return to in Chapter 18.

How many P values were calculated?

Now assume that everyone in a class of 200 students flipped a coin 20 times and recorded the results? Inspect the results of these 200 "experiments" and pick the one with the most heads (or most tails) for further analysis. It wouldn't be surprising at all to find 16 (or more) heads in 20 flips. You would expect to get 16 or more heads (or 16 or more tails) in 1.19% of the experiments. So with 200 different experiments, it would be surprising *not* to find one (or more) with 16 or more heads.

We'll return to the idea of multiple comparisons in Chapters 22 and 23. When judging how unusual a result is, you must take into account how many comparisons were made. When many comparisons are made, even if they weren't all reported, small P values are to be expected.

How was the P value calculated?

The *cumulative binomial distribution* computes the answer. The inputs to the calculation are the probability of success in the population (in our example, "success" is picking 16 or more heads or tails) and the number of trials. The binomial distribution then computes the probability of observing any particular number of successes. The cumulative binomial distribution sums up these individual probabilities to determine the chance (P value) of observing at least a specified number of successes (e.g., 16 or more). You would then double that value so as to also include the opposite possibility (four or fewer heads).

What about statistical significance?

P values can be, and should be, understood on their own. Applying the concept of statistical significance is entirely optional. Chapter 16 will explain.

EXAMPLE 2: BODY TEMPERATURE

Defining the P value

Many books (at least those written before 2000) will tell you that the average normal body temperature is 37.0°C. Many thermometers mark this value as the borderline between normal and abnormal. Continuing the body-temperature example used in the past few chapters: The mean temperature of 130 people is 36.82°C and the 95% CI ranges from 36.75 to 36.89°C. The 95% CI does not include 37.0°C. In other words, our data are inconsistent (with 95% confidence) with the hypothesis that the values were drawn from a population whose mean is 37.0°C.

The discrepancy between the sample mean and the hypothetical population mean is 0.18°C. A P value answers this question:

> If the population mean truly is 37.0°C, what is the chance that in a sample with n = 130 the absolute value of the discrepancy between sample mean and hypothetical population mean is 0.18°C or larger?

The P value equals 0.0000018. Many programs would simply report P<0.0001. This small P value tells us that if the population mean truly is 37.0°C, there is only a tiny chance that the mean of a sample of 130 will be as far from the hypothetical mean as actually observed. This doesn't prove that the null hypothesis is incorrect. It just says that if that hypothesis were correct, there is a very small chance of obtaining the data we observed.

Putting the P value in context

P values must always be interpreted in context. How firm are the data that the average temperature is 37.0°C? If this value were based on many studies of thousands of people, you'd need super strong data to reject it. In fact, this rule of thumb is not based on overwhelmingly convincing data, but rather on strong tradition. Because this is the case, the assertion that the true mean is not really 37.0°C seems more convincing. Chapter 18 will revisit this idea.

How many P values were calculated?

Is this a single sample of 130? Or did someone search a database to get the 130 lowest-recorded temperatures of many thousands collected? Or was the temperature measured multiple times in each subject, but only the lowest value recorded? In the latter cases the P value is irrelevant, because we already know that the values are not representative. This point hints at the problem of multiple comparisons, which we'll address again in Chapters 22 and 23.

Putting the P value in context—How large is the discrepancy?

The discrepancy between the hypothetical mean and the true mean is tiny—only about 1/4 of a degree centigrade, which is about 1/10 of a degree Fahrenheit. Such a tiny difference makes very little, if any, practical difference. Although statistical calculations prove that this discrepancy is very unlikely to be the result of chance, statistics has nothing to say about whether the size of the difference is large enough to care about.

The P value from the smaller n = 12 sample

For the smaller (n = 12) sample, the sample mean is 36.76°C and the 95% CI ranges from 36.51 to 37.02°C. The 95% CI includes 37.0°C. In other words, our data are consistent (with 95% confidence) with the hypothesis that the values were drawn from a population whose mean is 37.0°C. The P value answers this question:

> If the population mean truly is 37.0°C, what is the chance the absolute value of the discrepancy between sample mean (n = 12) and hypothetical population mean is 0.23°C or larger?

The P value is 0.0687. If a P value is greater than 0.05, people often say that the result is not statistically significant (see Chapter 16). This certainly doesn't prove the null hypothesis that the population mean is 37.0°C. All we can say is that if that hypothesis were true, the data we observed would not seem surprising (with n = 12).

Why are the conclusions different from the large and small studies?

With a smaller sample size (n = 12 vs. n = 130), the population mean is defined with less precision, and so the SEM is larger and the 95% CI is wider. If we only had this small sample, the data would seem to be consistent with a population mean of 37.0°C. With the larger sample, we can see that in fact the data are not consistent with that hypothesis.

Calculating the P value

The P value of 0.0000018 is calculated from a *one-sample t test*. This section will explain, in general, how that test works (using the n = 130 sample).

First, calculate the discrepancy between the observed sample mean and the hypothetical population mean: 36.82 − 37.00°C = −0.18°C. The minus sign just says that the sample mean was lower than the hypothetical population mean.

Next, divide the discrepancy by the SEM (see Chapter 14) to account for variability and sample size. The result is called a *t ratio*. Here, t = 0.18°C/ 0.036°C = −5.00. This unitless ratio tells us that the discrepancy between the hypothesized population mean and the actual sample mean is five times larger than the SEM.

The P value is the chance that random sampling would result in a t ratio greater than 5.0 or smaller than −5.0, with n = 130 (so df = 129). Computer programs can do the complicated calculation to find the P value.

Chapter 14 explained an alternative method to compute a CI using resampling. That approach can also compute a P value. We'll use the same set of 500 simulated, resampled data sets (from the n = 12 data set). Of those 500 sets, only 7 have a mean greater than 37.0°C. This means that the resampling P value (one-tailed) is 7/500, or 0.014. Double that value to get a two-tail P value, 0.028.

EXAMPLE 3: ANTIBIOTICS ON SURGICAL WOUNDS

Heal and colleagues (2009) tested whether applying an antibiotic (chloramphenicol) to surgical wounds would reduce the incidence of wound infection. They randomly assigned surgical patients to receive either an antibiotic ointment or an ointment with no active medication.

Infections occurred in 6.6% of the patients who received antibiotic, compared with 11.0% of the patients who received inactive ointment. They compared these two rates (using a method to be explained in Chapter 27) and reported that the P value is 0.010.

To interpret any P value, the null hypothesis must be defined. Here, the null hypothesis is that the risk of infections is the same in patients who receive an antibiotic ointment and those who receive an inactive ointment, so that any discrepancy in the incidence of infections is the result of chance. The P value answers this question:

> If the null hypothesis were true, what is the chance that random sampling would lead to a difference in incidence rates equal to or larger than the difference observed in this study?

EXAMPLE 4: ANGIOPLASTY
AND MYOCARDIAL INFARCTION

Cantor and colleagues (2009) studied the optimal way to treat patients who had myocardial infarctions (heart attacks), but were admitted to a hospital that could not do percutaneous-coronary intervention (PCI, also known as angioplasty). They randomized 1059 such patients into two groups. One group was immediately transferred to a different hospital and received PCI. The other half were given standard therapy at the admitting hospital. They assessed the fraction of patients who, within 30 days, died or had worsening heart disease (another myocardial infarction or worsened congestive heart failure).

By 30 days, one (or more) of these end points had occurred in 11.0% of the patients who were transferred and 17.2% of the patients who received standard therapy. The risk ratio was 11.0/17.0 = 0.64. The P value was 0.004.

To interpret any P value, the null hypothesis must be defined. Here, the null hypothesis is that the risk of death, reinfarction, or heart failure is the same in both populations of patients, so that any discrepancy observed in the particular patients in this study is the result of chance. In other words, the null hypothesis is that the risk ratio in the overall populations equals 1.0. The P value answers this question:

> If the null hypothesis were true, what is the chance that random sampling would lead to a risk ratio as far from 1.0 as observed in this study?

ONE- OR TWO-TAIL P VALUES

The body temperature example again

When comparing two groups, you must distinguish between one- and two-tail P values. Some books refer to *one-side* and *two-side* P values, which mean the same thing.

For the body-temperature data (n = 12), the two-tail P value answers this question:

> If the population mean truly is 37.0°C, what is the chance the absolute value of the discrepancy between the sample mean (n = 12) and the hypothetical population mean is 0.23°C or higher?

The P value is two-tailed, because it treats a sample mean greater than the hypothetical population mean the same as it treats a sample mean smaller than the hypothetical mean.

To compute a one-tail P value, you must specify the direction of your alternative hypothesis. The null hypothesis remains that the population mean is 37.0°C. To compute a one-tail P value, you must specify a directional alternative hypothesis. It is not fair to base this on what you actually observed in this experiment. The direction of the alternative hypothesis must be set in advance. Let's say we had reason to believe that the mean temperature is truly lower than 37.0°C. Now we can compute and interpret a one-tail P value that answers this question:

> If the population mean truly is 37.0°C, what is the chance the sample mean will be at least 0.23°C less than the hypothetical population mean?

The sample mean was indeed lower than the hypothetical population mean, so this P value is half the two-tail P value. Sticking with the standard approach (assume Gaussian distribution), the one-side P value is 0.0343.

Let's imagine that our experimental hypothesis was that the true mean temperature is greater than the hypothetical 37.0°C. Our sample mean was in fact lower than 37.0°C. In this case, there is no point computing a one-tail P value. It would be greater than 0.5.

Comparing two groups

Now let's imagine that you are comparing the mean of two groups (with an *unpaired t test*, which will be covered in Chapter 33). Both one- and two-tail P values are based on the same null hypothesis, that two populations really are the same, and that the observed discrepancy between sample means is caused by chance.

A two-tail P value answers this question:

Assuming the null hypothesis is true, what is the chance that randomly selected samples would have means as far apart as (or farther apart than) you observed in this experiment, with *either* group having the larger mean?

To interpret a one-tail P value, you must predict which group will have the larger mean before collecting any data. The one-tail P value then answers this question:

Assuming the null hypothesis is true, what is the chance that randomly selected samples would have means as far apart as (or farther apart than) those observed in this experiment, with the *specified* group having the larger mean?

If the observed difference went in the direction predicted by the experimental hypothesis, the one-tail P value is half the two-tail P value (with most, but not quite all, statistical tests).

A one-tail test is appropriate when previous data, physical limitations, or common sense tells you that the difference, if any, can only go in one direction. You should only choose a one-tail P value when both of the following are true:

- You predicted which treatment group will have the larger mean (or proportion) before you collected any data.
- If the other treatment group had ended up with the larger mean—even if it is quite a bit larger—you would have attributed that difference to chance and called the difference "not statistically significant."

Here is an example in which it might be appropriate to choose a one-tail P value: You are testing whether a new antibiotic impairs renal function, as measured by serum creatinine. Many antibiotics poison kidney cells, resulting in reduced glomerular filtration and increased serum creatinine. As far as I know, no antibiotic is known to decrease serum creatinine. Before collecting any data, it would not be unreasonable to state that there are two possibilities: Either the drug will not change the mean serum creatinine of the population, or it will increase the mean serum creatinine in the population. Accordingly, it makes sense to calculate a one-tail P value that tests the null hypothesis that the drug does not increase the creatinine level. If the creatinine level goes down, no matter how much, you'd attribute that decrease to chance.

The problem with this approach is that it assumes that it is completely impossible that a drug could improve kidney function, and thereby decrease creatinine. What if you happened to test such a drug? Given the rules of a one-side P value, you would attribute that decreased creatinine to chance and miss what might have been a truly important discovery.

When is a one-tail P value appropriate?

The issue in choosing between one- and two-tail P values is not whether you expect a difference to exist. If you already knew whether a difference existed, there would be no reason to collect the data.

You should only use a one-tail P value when you can state with certainty (before collecting any data) that between the overall populations there either is no difference, or there is a difference in a specified direction. If your data end up indicating a difference in the "wrong" direction, you should be willing to attribute that difference to random sampling, without even considering the notion that the difference in your samples might reflect a true difference between the overall populations. If a difference in the wrong direction would intrigue you (even a little), you should calculate a two-tail P value.

When in doubt, use two-tail P values

Two-tail P values are used more frequently than one-tail P values for the following reasons:

- The relationship between P values and CIs is more straightforward with two-tail P values.
- Two-tail P values are larger (more conservative). Because many experiments do not completely comply with all the assumptions on which the statistical calculations are based, many P values are smaller than they ought to be. Using the larger two-tail P value partially corrects for this.
- Some tests compare three or more groups, which makes the concept of tails inappropriate (more precisely, the P value has more than two tails). A two-tail P value is more consistent with P values reported by these tests.
- Choosing one-tail P values can put you in awkward situations. If you decided to calculate a one-tail P value, what would you do if you observed a large difference in the direction opposite to the experimental hypothesis? To be honest, you should state that the P value is large and that you found "no significant difference." But most people would find this difficult. Instead, they'd be tempted to switch to a two-tail P value or stick with a one-tail P value, but change the direction of the hypothesis. You avoid this temptation by choosing two-tail P values in the first place.

When interpreting published P values, note whether they are calculated for one or two tails. If the author doesn't say, the result is somewhat ambiguous.

WHY ARE P VALUES SO HARD TO UNDERSTAND?

Thinking about P values seems quite counterintuitive at first, except maybe to lawyers or Talmudic scholars used to this sort of argument by contradiction. Three aspects are awkward:

- The hypothesis tested (the null hypothesis) is usually opposite to the hypothesis the experimenter expects or hopes to be true.
- Although mathematicians are comfortable with the idea of probability distributions, clinicians and scientists find it strange to calculate the

probabilities of obtaining results that weren't actually obtained. The derivation of the theoretical probability distributions depends on mathematics beyond the ready reach of almost all scientists.

- The logic goes in a direction that seems intuitively backward. You observed a sample and want to make inferences about the population. Calculations of the P value start with an assumption about the population (the null hypothesis) and determine the probability of randomly selecting samples with as large a difference as you observed. This is a fundamental problem in statistics. The mathematical logic (albeit, not the details) is quite straightforward when making predictions about samples from a known population. This same logic must be twisted backward to make inferences about the population from a known sample.

Q & A: P Values

Is the P value the probability that the null hypothesis is true?	No. The P value is computed assuming that the null hypothesis is true, so it cannot be the probability that it is true.
Is the P value the probability that the result was the result of sampling error?	No. The P value is computed assuming the null hypothesis is true and that all differences are the result of random sampling. Therefore, the P value cannot tell you the probability that the result is caused by sampling error.
Is 1.0 minus the P value the probability that the alternative hypothesis is true?	No. If the P value is 0.03, it is very tempting to think: If there is only a 3% probability that my difference would have been caused by random chance, then there must be a 97% probability that it was caused by a real difference. The premise is not correct. It is not correct to interpret the P value of 0.03 as "the probability that my difference was caused by random chance." Because the premise is wrong, so is the conclusion. It is not correct to say that "there is a 97% probability that my difference is real."
	What you can say is that if the null hypothesis were true, then 97% of experiments would result in a difference smaller than the one you observed, and 3% of experiments would lead to a difference as large as, or larger than, the one you observed.
Is 1.0 minus the P value the probability that the results will hold up when the experiment is repeated?	No. If the P value is 0.03, it is tempting to think that this means there is a 97% chance of getting "similar" results in a repeated experiment. Not so.

Continued

Q&A Continued

Does a high P value prove that the null hypothesis is true?	No. A high P value means that if the null hypothesis were true, it would not be surprising to observe the difference or effect seen in this experiment. But that does not prove the null hypothesis is true.
Can P values be negative?	No. P values are fractions, so they are always between 0.0 and 1.0.
Should P values be reported as fractions or percentages?	A P value is a fraction, with a value between 0.0 and 1.0. Equivalently, it is a percentage with a value between 0.0 and 100.0%. By tradition, however, P values are presented as fractions, not percentages.

Is a one-tail P value always equal to half the two-tail P value?	Not always.
	    Some distributions are asymmetrical. For example, a one-tail P value from a Fisher's exact test (see Chapter 27) is usually not exactly equal to half the two-tail P value. With some data, in fact, the one- and two-tail P values can be identical. This is rare.
	    Even if the distribution is symmetrical (as most are), the one-tail P value is only equal to half the two-tail value if you correctly predicted the direction of the difference (association, etc.) in advance. If the effect actually went in the opposite direction to your prediction, the one-tail P is not equal to half the two-tail P value. If you were to calculate it, it would be greater than 0.5 and greater than the two-tail P value.

Can a one-tail P value always be computed?	No. It only makes sense to talk about one- or two-tail P values when the effect has two possible directions. With some analyses, such as ANOVA, this is not the case, so the distinction between one- and two-tail P values really doesn't make any sense.
Is a P value always associated with a null hypothesis?	Yes. If you aren't sure what the null hypothesis is, then you can't interpret the P value.
Shouldn't P values always be presented with a conclusion about whether the results are statistically significant?	No. A P value should be interpreted on its own. In some situations, it can make sense to go one step further and report whether the results are statistically significant (as will be explained in Chapter 16). But this is an optional step.
I chose to use a one-tail P value, but the results came out in the direction opposite to my prediction. Can I report the one-tail P value calculated by a statistical program?	Probably not. Most statistical programs don't ask you to specify the direction of your hypothesis, so you can report the one-tail P value only if you correctly predicted the direction of the difference (or association). If the data indicated a difference in the direction opposite to your prediction (i.e., you predicted an increase, but

Continued

	the data indicate a decrease), then the correct one-tail P value equals 1.0 minus the P value reported by the program. For example, if the program reports a one-tail P value of 0.04, and assuming you predicted the direction incorrectly, the true one-tail P value (given your incorrect prediction) is 1.0 – 0.04 = 0.96. If your prediction is opposite to the actual effect, the correct one-tail P value will always be between 0.5 and 1.0.

Is the null hypothesis ever true?	Rarely.
	    P values always answer a question that begins, "If the null hypothesis were true." But in many cases, you already can be quite sure the null hypothesis is not true. Whenever you compare two groups, it is very unlikely that the two population means (or proportions, etc.) will be *exactly* the same. When you apply a treatment, it is very unlikely that the treatment has zero effect.
	    The practical or scientific question is whether the differences between the groups are large enough to matter. In some situations, the groups might be very similar or the treatment may have only a trivial effect. But even in those cases, the null hypothesis is not quite true.
	    Even if you know the null hypothesis can't actually be true, you can use the P value as a measure of the strength of evidence.

P VALUES OR CIs?

Many statistical analyses generate both P values and CIs. Many scientists report the P value and ignore the CI. I think this is a mistake.

Interpreting P values is tricky, requiring defining a null hypothesis and thinking about the distribution of the results of hypothetical experiments.

Interpreting CIs, in contrast, is quite simple. You collect some data and do some calculations to quantify a treatment effect such as a difference, ratio, or best-fit value. Then you report that value along with a CI that quantifies the precision of that value. This approach is very logical and intuitive. You report what you calculated along with a CI that shows how sure you are.

The underlying theory is identical for CIs and P values. If both are interpreted correctly, the conclusions will be identical. But what a big "if"! P values are often interpreted incorrectly (by people who haven't read this book).

CHAPTER 16

Statistical Significance and Hypothesis Testing

For the past eighty years, it appears that some of the sciences have made a mistake by basing decisions on statistical significance.

S. ZILIAK AND D. MCCLOSKEY (2008)

The phrase "statistically significant" is commonly misunderstood, because this use of the word "significant" has almost no relationship to the conventional meaning of the word as used to describe something that is important or consequential. This chapter explains that the concept is quite straightforward once you get past the confusing terminology.

STATISTICAL HYPOTHESIS TESTING

Making a decision is the primary goal when analyzing some kinds of data. In a pilot experiment of a new drug, the goal may be to decide whether the results are promising enough to merit a second experiment. In a Phase III drug study, the goal may be to decide whether the drug should be recommended.

Statistical hypothesis testing automates decision making. First, define a threshold P value for declaring whether a result is statistically significant. This threshold is called the *significance level* of the test; it is denoted by α (alpha) and is commonly set to 0.05. If the P value is less than α, conclude that the difference is *statistically significant* and decide to *reject the null hypothesis*. Otherwise, conclude that the difference is not statistically significant and decide to not reject the null hypothesis.

Note that statistics gives the term *hypothesis testing* a unique meaning, that is very different than what most scientists think of when they go about testing a scientific hypothesis.

ANALOGY: INNOCENT UNTIL PROVEN GUILTY

The steps that a jury must follow to determine criminal guilt are very similar to the steps that a scientist follows to determine statistical significance.

A jury starts with the presumption that the defendant is innocent. A scientist starts with the presumption that the null hypothesis of "no difference" is true.

A jury bases its decision only on factual evidence presented in the trial and should not consider any other information, such as newspaper stories. A scientist bases the decision about statistical significance only on data from one experiment, without considering what other experiments have concluded.

A jury reaches the verdict of guilty when the evidence is inconsistent with the assumption of innocence. Otherwise, the jury reaches a verdict of not guilty. When performing a statistical test, a scientist reaches a conclusion that the results are statistically significant when the P value is small enough to make the null hypothesis unlikely. Otherwise, a scientist concludes that the results are not statistically significant.

A jury does not have to be convinced that the defendant is innocent to reach a verdict of not guilty. A jury reaches a verdict of not guilty when the evidence is consistent with the presumption of innocence. A scientist reaches the conclusion that results are not statistically significant whenever the data are consistent with the null hypothesis. The scientist does not have to be convinced that the null hypothesis is true.

A jury can never reach a verdict that a defendant is innocent. The only choices are guilty or not guilty. A statistical test never concludes the null hypothesis is true, only that there is insufficient evidence to reject it.

A jury must try to reach a conclusion of guilty or not guilty and can't conclude "we are not sure." Similarly, each statistical test leads to a crisp conclusion of statistically significant or not statistically significant. A scientist who strictly follows the logic of statistical hypothesis testing cannot conclude, "Let's wait for more data before deciding."

TRIAL BY JURY VERSUS TRIAL BY JOURNALISTS

Jurors aren't the only people who evaluate evidence presented at a criminal trial.

Journalists also evaluate evidence presented at a trial, but they follow very different rules than jurors. A journalist's job is not to reach a verdict of guilty or not guilty, but rather to summarize the proceedings.

Many scientists find themselves in the role of a journalist more often than they find themselves in the role of a juror. The goal of a scientist often is to summarize the data. It is not always necessary to make a crisp decision from one experiment. Focusing on whether or not a result is statistically significant can get in the way of good science.

WHEN IS HYPOTHESIS TESTING USEFUL?

The whole point of statistical hypothesis testing is to make a crisp decision from one result. Make one decision when the results are statistically significant and another decision when the results are not statistically significant. This situation is common in quality control, but is rare in exploratory basic research.

SYMBOLS	PHRASE	P VALUE
NS	Not significant	$P > 0.05$
*	Significant	$P < 0.05$
**	Highly significant	$P < 0.01$
***	Extremely significant	$P < 0.001$

Table 16.1. Using asterisks to denote statistical significance.
The scheme shown here is commonly used, but is not universal.
If you see graphs decorated with asterisks to denote statistical
significance, be sure to check the legend to see how the authors
defined the symbols.

In many scientific situations, it is not necessary—and can even be counter-productive—to reach a crisp conclusion of statistically significant or not statistically significant. P values and CIs can help you assess and present scientific evidence without ever using the phrase "statistically significant".

When reading the scientific literature, don't let a conclusion about statistical significance stop you from trying to understand what the data really show. Don't let the rubric of statistical hypothesis testing get in the way of clear scientific thinking.

SIGNIFICANT, VERY SIGNIFICANT, OR EXTREMELY SIGNIFICANT?

Is a result with $P = 0.004$ more statistically significant than a result with $P = 0.04$?

Some statisticians say no. Once you have established a significance level, every result is either statistically significant or not statistically significant. It doesn't matter whether the P value is very close to α or far away. Because the goal of statistical hypothesis testing is to make a crisp decision, only two conclusions are needed.

Most scientists are less rigid and refer to *very significant* or *extremely significant* results when the P value is tiny.

When showing P values on graphs, investigators commonly use asterisks to create a "Michelin Guide" scale (Table 16.1). When you read this kind of graph, make sure that you look at the key that defines the symbols, because different investigators use different threshold values.

BORDERLINE STATISTICAL SIGNIFICANCE

If you follow the strict paradigm of statistical hypothesis testing and set α to its conventional value of 0.05, then a P value of 0.049 denotes a statistically significant difference and a P value of 0.051 does not. This arbitrary distinction is

	DECISION: REJECT NULL HYPOTHESIS	DECISION: DO NOT REJECT NULL HYPOTHESIS
Null hypothesis is true	Type I error	(No error)
Null hypothesis is false	(No error)	Type II error

Table 16.2. Definition of Type I and Type II errors.

unavoidable, because the whole point of statistical hypothesis testing is to reach a crisp conclusion from every experiment, without exception.

When a P value is just slightly greater than α, some scientists refer to the result as *marginally significant* or *almost significant*. Rather than deal with linguistic tricks, it is often better to just report the actual P value and not worry about whether it is above or below some arbitrary threshold value.

When a two-tail P value is between 0.05 and 0.10, some are tempted to switch to a one-tail P value. The one-tail P value is (with rare exceptions) equal to half the two-tail P value, and so it is less than 0.05. Switch to a one-tail P value and the results become statistically significant, as if by magic. Obviously, this is not an appropriate reason to choose a one-tail P value! The choice should be made before the data are collected.

One way to deal with borderline P values would be to choose among three decisions rather than two. Rather than decide whether a difference is statistically significant, or not add a middle category of *inconclusive*. This approach is not commonly used.

LINGO: TYPE I AND TYPE II ERRORS

Statistical hypothesis testing makes a decision based on the results of one comparison. When you make this decision, there are two kinds of mistakes you can make (Table 16.2).

Type I error
When there really is no difference (association, correlation) between the populations random sampling can result in data with a statistically significant difference (association, correlation). This is a Type I error. It occurs when you decide to reject the null hypothesis when in fact the null hypothesis is true.

Type II error
When there really is a difference (association, correlation) between the populations, random sampling (and small sample size) may cause your samples of data to not show a statistically significant difference. You will therefore decide not to reject the null hypothesis, but that decision is based on an erroneous conclusion. This is a Type II error. It occurs when you decide not to reject the null hypothesis when in fact the null hypothesis is false.

	DECISION: DELETE AS JUNK	DECISION: PLACE IN INBOX
Good email	Type I error	(No error)
Spam	(No error)	Type II error

Table 16.3. Type I and Type II errors in the context of spam filters.

You won't know

Type I and II errors are theoretical concepts. When you analyze any particular set of data, you don't know whether the populations are identical. You only know the data in your particular samples. You will never know whether you made a Type I or Type II error as part of any particular analysis.

CHOOSING A SIGNIFICANCE LEVEL

The trade-off

A result is deemed statistically significant when the P value is less than a significance level (α) set in advance. By tradition, α is usually set to equal 0.05. Why not reduce that probability by setting α to a much lower value, say 0.01? Or 0.0001?

If you choose a stricter significance level, it is also harder to find real effects. When choosing a significance level, therefore, you confront a trade-off.

If you set α to a very low value, you will make few Type I errors. That means that if the null hypothesis were true, there would be only a small chance that you will mistakenly call a result statistically significant. However, there is also a larger chance that you will not find a significant difference, even if the null hypothesis were false. In other words, reducing the value of α will decrease your chance of making a Type I error, but increase the chance of a Type II error.

If you set α to a very large value, you will make many Type I errors. If the null hypothesis is true, there is a large chance that you will mistakenly find a significant difference. But there is a small chance of missing a real difference. In other words, increasing the value of α will increase your chance of making a Type I error, but decrease the chance of a Type II error. The only way to reduce the chances of both a Type I error and a Type II error is to collect bigger samples (see Chapter 43).

Ideally, scientists should balance the costs or consequences of Type I and Type II errors and alter the value of α accordingly. However, the standard threshold of 0.05 is almost always used.

Detecting spam

Table 16.3 recasts Table 16.2 in the context of detecting spam (junk) email. Spam filters use various criteria to evaluate the likelihood that a particular email is spam and to deliver that message to the inbox or route it to the spam box (or delete it).

	VERDICT: GUILTY	VERDICT: NOT GUILTY
Did not commit the crime	Type I error	(No error)
Did commit the crime	(No error)	Type II error

Table 16.4. Type I and Type II errors in the context of trial by jury in a criminal case.

The null hypothesis is that an email is good (not spam). A Type I error occurs when a good email is mistakenly sent to the spam mailbox. A Type II error occurs when spam is delivered to the inbox.

Here, the consequence of a Type I error is pretty bad—a real email gets ignored in the junk folder or is deleted. The consequence of a Type II error is not so bad—one more spam email in the inbox. Spam filters tend to be designed to have low Type I errors, even at the expense of high Type II errors. Some spam-filtering software lets you adjust the criteria used, so that you can choose to have more Type I or more Type II errors.

Trial by jury

Table 16.4 continues the analogy between statistical significance and the legal system. The relative consequences of Type I and Type II errors depend on the type of trial.

In the United States (and many other countries), a defendant in a criminal trial is considered innocent until proven guilty "beyond a reasonable doubt." This system is based on the belief that it is better to let many guilty people go free than to falsely convict one innocent person. The system is designed to avoid Type I errors in criminal trials, even at the expense of many Type II errors. You could say that α is set to a very low value.

In civil trials, the court or jury rules in favor of the plaintiff if the evidence shows that the plaintiff is "more likely than not" to be right. The thinking is that it is no worse to falsely rules in favor of the plaintiff than to falsely rules in favor of the defendant. The system attempts to equalize the chances of Type I and Type II errors in civil trials.

Phase III clinical trial

A Phase III clinical trial is testing a drug for a disease (like hypertension) for which there are good existing therapies. If the results are statistically significant, you will market the drug. If the results are not statistically significant, work on the drug will cease. In this case, the null hypothesis is that the drug doesn't work at all, and a Type I error results in treating some future patients with a drug that is ineffective. A Type II error results in aborting development of a good new drug for a condition that can be treated adequately with existing drugs. Thinking scientifically (not commercially), it makes sense to minimize the risk of a Type I error, even at the expense of a higher chance of a Type II error.

But let's say the trial is for a drug that purportedly treats a disease for which there is no good existing therapy. If the results are statistically significant, you will market the drug. If the results are not statistically significant, work on the drug will cease. In this case, a Type I error results in treating future patients with a useless drug, instead of nothing. A Type II error results in canceling development of a good drug for a condition that is currently not treatable. It makes sense to set α to a relatively high value because a Type I error isn't so bad, but a Type II error would be awful. It might make sense to set α to 0.10 or even higher.

Of course, these scenarios are simplistic. Difficult decisions about drug development rarely depend on a single conclusion about statistical significance. The scenarios above are designed to help you understand the trade-offs between Type I and Type II errors, and not to provide guidance in how to make those difficult decisions.

Q & A: Statistical Significance and Hypothesis Testing

Is it possible to report scientific data without using the word *significant*?	Yes. Report the data, along with CIs and P values. Decisions about statistical significance are often not needed and not helpful.
Is the concept of statistical hypothesis testing about making decisions or about making conclusions?	Decision making. The system of statistical-hypothesis testing makes perfect sense when it is necessary to make a crisp decision based on one statistical analysis. If you have no need to make a decision from one analysis, then it may not be helpful to use the term *statistically significant*.
But isn't the whole point of statistics to decide when an effect is statistically significant?	No. The whole point of statistics is to quantify scientific evidence and uncertainty.
Why is statistical hypothesis testing so popular?	There is a natural aversion to ambiguity. The crisp conclusion "the results are statistically significant" is more satisfying to many than the wordy conclusion that "random sampling would create a difference this big or bigger in 3% of experiments if the null hypothesis were true."
Who invented the threshold of P < 0.05 as meaning statistically significant?	That threshold, like much of statistics, came from the work of Ronald Fisher. He did not intend for it to become a firmly entrenched value.
Are the P value and α the same?	No. A P value is computed from the data and is a measure of the strength of evidence. The significance level α is set as part of the experimental design, before collecting any data, so that it is not influenced by the data. A difference is termed *statistically significant* if the P value computed from the data is less than the value of α set in advance.

Continued

Q&A Continued

Is the P value the probability of rejecting the null hypothesis?	No. You reject the null hypothesis (and deem the results statistically significant) when a P value from a particular experiment is less than the significance level α, which you (should have) set in advance as part of the experimental design. If the null hypothesis is true, α is the probability of rejecting the null hypothesis. It is set in advance by the scientist. The P value, in contrast, is computed from the data.
If I perform many statistical tests, is it true that the conclusion "statistically significant" will be incorrect 5% of the time?	No! That would only be true if the null hypothesis is, in fact, true in every single experiment. Of course, the null hypothesis is not always true, so you don't know what fraction of the "statistically significant" conclusions are incorrect. Chapter 18 explains further.
My two-tail P value is not low enough to be statistically significant, but the one-tail P value is. What do I conclude?	Stop playing games with your data. It is only OK to compute a one-tail P value when you decided to do so as part of the experimental protocol (see Chapter 15).
Isn't it possible to look at statistical hypothesis testing as a way to choose between alternative models?	Yes. See Chapter 35.

CHAPTER 17

Relationship Between Confidence Intervals and Statistical Significance

> Reality must take precedence over public relations, for Nature cannot be fooled.
>
> *Richard Feynman*

This book has presented the concepts of CIs and statistical hypothesis testing in separate chapters. The two approaches are based on the same assumptions and the same mathematical logic. This chapter explains how they are related.

CIs AND STATISTICAL HYPOTHESIS TESTING ARE CLOSELY RELATED

CIs and statistical hypothesis testing are based on the same statistical theory and assumptions, so they are closely linked.

The CI computes a range that you can be 95% sure contains the population value (given some assumptions).

The hypothesis testing approach computes a range that you can be 95% sure would contain experimental results if the null hypothesis were true. Any result within this range is considered not statistically significant, and any result outside this range is considered statistically significant.

WHEN A CI INCLUDES THE NULL HYPOTHESIS

Figure 17.1 shows the results of comparing observed body temperatures (n = 12) with the hypothetical mean value of 37°C (see Chapter 15).

The bottom bar of Figure 17.1 shows the 95% CI of the mean. It is centered on the sample mean. It extends in each direction a distance computed by multiplying the SEM times the critical value of the t distribution from Appendix D (for 95% confidence).

The top bar in Figure 17.1 shows the range of results that would not be statistically significant (P > 0.05). It is centered on the null hypothesis, in this case that the mean body temperature is 37°C. It extends in each direction exactly the

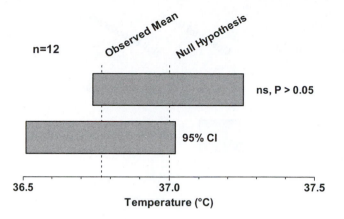

Figure 17.1. Comparing observed body temperatures (n = 12) with the hypothetical mean value of 37°C.

The top bar shows the range of results that are not statistically significant (P > 0.05). The bottom bar shows the 95% CI of the mean. It is centered on the sample mean. The lengths of the two bars are identical. Because the 95% CI contains the null hypothesis, the zone of statistically not significant results must include the sample mean.

same distance as the other bar, equal to the product of the SEM times the critical value of the t distribution.

The two bars have identical widths, but different centers. The CI is based on the observed value and shows you the zone of results that are consistent with the population mean (bottom bar in Figure 17.1) . The not statistically significant zone is based on the null hypothesis and shows you the range of sample means that are consistent with that null hypothesis (top bar in Figure 17.1).

In this example, the 95% CI contains the null hypothesis. Therefore, the zone of statistically not significant results must include the sample result (in this case, the mean).

WHEN A CI DOES NOT INCLUDE THE NULL HYPOTHESIS

Figure 17.2 shows the n = 130 data, but is otherwise similar to Figure 17.1.

The bottom bar of Figure 17.2 shows the 95% CI of the mean. It is centered on the sample mean. It extends in each direction a distance computed by multiplying the SEM times the critical value of the t distribution from Appendix D (for 95% confidence). This bar is much shorter than the corresponding bar in Figure 17.1. The main reason for this is that the SEM is much smaller because of the much larger sample size. Another reason is that the critical value from the t distribution is a bit smaller (1.98 instead of 2.20).

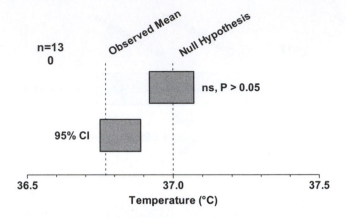

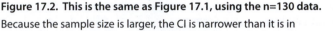

Figure 17.2. This is the same as Figure 17.1, using the n=130 data.
Because the sample size is larger, the CI is narrower than it is in
Figure 17.1, as is the zone of possible results that would not be
statistically significant. Because the 95% CI does not contain the null
hypothesis, the zone of not statistically significant results cannot contain
the sample mean. Whether the two boxes overlap is not relevant.

The top bar in Figure 17.2 shows the range of results that would not be statistically significant (P > 0.05). It is centered on the null hypothesis, in this case
that the mean body temperature is 37°C. It extends in each direction exactly the
same distance as the other bar, equal to the product of the SEM times the critical
value of the t distribution.

In this example, the 95% CI does not contain the null hypothesis.
Therefore, the zone of statistically not significant results cannot include the
sample mean.

A RULE THAT LINKS CONFIDENCE INTERVALS AND STATISTICAL SIGNIFICANCE

Here is a general rule that you should remember:

- If a 95% CI does not contain the value of the null hypothesis, then the
  result must be statistically significant with P < 0.05.
- If a 95% CI does contain the value of the null hypothesis, then the result
  must not be statistically significant (P > 0.05).

There is nothing special about 95% CIs and a significance level of 5%. The
rule also works like this: If the 99% CI does not contain the null hypothesis value,
then the P value must be less than 0.01.

In the examples, the "result" represented the comparison of a sample mean with a hypothetical population mean. The rule works for many other kinds of data. For example:

- If the CI for the difference between two means does not include zero (the null hypothesis), then the result must be statistically significant ($P < 0.05$).
- If the CI for the ratio of two proportions does not include 1.0 (the null hypothesis), then the result must be statistically significant ($P < 0.05$).

CHAPTER 18

Interpreting a Result That Is Statistically Significant

Facts do not "speak for themselves," they are read in the light of theory.

STEPHEN JAY GOULD

When you see a result that is "statistically significant," don't stop thinking. That phrase is often misunderstood, as this chapter explains. All it means is that the calculated P value is less than a preset threshold you set. This means that the results would be surprising (but not impossible) if the null hypothesis were true. A conclusion of statistical significance does not mean the difference is large enough to be interesting or worthy of follow-up, and does not mean that the finding is scientifically or clinically significant.

DISTINGUISH STATISTICAL SIGNIFICANCE FROM SCIENTIFIC IMPORTANCE

A result is said to be statistically significant when the calculated P value is less than a preset value of α. This means that the results are surprising and would not commonly occur if the null hypothesis were true. In other words, the conclusion "statistically significant" means only that a number (P value) you calculate from data is smaller than a threshold that you previously set. That's it!

A conclusion of statistical significance does not mean the difference is large enough to be interesting, does not mean the results are intriguing enough to be worthy of further investigations, and does not mean that the finding is scientifically or clinically significant.

The example in Chapter 15 asked whether the mean body temperature differed from the value of 37.0°C (which was commonly believed to be the average body temperature). With the large (n = 130) sample, the P value is tiny, only 0.0000018. But the discrepancy between the hypothetical mean and the true mean is also tiny and makes very little, if any, practical difference. The discrepancy is extremely statistically significant, but not even close to being clinically significant.

	DECISION: REJECT NULL HYPOTHESIS	DECISION: DO NOT REJECT NULL HYPOTHESIS	TOTAL
Null hypothesis is true	A	B	A+B
Null hypothesis false	C	D	C+D
Total	A+C	B+D	A+B+C+D

Table 18.1. The results of many hypothetical statistical analyses, each analyzed to reach a decision to reject or not reject the null hypothesis.

The top row tabulates results for experiments where the null hypothesis is really true. The second row tabulates experiments where the null hypothesis is not true. When you analyze data, you don't know whether the null hypothesis is true, so you could never create this table from an actual series of experiments. A, B, C, and D are integers (not proportions) that count the number of analyses.

Once some people hear the word *significant*, they stop thinking about the data. Belief in the usefulness of statistical significance has been called a cult (Ziliak & McCloskey, 2008). I suggest the following:

- When describing the conclusion from statistical hypothesis testing, always use the phrase "statistically significant." Don't use the word *significant* by itself. Even better, use the phrase "reject the null hypothesis" and avoid the term *significant* entirely. In many cases, it makes more sense to simply report the P value.
- When discussing the importance or impact of data and you feel an uncontrollable urge to use that word, use it as part of a phrase, like "scientifically significant" or "clinically significant." But try to avoid that word entirely and instead use one of these alternatives terms: consequential, eventful, meaningful, momentous, large, big, substantial, remarkable, valuable, worthwhile, impressive, major, or prominent.

A COMMON MISCONCEPTION

Many scientists and students misunderstand the definition of statistical significance (and P values).

Table 18.1 shows the results of many hypothetical statistical analyses, each analyzed to reach a decision to reject or not reject the null hypothesis. The top row tabulates results for experiments where the null hypothesis is really true. The second row tabulates experiments where the null hypothesis is not true. This kind of table is only useful for understanding statistical theory. When you analyze data, you don't know whether the null hypothesis is true, so you could never create this table from an actual series of experiments. Table 18.2 reviews the definitions of Type I and Type II errors.

	DECISION: REJECT NULL HYPOTHESIS	DECISION: DO NOT REJECT NULL HYPOTHESIS
Null hypothesis is true	Type I error	
Null hypothesis is false		Type II error

Table 18.2. Definition of Type I and Type II errors.

The significance level (usually set to 5%) is defined to equal the ratio $A/(A + B)$. The significance level is the answer to these two equivalent questions:

> If the null hypothesis is true, what is the probability of incorrectly rejecting that null hypothesis?

> Of all experiments you could conduct when the null hypothesis is true, in what fraction will you reach a conclusion that the results are statistically significant?

Many people mistakenly think that the significance level is the ratio $A/(A + C)$. This ratio, called the *false discovery rate* (FDR), is quite different.

The FDR, which we'll return to in Chapter 22, answers these two equivalent questions:

> If a result is statistically significant, what is the probability that the null hypothesis is really true?

> Of all experiments that reach a statistically significant conclusion, in what fraction is the null hypothesis true?

PRIOR PROBABILITY INFLUENCES THE FDR

The FDR is influenced by your choice of significance level. But it also is influenced by the context of the experiment.

Imagine that you work at a drug company and are screening drugs as possible treatments for hypertension. You test the drugs in a group of animals. You have decided that you are interested in a mean decrease in blood pressure of 10 mm Hg, and are using large enough samples so that there is an 80% chance of finding a statistically significant difference ($P < 0.05$) if the true difference between population means is 10 mmHg. (You will learn how to calculate the sample size in Chapter 43.)

You test a new drug and find a statistically significant drop in mean blood pressure. You know that there are two possibilities. Either the drug really works to lower blood pressure or the drug doesn't alter blood pressure at all and you just happened to get lower pressure readings on the treated animals. How likely are the two possibilities?

Because you set α to 0.05, you know that 5% of studies done with inactive drugs will demonstrate a statistically significant drop in blood pressure. But that isn't the question you are asking. You want to know the answer to a different question: In

	DECISION: REJECT NULL HYPOTHESIS	DECISION: DO NOT REJECT NULL HYPOTHESIS	TOTAL
Drug is ineffective	45	855	900
Drug works	80	20	100
Total	125	875	1,000

Table 18.3. Distribution of results with 80% power, 5% significance level, and prior probability = 10%.

what fraction of experiments in which you observe a statistically significant drop in pressure is the drug really effective? The answer is not necessarily 5%.

The answer depends on what you knew about the drug before you started the experiment, expressed as the prior probability that the drug works. This point is illustrated in the following three examples.

Drug A

This drug is known to weakly block angiotensin receptors, but the affinity is low and the drug is unstable. From your experience with such drugs, you estimate that there is about a 10% chance that it will depress blood pressure. In other words, the prior probability that the drug works is 10%. What will happen if you test 1,000 such drugs? The number 1,000 is arbitrary, because we only care about ratios. The answer is shown in Table 18.3.

These are the steps you need to follow to create the table:

1. We are predicting the results of 1,000 experiments with 1,000 different drugs, so the grand total is 1,000. This number is arbitrary, because the important conclusions will be expressed as ratios.
2. Of those 1,000 drugs we screen, we expect that 10% will really work. In other words, the prior probability equals 10%. So we place 10% of 1,000, or 100, as the total of the second row, leaving 900 for the sum of the first row.
3. Of the 100 drugs that really work, we will obtain a statistically significant result in 80% (because our experimental design has 80% power; see Chapter 20). So we place 80% of 100, or 80, into the bottom left cell of the table. This leaves 20 experiments with a drug that really works, but $P > 0.05$ so we conclude that the drug is not effective.
4. Of the 900 drugs that are really ineffective, we will by chance obtain a statistically significant reduction in blood pressure in 5% (because we set α equal to 0.05). Thus, the top left cell is 5% × 900, or 45. That leaves 855 experiments in which the drug is ineffective, and we correctly observe no statistically significant difference.
5. Determine the row totals by addition.

Of 1,000 tests of different drugs, we expect to obtain a statistically significant difference ($P < 0.05$) in 125 of them. Of those, 80 drugs are really effective and

	DECISION: REJECT NULL HYPOTHESIS	DECISION: DO NOT REJECT NULL HYPOTHESIS	TOTAL
Drug is ineffective	10	190	200
Drug works	640	160	800
Total	650	350	1,000

Table 18.4. Distribution of results with 80% power, 5% significance level, and prior probability = 80%.

	DECISION: REJECT NULL HYPOTHESIS	DECISION: DO NOT REJECT NULL HYPOTHESIS	TOTAL
Drug is ineffective	50	940	990
Drug works	8	2	10
Total	58	942	1,000

Table 18.5. Distribution of results with 80% power, 5% significance level, and prior probability = 1%.

45 are not. When you see a statistically significant result for any particular drug (where the prior probability is 10%), you can conclude that there is a 64% chance (80/125) that the drug is really effective and a 36% chance (45/125) that it is really ineffective. In other words, you expect the FDR to equal 36%.

Drug B

Here the pharmacology is much better characterized. Drug B blocks the right kinds of receptors with reasonable affinity and the drug is chemically stable. From your experience with such drugs, you estimate that the prior probability that the drug is effective equals 80%. What would happen if you tested 1,000 such drugs? The calculations are similar to those for Drug A, and the results are shown in Table 18.4.

If you test 1,000 drugs like this one, you expect to see 650 statistically significant results. Of those, 98.5% (640/650) will be truly effective. When you see a statistically significant result for any particular drug (where the prior probability is 80%), you can conclude that there is a 98.5% chance that it really lowered blood pressure and a 1.5% chance that it is really ineffective.

Drug C

This drug was randomly selected from the drug company's inventory of compounds. Nothing you know about this drug suggests that it affects blood pressure. Your best guess is that about 1% of such drugs will lower blood pressure. What would happen if you screen 1,000 such drugs? The answer is shown in Table 18.5.

If you test 1,000 drugs like this one, you expect to see 58 statistically significant results. Of those, you expect that 14% (8/58) will be truly effective and that 86% (50/58) will be ineffective. When you see a statistically significant result for any particular drug (where the prior probability is only 1%), you can conclude that there is a 14% chance that it will really lower blood pressure and an 85% chance that it is really ineffective.

BAYESIAN LOGIC

These examples demonstrate that your interpretation of a statistically significant result appropriately depends on what you knew about the drug before you started. Understanding the results requires combining the P value obtained from the experiment with the prior probability based on the context of the experiment. This approach is called *Bayesian inference*, named after Thomas Bayes, who first published work on this problem in the mid- 18th century. The idea of Bayesian thinking is to combine the experimental evidence with your prior knowledge.

There are some situations where the prior probabilities are well defined, for example in analyses of genetic linkage. The prior probability that two genetic loci are linked is known, so Bayesian statistics are routinely used in analysis of genetic linkage. There is nothing controversial about using Bayesian inference when the prior probabilities are known precisely.

However, as in the example above, the prior probability can be no more than a subjective feeling. Some statisticians think it is OK to convert these feelings to numbers ("99% sure" or "70% sure"), which they define as the prior probability. Other statisticians think that you should never equate subjective feelings with probabilities.

The Bayesian approach explains why you must interpret P values and conclusions of statistical significance in the context of what you already know or believe, and why you must think about biological plausibility when interpreting data.

When scientific theory changes, it is appropriate to change your perception of the prior probability and your interpretation of data. Accordingly, different people can honestly reach different conclusions from the same data. All statistically significant results are not created equal.

APPLYING BAYESIAN THINKING INFORMALLY

When reading biomedical research, you'll rarely (if ever) see Bayesian calculations used to interpret P values. However, many scientists use Bayesian thinking in a more informal way, without stating the prior probability explicitly and without performing any additional calculations. When reviewing three different studies, the thinking might go like this:

- This study tested a hypothesis that is biologically sound and supported by previous data. The P value is 0.04, which is marginal. I have a choice of believing that the results occurred by a coincidence that will happen 1 time in 25 under the null hypothesis, or of believing that the experimental hypothesis is true. Because the experimental hypothesis makes so much sense, I'll believe it. The null hypothesis is probably false.

- This study tested a hypothesis that makes no biological sense and has not been supported by any previous data. The P value is 0.04, which is lower than the usual threshold of 0.05, but not by very much. I have a choice of believing that the results occurred by a coincidence that will happen 1 time in 25 under the null hypothesis, or of believing that the experimental hypothesis is true. Because the experimental hypothesis is so crazy, I find it easier to believe that the results are the result of coincidence. The null hypothesis is probably true.

- This study tested a hypothesis that makes no biological sense and has not been supported by any previous data. I'd be amazed if it turned out to be true. The P value is incredibly low (0.000001). I've looked through the details of the study and cannot identify any biases or flaws. These are reputable scientists, and I believe that they've reported their data honestly. I have a choice of believing that the results occurred by a coincidence that will happen 1 time in a million under the null hypothesis, or of believing that the experimental hypothesis is true. Although the hypothesis seems crazy to me, the data force me to believe it. The null hypothesis is probably false.

You *should* interpret experimental data in the context of scientific theory and previous data. That's why different people can legitimately reach different conclusions from the same data.

CHAPTER 19

Interpreting a Result That Is Not Statistically Significant

I was gratified to be able to answer promptly, and I did. I said I didn't know.

MARK TWAIN

*W*hen you see a result that is not statistically significant, don't stop thinking. "Not statistically significant" only says only that the P value is larger than a preset threshold. Thus, a difference (correlation, association...) as large as what you observed would not be unusual due to random sampling if the null hypothesis is true. This does not prove that the null hypothesis is true. This chapter explains how to use confidence intervals to help interpret the findings that are not statistically significant.

"NOT SIGNIFICANTLY DIFFERENT" DOES NOT MEAN "NO DIFFERENCE"

A large P value means that a difference (correlation, association...) as large as what you observed would happen frequently as a result of random sampling. But this does not necessarily mean that the null hypothesis of no difference is true or that the difference you observed is definitely the result of random sampling.

Vickers (2006a) told a great story that illustrates this point:

> The other day I shot baskets with [the famous basketball player] Michael Jordan (remember that I am a statistician and never make things up). He shot 7 straight free throws; I hit 3 and missed 4 and then (being a statistician) rushed to the sideline, grabbed my laptop, and calculated a *P* value of .07 by Fisher's exact test. Now, you wouldn't take this *P* value to suggest that there is *no* difference between my basketball skills and those of Michael Jordan, you'd say that our experiment hadn't *proved* a difference.

A high P value does not prove the null hypothesis. Deciding not to reject the null hypothesis is not the same as believing that the null hypothesis is definitely true. The absence of evidence is not evidence of absence (Altman & Bland, 1995).

	CONTROLS	HYPERTENSION
Number of subjects	17	18
Mean receptor number (receptors/platelet)	263	257
SD	87	59

Table 19.1. Number of α_2-adrenergic receptors on the platelets of controls and people with hypertension.

EXAMPLE: α_2-ADRENERGIC RECEPTORS ON PLATELETS

Epinephrine, acting through α_2-adrenergic receptors, makes blood platelets stickier and thus helps blood clot. We counted these receptors and compared people with normal and high blood pressure (Motulsky, O'Connor, & Insel, 1983). The idea was that the adrenergic signaling system might be abnormal in high blood pressure (hypertension). We were most interested in the effects on the heart, blood vessels, kidney, and brain, but obviously couldn't access those tissues in people, so we counted receptors on platelets instead. Table 19.1 shows the results.

The results were analyzed with an unpaired t test (see Chapter 30). The average number of receptors per platelet was almost the same in both groups, so of course the P value was high, 0.81. If the two populations had identical means, you'd expect to see a difference as large or larger than that observed in this study in 81% of studies of this size.

Clearly, these data provide no evidence that the mean receptor number differs in the two groups. When I published this study 25 years ago, I stated that the results were not statistically significant and stopped there, implying that the high P value proves that the null hypothesis is true. But that was not a complete way to present the data. We should have interpreted the CI.

The 95% CI for the difference between group means extends from -45 to 57 receptors/platelet. To put this in perspective, you need to know that the average number of receptors per platelet is about 260. Therefore, the 95% confidence interval extends approximately plus or minus 20%.

It is only possible to properly interpret the confidence in a scientific context. Here are two alternative, contradictory, ways to think about these results:

- A 20% change in receptor number could have a huge physiological impact. With such a wide CI, the data are inconclusive, because they are consistent with no difference, substantially more receptors on platelets from people with hypertension, or substantially fewer receptors on platelets of people with hypertension.
- The CI convincingly shows that the true difference is unlikely to be more than 20% in either direction. This experiment counts receptors on a convenient tissue (blood cells) as a marker for other organs, and we know the number of receptors per platelet varies a lot from individual to individual. For these reasons, we'd only be intrigued by the results (and want

	ADVERSE OUTCOME	TOTAL	RISK	RELATIVE RISK
Routine ultrasound	383	7,685	0.050%	1.020
Only when indicated	373	7,596	0.049%	
Total	756	15,281		

Table 19.2. Relationship between fetal ultrasounds and outcome.

The risks in column 4 are computed by dividing the number of adverse outcomes by the total number of pregnancies. The relative risk is computed by dividing one risk by the other (see Chapter 27 for more details).

to pursue this line of research) if the receptor number in the two groups differed by at least 50%. Here, the 95% CI extended about 20% in each direction. Therefore, we can reach a solid negative conclusion that either there is no change in receptor number in individuals with hypertension, or any such change is physiologically trivial and not worth pursuing.

Those two conclusions contradict each other. The difference is a matter of scientific judgment. Would a difference of 20% in receptor number be scientifically relevant? The answer depends on scientific (physiological) thinking. Statistical calculations have nothing to do with it. Statistical calculations are only a small part of interpreting data.

EXAMPLE: FETAL ULTRASOUNDS

Ewigman et al. (1993) investigated whether the routine use of prenatal ultrasound would improve perinatal outcome. They randomly divided a large group of pregnant women into two groups. One group received routine ultrasound exams (or, *sonograms*) twice during the pregnancy. The other group received sonograms only if there was a clinical reason to do so. The physicians caring for the women knew the results of the sonograms and cared for the women accordingly. The investigators looked at several outcomes. Table 19.2 shows the total number of adverse events, defined as fetal or neonatal deaths (mortality) or moderate to severe morbidity.

The null hypothesis is that the risk of adverse outcomes is identical in the two groups. In other words, the null hypothesis is that routine use of ultrasound neither prevents nor causes perinatal mortality or morbidity, so the relative risk equals 1.00. Chapter 27 will explain the concept of relative risk in more detail.

Table 19.2 shows that the relative risk is 1.02. That isn't far from the null hypothesis value of 1.00. The two-tail P value is 0.86.

Interpreting the results requires knowing the 95% CI for the relative risk, which a computer program can calculate. For this example, the 95% CI ranges from 0.88 to 1.17.

Our data are certainly consistent with the null hypothesis, because the CI includes 1.0. This does not mean that the null hypothesis is true. Our CI tells us that the data are also consistent (within 95% confidence) with relative risks ranging from 0.88 to 1.17.

Here are three approaches to interpreting the results:

- The CI is centered on 1.0 (no difference) and is quite narrow. These data convincingly show that the routine use of ultrasound is neither helpful nor harmful.
- The CI is narrow, but not all that narrow. It certainly makes clinical sense that the extra information provided by ultrasound will help obstetricians manage the pregnancy and might decrease the chance of a major problem. The CI goes down to 0.88, a risk reduction of 12%. If I were pregnant, I'd certainly want to use a risk-free technique that reduces the risk of a sick or dead baby by as much as 12%! The data certainly don't prove that routine ultrasound is beneficial, but the study leaves open the possibility that routine use of ultrasound might reduce the rate of truly awful events by as much as 12%.
- The CI goes as high as 1.17. That is a 17% increase in problems. Without data from a much bigger study, these data do not convince me that ultrasound is helpful and makes me worry that they might be harmful.

Statistics can't help resolve the difference among these three approaches. It all depends on how you interpret a relative risk of 0.88 and 1.17, how worried you are about possible risks of ultrasound, and how you combine the data in this study with data from other studies (I have no expertise in this field and have not looked at other studies).

In interpreting the results of this example, you also need to think about benefits and risks that don't show up as a reduction of adverse outcomes. The ultrasound picture helps reassure parents that their baby is developing normally and gives them a picture to bond with and to show relatives. This can be valuable regardless of whether it reduces the chance of adverse outcomes. Although statistical analyses focus on one outcome at a time, you must consider all the outcomes when evaluating the results.

HOW TO GET NARROWER CIs

Both examples presented above demonstrate the importance of interpreting the CI in the scientific context of the experiment. Different people will appropriately have different opinions about how large a difference (or relative risk) is scientifically or clinically important, and will interpret a not significant result differently.

If the CI is wide enough to include values you consider clinically or scientifically important, then the study is inconclusive. In some cases, you might be able to narrow the confidence intervals by improving the methodology and thereby reduce the SD. But in most cases, increasing the sample size is the only approach to narrowing the CI in a repeat study. This rule of thumb can help: If sample size is increased by a factor of 4, the CI is expected to narrow by a factor of 2. More generally, the width of a CI is inversely proportional to the square root of sample size.

WHAT IF THE P VALUE IS REALLY HIGH?

If you ran many experiments where the null hypothesis was really true, you'd expect the P values to be uniformly distributed between 0.0 and 1.0. Half of the P values would have values greater than 0.5 and 10% would have values greater than 0.9. But what do you conclude when the P value is really high?

In 1865, Mendel published a paper on heredity in pea plants. This was the first explanation of heredity and recessive traits and really founded the field of genetics. Mendel proposed a model of recessive inheritance, designed an experiment with peas to test the model, and showed that the data fit the model very well. Extremely well! Fisher (1936) reviewed these data and then pooled all of Mendel's published data to calculate a P value that answered this question:

> Assuming that Mendel's genetic theory is correct and every plant was classified correctly, what is the probability that the deviation between expected and observed would be as great or greater than actually observed?

The answer (the P value) is 0.99993. In other words, if all the data were honestly reported, there is only a 0.007% chance that the data would match the theory this well. You'd expect more random discrepancies between theory and data. If 100,000 scientists were to repeat the work, only 7 would be expected to gather observed data that match the theory so well.

Although it is possible that Mendel was extremely lucky, Fisher concluded that Mendel's data are simply too good to be true. Explanations include his unintentional bias when doing the classification, and his not publishing experiments with data that strayed from expectations. The incredibly close match between theory and observations is most likely the result of data massaging by Mendel or his assistants.

CHAPTER 20

Statistical Power

There are two kinds of statistics, the kind you look up, and
the kind you make up.

REX STOUT

*The power of an experimental design answers this question: If the true
effect is of a specified size and the experiment is repeated many times,
what fraction of the results will be statistically significant? The concept of
power can help when deciding how large a sample size to use (Chapter 43)
and can help interpret results that are not statistically significant.*

WHAT IS POWER?

The definition of a P value begins with "If the null hypothesis is true…"

But what if the null hypothesis is false, and the treatment really does affect
the outcome? Even so, your data may reach the conclusion that the effect is not
statistically significant. Just by chance, your data may yield a P value greater than
0.05 (or whatever significance level you chose). This question becomes relevant:

> If there really were a difference (or relative risk or correlation) of a specified
> value in the overall population, what is the chance of obtaining a difference
> (etc.) that is statistically significant in one particular sample?

The answer, called the *power* of the experiment, depends on the sample size,
on the amount of scatter, and on the size of the difference you hypothesize exists.
Given these values, power is the fraction of experiments that you would expect to
yield a statistically significant result.

Table 20.1 (which repeats Table 18.1) shows the results of many hypothetical
statistical analyses, each analyzed to reach a conclusion of "statistically significant" or "not statistically significant." Assuming the null hypothesis is not true,
power is the fraction of experiments that reach a statistically significant conclusion. So power equals C/(C+D). Beta (β) is 1.0 minus power, so it equals D/
(C+D).

Note the similarity in the definitions of α and β. If the null hypothesis is true,
then α is the chance of making the wrong decision (rejecting the null hypothesis).
If the null hypothesis is false (with a specified alternative hypothesis), β is the
chance of making the wrong decision (not rejecting the null hypothesis).

	DECISION: REJECT NULL HYPOTHESIS	DECISION: DO NOT REJECT NULL HYPOTHESIS	TOTAL
Null hypothesis is true	A	B	A+B
Null hypothesis is false	C	D	C+D

Table 20.1. Definition of power.
This shows the results of A+B+C+D experiments. In some cases, the null hypothesis is true (top row), whereas in other cases it is not (bottom row). The first column tabulates results that are statistically significant (so you decide to reject the null hypothesis), whereas the second column tabulates results that are not statistically significant. Power is the fraction of experiments, when the null hypothesis is false, that achieve a statistically significant result. Thus, power is defined as C/(C+D).

AN ANALOGY TO UNDERSTAND POWER

This analogy helps illustrate the concept of statistical power (Hartung, 2005). You send your child into the basement to find a tool. He comes back and says, "It isn't there." What do you conclude? Is the tool there or not?

There is no way to be sure, so the answer must be a probability. The question you really want to answer is, "What is the probability that the tool is in the basement?" But that question can't really be answered without knowing the prior probability and using Bayesian thinking (see Chapter 18). Instead, let's ask a different question: "If the tool really is in the basement, what is the chance your child would have found it?" The answer, of course, is "it depends." To estimate the probability, you'd want to know three things:

- How long did he spend looking? If he looked for a long time, he is more likely to have found the tool. This is analogous to sample size. An experiment with a large sample size has high power to find an effect.
- How big is the tool? It is easier to find a snow shovel than the tiny screwdriver used to fix eyeglasses. This is analogous to the size of the effect you are looking for. An experiment has more power to find a big effect than a small one.
- How messy is the basement? If the basement is a real mess, he was less likely to find the tool than if it is carefully organized. This is analogous to experimental scatter. An experiment has more power when the data are very tight (little variation).

If the child spent a long time looking for a large tool in an organized basement, there is a high chance that he would have found the tool if it were there. So you can be quite confident of his conclusion that the tool isn't there. Similarly, an experiment has high power when you have a large sample size, are looking for a large effect, and have data with little scatter (small standard deviation). In this situation, there is a high chance that you would have obtained a statistically significant effect if the effect existed.

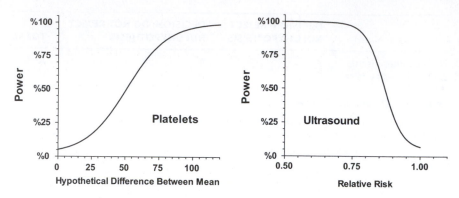

Figure 20.1. The power of the two experiments.

The graph on the left summarizes the experiment in Table 19.1, which compared a_2-receptor number in controls and people with hypertension. The graph on the right summarizes the data in Table 19.2, evaluating the advantages of fetal ultrasound. For any hypothetical difference between means (X-axis), this graph shows the power of the study to find a statistically significant difference (P < 0.05). Note that an increasing effect for the platelet example (larger difference in receptor number) goes from left to right, whereas an increasing effect for the ultrasound example (smaller relative risk) goes from right to left.

If the child spent a short time looking for a small tool in a messy basement, his conclusion that "the tool isn't there" doesn't really mean very much. Even if the tool were there, he probably would have not found it. Similarly, an experiment has little power when you use a small sample size, are looking for a small effect, and the data have lots of scatter. In this situation, there is a high chance of obtaining a conclusion of "statistically significant" even if the effect exists.

POWER OF THE TWO EXAMPLE STUDIES

The power of an experimental design can be computed to detect various hypothetical differences. The left side of Figure 20.1 shows the power of the platelet study (described in Chapter 19) to detect various hypothetical differences between means. The power was calculated using the program GraphPad StatMate from the sample size of the study, the SDs in the two groups, and the definition of significance (P < 0.05).

If there really is no difference between population means, there is a 5% chance of obtaining a statistically significant result. That is the definition of statistical significance (using the traditional 5% significance level). So the curve intersects the Y-axis at 5%. If there is a difference between population means, the power of this study depends on the size of that difference. If the difference is tiny (left side of the graph), then the power is low. If the difference is large, then so is the power, which approaches 100% with very large differences.

The right side of Figure 20.1 shows the power of the ultrasound study. If the relative risk is really 1.0 (no effect), there is a 5% chance of obtaining a statistically significant result, because that is the definition of statistical significance. So the curve shows 5% power with a relative risk of 1.00, and more power as the effect gets more pronounced (lower relative risk, showing that ultrasound is beneficial).

The shapes in Figure 20.1 are universal. All experimental designs have little power to detect small differences and high power to detect huge differences. What varies between studies is the horizontal location of the curve.

These graphs help explain the concepts of statistical power and nonsignificant results. You can see that the platelet study had huge power to detect a difference in receptor number of 100 or more, and that the ultrasound study had enormous power to detect a relative risk of 0.75 or less. You'd reach the same conclusion by interpreting the CIs, so these kinds of power graphs are rarely used when interpreting nonsignificant results.

POST HOC POWER ANALYSIS IS NOT HELPFUL

Some software programs try to make things easy and remove the need to think in a scientific context. These programs compute the power to detect the effect size (or difference, relative risk, etc.) actually observed in a particular experiment. The result is sometimes called *observed power*, and the procedure is sometimes called a *post hoc power analysis* or *retrospective power analysis*.

This approach is not helpful (Hoenig & Heisey, 2001; Lenth, 2001; Levine & Ensom, 2001). If your study reached a conclusion that the difference is not statistically significant, then by definition, its power to detect the effect actually observed is very low. You learn nothing new by calculating the observed power.

In contrast, it does make sense to ask how much power an experiment had to detect an effect of some specified size. That effect size must be chosen based on scientific goals and is unrelated to the effect actually observed in a particular experiment.

CHAPTER 21

Testing for Equivalence or Noninferiority

The problem is not what you don't know, but what you know that ain't so.

WILL ROGERS

In many scientific and clinical investigations, the goal is not to find out whether one treatment causes a substantially different effect than another treatment. Instead, the goal is to find out whether the effects of a new treatment are equivalent to (or not inferior to) that of a standard treatment. This chapter explains how the usual approach of statistical hypothesis testing is not useful. A conclusion that the difference between two treatments is statistically significant does not answer the question about equivalence, and neither does a conclusion that the difference is not statistically significant.

EQUIVALENCE MUST BE DEFINED SCIENTIFICALLY, NOT STATISTICALLY

You've created a generic drug and want to prove it works just the same as a standard drug. There are many aspects of drug action that can be compared, and we'll focus on one question: Is the peak blood-plasma concentration of the two formulations of the drug equivalent? Patients are given first one drug formulation and then (after a washout period) the other, randomizing the order. The peak concentration of each drug formulation is measured in each subject.

When you compare the two drugs, you will always see some difference in peak plasma concentration. It doesn't make sense to ask whether the two give precisely the same outcome. When asking about equivalence, the question is whether the outcomes are *close enough* to be clinically or scientifically indistinguishable.

How close is close enough? It must be defined as a range of treatment effects considered scientifically or clinically trivial. This requires thinking about the scientific or clinical context of your experiment. Statistical calculations and conclusions about statistical significance are completely irrelevant in defining this range, or *equivalence zone* also called the *equivalence margin*.

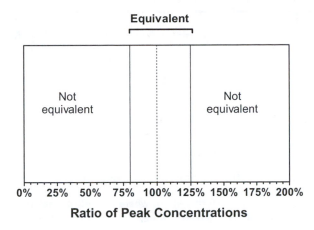

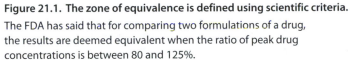

Figure 21.1. The zone of equivalence is defined using scientific criteria.
The FDA has said that for comparing two formulations of a drug,
the results are deemed equivalent when the ratio of peak drug
concentrations is between 80 and 125%.

When testing a generic drug, the U.S. Food and Drug Administration (FDA) defines two drug formulations to be equivalent when the ratio of their peak concentrations in blood plasma is between 0.80 and 1.25. This definition is based on clinical understanding of drug action, and statistical thinking had nothing to do with setting the limits. In addition, the FDA specifies that the entire 90% CI of that ratio should be within the 0.80 to 1.25 range.

Figure 21.1 shows this definition. Make sure you understand Figure 21.1, because it is the basis for Figures 21.2 and 21.3.

Note that the zone of equivalence does not appear to be symmetrical around 100%, but in fact it is. It is fairly arbitrary whether you calculate the ratio of peak levels as the peak level of the new formulation divided by the peak level of the standard formulation, or as the peak level of the standard formulation divided by the peak level of the new formulation. The reciprocal of 80% is 125% (1/0.8 = 1.25) and the reciprocal of 125% is 80% (1/1.25 = 0.80). So the zone of equivalence is, in a practical sense, symmetrical.

MEAN WITHIN THE EQUIVALENCE ZONE

Figure 21.2 shows data from three drugs where the mean ratio of peak concentrations is within the zone of equivalence. The fact that the mean value is within the zone does not prove equivalence. Two drugs are defined to be bioequivalent (by the FDA) only when the entire CI for the ratio of peak concentrations lies within the equivalence zone.

This is the case for drugs B and C. Those CIs lie entirely within the equivalence zone, so the data demonstrate that drugs B and C are equivalent to the standard drug they are being compared with.

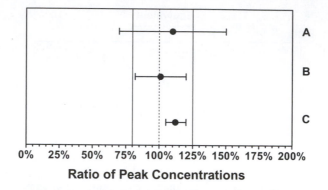

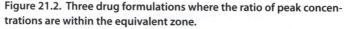

Ratio of Peak Concentrations

Figure 21.2. Three drug formulations where the ratio of peak concentrations are within the equivalent zone.

For drug A, the CI extends outside of the equivalent zone, so the results are inconclusive. The results are consistent with the two drugs being equivalent or not equivalent. In experiments B and C, the CIs lie completely within the equivalent zone, so the data demonstrate that the two drugs are equivalent to the standard drug.

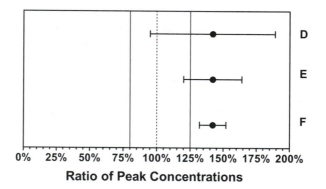

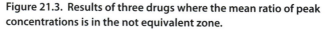

Ratio of Peak Concentrations

Figure 21.3. Results of three drugs where the mean ratio of peak concentrations is in the not equivalent zone.

With drugs D and E, the CI includes both equivalent and not equivalent zones, so the data are not conclusive. The CI for drug F is entirely outside the equivalence zone, proving that it is not equivalent to the standard drug.

In contrast, the CI for drug A is partly in the equivalence zone and partly outside of it. The data are inconclusive.

MEAN OUTSIDE OF THE EQUIVALENCE ZONE

Figure 21.3 shows data from three drugs where the mean ratio of peak concentrations is in the not equivalent zone. This does not prove the drugs are not equivalent. You must look at the entire CI.

The CIs for drugs D and E are partly within the equivalent zone and partly outside it. The data are not conclusive.

The CI for drug F lies totally outside the equivalence zone. These data prove that the drug F is not equivalent to the standard drug.

THE USUAL APPROACH OF STATISTICAL HYPOTHESIS TESTING IS NOT HELPFUL

A common mistake is to simply compare the peak blood concentration of the two drugs using a paired t test (Chapter 31). It seems as though the P value ought to be informative, but this approach is not helpful. If the results are not statistically significant, it is a mistake to conclude that the blood concentrations of the two drugs are equivalent. Similarly, if the results are statistically significant, it is a mistake to conclude that the two drugs are not equivalent.

A paired t test would test the null hypothesis that the two drugs have the same mean peak levels, so the ratio of peak concentrations equals 1.0. All three figures have a vertical dotted line marking that point.

You can look at the data shown in Figures 21.2 and 21.3 and instantly know whether the difference between peak levels is statistically significant. A result is statistically significant with a P value less than 0.05 when the 95% CI does not include the value that defines the null hypothesis. Data from drug C (Figure 21.1) and drugs E and F (Figure 21.2) meet this criterion, because their CIs do not include 100%. The difference between the peak concentrations of each of these drugs and the standard drug is statistically significant. However, (as explained above) drug C is equivalent to the standard drug, drug F is not equivalent, and the data for drug E are inconclusive.

A result is not statistically significant (P>0.05) when the 95% CI includes the value defined by the null hypothesis. The data for drugs A, B, and D meet this criterion, because the CIs include 100%. The difference between the peak concentration of each of these drugs and the standard drug is not statistically significant. But this tells us nothing about equivalence. The data for drug B demonstrate equivalence, whereas the data for drugs A and D are inconclusive about whether the drugs are equivalent to the standard drug.

BENDING OVER BACKWARD TO ADAPT HYPOTHESIS TESTING TO EQUIVALENCE

It is possible to apply the ideas of statistical hypothesis testing to testing for equivalence, but it is tricky (Wellek, 2002). The approach is to pose two distinct null hypotheses and define statistical significance using two distinct one-tail tests.

Let's continue the example of comparing peak drug concentrations for two drugs. The two drugs are shown to be equivalent when both of the following conditions are true (Figure 21.4).

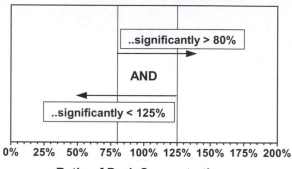

Figure 21.4. Applying the idea of statistical hypothesis testing to equivalence testing.

A conclusion of equivalence requires a statistically significant finding from two different tests of two different null hypotheses, shown by the vertical lines. Each null hypothesis is tested with a one-side alternative hypothesis, shown by the arrows. Two drugs are considered equivalent when the ratio of peak concentrations is significantly greater than 80% and also significantly less than 125%.

- The mean value of the ratio is *greater* than 0.80 (the lower limit that defines equivalence), and this increase is statistically significant.
- The mean value of the ratio is *less* than 1.25 (the upper limit that defines equivalence), and this decrease is statistically significant.

Each null hypothesis is tested with a one-tail P value (Chapter 15). If both P values are less than a threshold set in advance, the results demonstrate equivalence.

Juggling two null hypothesis and two P values (each one-tailed) is not for the statistical novice. The results are the same as those obtained using the CI approach described above. The CI approach is much easier to understand.

NONINFERIORITY TRIALS

Equivalence trials attempt to prove that a new treatment or drug works about the same as the standard treatment. Noninferiority trials attempt to prove that a new treatment is not worse than the standard treatment.

To prove equivalence, all parts of the CI must be *within* the equivalence zone. To prove noninferiority, all parts of the CI must be to the right of the lower border of the equivalence zone. The entire CI, therefore, is in a range that either shows the new drug is superior, or shows that the new drug is slightly inferior, but still in the zone defined to be practically equivalent.

YOU MUST BE SURE THE STANDARD
TREATMENT WORKS

Snapinn (2000) and Kaul and Diamond (2006) reviewed the many issues one must think about when interpreting data that purport to demonstrate equivalence or noninferiority.

The most important issue is this: You must be 100% sure the standard drug works. A conclusion that a new treatment is equivalent (or not inferior) to a standard treatment is only useful when you are absolutely, positively sure that the standard treatment actually works better than placebo. If the data from other studies leave any doubts about whether the standard treatment works, then it really doesn't make any sense to ask whether a new treatment is equivalent (or not inferior) to it.

PART E

Challenges in Statistics

CHAPTER 22

Multiple Comparisons Concepts

> If you torture your data long enough, they will tell you what-
> ever you want to hear.
>
> JAMES L. MILLS (1993)

*C*oping with multiple comparisons is one of the biggest challenges in
data analysis. If you calculate many P values, some are likely to be
small just by random chance. Therefore, it is impossible to interpret small
P values without knowing how many comparisons were made. This chapter explains three approaches to cope with multiple comparisons.

THE PROBLEM OF MULTIPLE COMPARISONS

If you make two independent comparisons, what is the chance of that one or both
comparisons will result in a statistically significant conclusion just by chance?
It is easier to answer the opposite question. Assuming both null hypotheses are
true, what is the chance that both comparisons will be not statistically significant? The answer is the chance that the first comparisons will be not significant
(0.95) times the chance that the second one will be not significant (also 0.95),
or 0.9025. That leaves about a 10% chance of obtaining at least one statistically
significant conclusion by chance.

It is easy to generalize that logic to more comparisons. With K independent
comparisons (where K is some positive integer), the chance that all will be not
significant is 0.95^K, so the chance that one or more comparison will be statistically significant is $1.0 - 0.95^K$. Figure 22.1 plots this probability for various numbers of independent comparisons.

Remember the unlucky number 13. If you perform 13 independent comparisons (with the null hypothesis true in all cases), the chance is about 50% that one
or more of these P values will be less than 0.05, and thus lead to a conclusion of
statistically significant.

With more than 13 comparisons, it is more likely than not that one or more conclusions will be significant just by chance. With 100 independent null hypotheses
that are all true, the chance of obtaining at least one significant P value is 99%.

The multiple-comparisons problem is clear. If you make lots of comparisons
(and make no special correction for the multiple comparisons), you are likely to
find some statistically significant results just by chance.

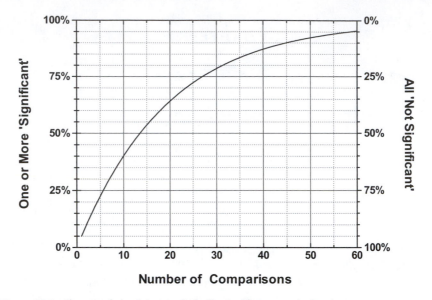

Figure 22.1. Chance of obtaining statistically significant results by chance.
The X-axis shows various numbers of statistical comparisons, each assumed to be independent of the others. The left Y-axis shows the chance of obtaining one or more statistically significant results (P < 0.05) by chance.

CORRECTING FOR MULTIPLE COMPARISONS IS NOT ALWAYS NEEDED

Corrections for multiple comparisons are not needed if the people reading the data take into account the number of comparisons

Some statisticians recommend never correcting for multiple comparisons (Rothman, 1990). The alternative is to report all of the individual P values and CIs and make it clear that no mathematical correction was made for multiple comparisons. This approach requires that all comparisons (or at least the *number* of comparisons) be reported. When you interpret these results, you must informally account for multiple comparisons. If all the null hypotheses are true, you'd expect 5% of the comparisons to have uncorrected P values less than 0.05. Compare this number with the actual number of small P values.

Corrections for multiple comparisons may not be needed if you make only a few planned comparisons

Even if a study collects lots of data, you may want to focus on only a few scientifically sensible comparisons, rather than every possible comparison. The term *planned comparison* is used to describe this situation. These comparisons must be designed into the experiment and cannot be decided upon after inspecting the data. When you make only a few planned comparisons, many statisticians think it is OK to not correct for multiple comparisons.

Corrections for multiple comparisons are not needed when the comparisons are complementary

Ridker and colleagues (2008) asked whether lowering LDL cholesterol would prevent heart disease in patients who did not have high LDL concentrations and did not have a prior history of heart disease (but did have an abnormal blood test suggesting the presence of some inflammatory disease). The study included almost 18,000 people. Half received a statin drug to lower LDL cholesterol and half received a placebo.

The investigators' primary goal (planned as part of the protocol) was to compare the number of "end points" that occurred in the two groups, including deaths from a heart attack or stroke, nonfatal heart attacks or strokes, and hospitalization for chest pain. These events happened about half as often to people treated with the drug, compared with people taking placebo. The drug worked.

The investigators also analyzed each of the end points separately. Those taking the drug (compared with those taking placebo) had fewer deaths, fewer heart attacks, fewer strokes, and fewer hospitalizations for chest pain.

The data from various demographic groups were then analyzed separately. Separate analyses were done for men and women, old and young, smokers and nonsmokers, people with hypertension and those without, people with a family history of heart disease and those without, etc. In each of 25 subgroups, patients receiving the drug experienced fewer primary end points than those taking placebo, and all of these effects were statistically significant.

The investigators made no correction for multiple comparisons for all these separate analyses of outcomes and subgroups. No corrections were needed, because the results are so consistent. The multiple comparisons each ask the same basic question, and all the comparisons lead to the same conclusion—people taking the drug had fewer cardiovascular events than those taking placebo.

IF YOU DON'T ACCOUNT FOR MULTIPLE COMPARISONS

Table 22.1 shows the results of many comparisons. You can't create this table with actual data, because the entries in the rows assume that you are "mother nature" and therefore know whether each null hypothesis is actually true. In fact, you never know that, so this table is conceptual.

The top row represents the results of comparisons where the null hypothesis is in fact true—the treatment really doesn't work. The second row shows the results of comparisons where there truly is a difference. The first column tabulates comparisons where the P value was low enough to be deemed statistically significant (or a "discovery" in the lingo of the FDR method discussed below).

	DECISION: "STATISTICALLY SIGNIFICANT" OR "DISCOVERY"	DECISION: "NOT STATISTICALLY SIGNIFICANT" OR "NOT A DISCOVERY"	TOTAL
Null hypothesis: True	A	B	A+B
Null hypothesis: False	C	D	C+D
Total	A+C	B+D	A+B+C+D

Table 22.1. This table (identical to Table 18.1) shows the results of many statistical analyses, each analyzed to reach a decision to reject or not reject the null hypothesis.

The top row tabulates results for experiments where the null hypothesis is really true. The second row tabulates experiments where the null hypothesis is not true. When you analyze data, you don't know whether the null hypothesis is true, so you could never create this table from an actual series of experiments. A, B, C, and D are integers (not proportions) that count the number of analyses.

The second column tabulates comparisons where the P value was high enough to

APPROACH	WHAT YOU CONTROL	FROM TABLE 22.1
Significance level (α) with no correction for multiple comparisons	α = If all null hypotheses are true, the fraction of all experiments where the conclusion is statistically significant	$\alpha = A/(A+B)$
Familywise significance level	α = The chance of obtaining one or more statistically significant conclusions if all null hypotheses are true	$\alpha = \text{probability}(A>0)$
False Discovery Rate (FDR)	Q = The fraction of all the discoveries where the null hypothesis really true	$Q = A/(A+C)$

Table 22.2. Three approaches to handling multiple comparisons.

be deemed not statistically significant (or not a discovery).

It would be nice if all comparisons ended up in cells B or C, leaving A and D empty. This is rarely the case. Even if the null hypothesis is true, random sampling will ensure that some comparisons will mistakenly yield a statistically significant conclusion and contribute to box A. And even if the null hypothesis is false, random sampling will ensure that some results will be not statistically significant and will contribute to box D.

A, B, C, and D each represent a number of comparisons, so the sum of A + B + C + D equals the total number of comparisons you are making.

What happens if you make no correction for multiple comparisons and set α to its conventional value of 5%? Of all experiments done when the null hypothesis is true, you expect 5% to be statistically significant just by chance. You expect the ratio A/(A + B) to equal 5%. This 5% value applies to each comparison separately, so is called *a per-comparison error rate*. In any particular set of comparisons, that ratio might be greater than 5% or less than 5%. But on average, if you make many comparisons, that is the value you'd expect. Table 22.2 summarizes three methods of dealing with multiple comparisons.

NO. OF "SIGNIFICANT" FINDINGS	NO CORRECTION (%)	BONFERRONI (%)
Zero	35.8	95.1
One	37.7	4.8
Two or more	26.4	0.1

Table 22.3. How many significant results will you find in 20 comparisons?
This table assumes you are making 20 comparisons, and all 20 null hypotheses are true. If there is no correction for multiple comparisons, there is only a 36% chance of observing no statistically significant findings. With the Bonferroni correction, this probability goes up to 95%.

THE TRADITIONAL APPROACH TO CORRECTING FOR MULTIPLE COMPARISONS

The Familywise Error Rate

When each comparison is made individually without any correction for multiple comparisons, the traditional 5% significance level applies to each individual comparison so it is known as *the per-comparison error rate*. It is the chance that random sampling would lead *this particular comparison* to an incorrect conclusion that the difference is statistically significant when this particular null hypothesis is true.

With multiple comparisons, the significance level is redefined to be the chance of obtaining *one or more* statistically significant conclusions if the *all* of the null hypotheses are actually true. The idea is to make a stricter threshold for defining significance. If α is set to the usual value of 5% and all the null hypotheses are true, then the goal is to have a 95% chance of obtaining zero statistically significant results and a 5% chance of obtaining one or more statistically significant results. That 5% chance applies to the entire family of comparisons performed in the experiment, so it is called a *familywise error rate* or the *per-experiment error rate*.

The Bonferroni correction

The simplest approach to achieve a family wise error rate is to divide the value of α (often 5%) by the number of comparisons. Then define any of the comparisons to be statistically significant only when its P value is less than that ratio. This is called the *Bonferroni method*.

Imagine that an experiment makes 20 comparisons. If all 20 null hypotheses are true and there are no corrections for multiple comparisons, about 5% of these comparisons are expected to be statistically significant (using the usual definition of α). Table 22.3 shows that there is about a 65% chance of obtaining one (or more) statistically significant result.

If the Bonferroni correction is used, a result is only declared to be statistically significant when its P value is less than $0.05/20 = 0.0025$. This ensures there is a 95% chance of seeing no statistically significant results among all 20 comparisons and only a 5% chance of seeing one (or more) statistically significant result.

The 5% significance level applies to the entire family of comparisons, rather than to each of the 20 individual comparisons.

Example of Bonferroni correction

Hunter and colleagues (1993) investigated whether vitamin supplementation could reduce the risk of breast cancer. The investigators sent dietary question-naires to over 100,000 nurses in 1980. From the questionnaires, they determined the participants' intake of vitamins A, C, and E, and divided the women into quintiles for each vitamin (i.e., the first quintile contains 20% of the women who consumed the smallest amount). They then followed these women for 8 years to determine the incidence rate of breast cancer. Using a test called the chi-square test for trend, the investigators calculated a P value to test the null hypothesis that there is no linear trend between vitamin-intake quintile and the incidence of breast cancer. There would be a linear trend if increasing vitamin intake was associated with increasing (or decreasing) incidence of breast cancer. There would not be a linear trend if (for example) the lowest and highest quintiles had a low incidence of breast cancer compared with the three middle quintiles. The authors determined a different P value for each vitamin. For vitamin C, $P = 0.60$; for vitamin E, $P = 0.07$; and, for vitamin A, $P = 0.001$.

Interpreting each P value is easy: If the null hypothesis is true, the P value is the chance that random selection of subjects would result in as large (or larger) a linear trend as was observed in this study. If the null hypothesis is true, there is a 5% chance of randomly selecting subjects such that the trend is statistically significant.

If no correction is made for multiple comparisons, there is a 14% chance of observing one or more significant P values, even if all three null hypotheses were true. The Bonferroni method sets a stricter significance threshold by dividing the significance level (0.05) by the number of comparisons (3), so a difference is declared statistically significant only when its P value is less than 0.050/3, or 0.0170. With this criterion, the relationship between vitamin A intake and the incidence of breast cancer is statistically significant, but the intakes of vitamins C and E are not significantly related to the incidence of breast cancer.

The terminology can be confusing. The significance level is still 5%, so α still equals 0.05. But now the significance level applies to the family of comparisons. The lower threshold (0.017) is used to decide whether each particular comparison is statistically significant, but α (now the familywise error rate) remains 0.05.

With the Bonferroni approach, it doesn't make sense to report individual P values. Because the whole point of multiple comparisons is to apply a family-wise significance level, it only makes sense to classify each comparison as being statistically significant or not. It does not make sense to ask about the individual P values.

Bonferroni method with a huge family of comparisons

The Bonferroni method is not very useful when you are analyzing a large number of comparisons at once. For example, suppose you are comparing gene expression between normal cells and cancer cells. Using gene chips, you are able to measure the expression of more than 10,000 genes. If you used the Bonferroni method and kept the traditional 5% definition of statistical significance, you'd only declare a change in gene expression significant when a P value is less than 0.05/10,000, or 0.000005. If none of the genes is differentially expressed, you will have only a 5% chance of finding any (one or more) differences that are statistically significant. But by making the threshold so strict, you will have very little power to detect any real differences. This approach is simply not practical. You can increase the value of α. But even if you increase it to 0.5, you'd still have little power.

An extension to the Bonferroni test, Holm's test, doesn't lose quite as much power, but has the same general problem. The next section explains an entirely different way of dealing with multiple comparisons that is especially useful with large families of comparisons.

CORRECTING FOR MULTIPLE COMPARISONS WITH THE FALSE DISCOVERY RATE

The false discovery rate (FDR) approach is an alternative approach to multiple comparisons that is especially useful when the number of simultaneous comparisons is large (Benjamini & Hochberg, 1995).

Lingo: FDR

First, some terminology. This approach does not use the term statistically significant, but instead uses the term "discovery." A finding is deemed to be a discovery when its P value is lower than a threshold.

A discovery is false when in fact the null hypothesis is true for that comparison. The False Discovery Rate (FDR) is the answer to these two equivalent questions:

> If a comparison is classified as a discovery, what is the chance that the null hypothesis is in fact true?

> What fraction of all the discoveries are expected to be false?

This definition actually defines the positive FDR, or pFDR, but the distinction between the pFDR and the FDR is subtle.

Controlling the FDR

When analyzing a set of P values, you can set the FDR to a desired value, abbreviated Q. If you set Q to 10%, then your goal is for 90% of the discoveries to be true and 10% to be false discoveries (where the null hypothesis is actually true). Of course, you can't know which are which.

A method developed by Benjamini and Hochberg (1995) sets the threshold values for deciding when a P value is low enough to be deemed a discovery. The method actually sets a different threshold value for each comparison. The threshold is tiny for the comparison with the smallest P value, and much larger for the largest P value. This makes sense. Imagine that you computed 100 P values, and all the null hypotheses were true. You'd expect the P values to be randomly distributed between 0.0 and 1.0. It would not be at all surprising for the smallest P value to equal 0.01. You'd expect that. But it would be surprising (if all null hypotheses were true) for the median P value to be 0.01. You'd expect that value to be about 0.5. So it makes perfect sense to rank the P values from low to high and use that rank when choosing the threshold that defines a discovery.

Here is a brief explanation of how those thresholds are determined. If all the null hypotheses are true, you'd expect the P values to be randomly scattered between 0 and 1. Half would be less than 0.50, 10% less than 0.10, etc. Let's imagine that you are making 100 comparisons and you have set Q (the desired FDR) to 5%. If all the null hypotheses were true, you'd expect that the smallest P value would be about 1/100, or 1%. Multiply that value by Q. So you declare the smallest P value to be a discovery if its P value is less than 0.0005. You'd expect the second smallest P value to be about 2/200, or 0.02. So you'd call that comparison a discovery if its P value is less than 0.0010. The threshold for the third smallest P value is 0.0015. And, finally, the discovery with the largest P value is called a discovery only if its value is less than 0.05. This description is a bit simplified, but gives the idea behind the method.

Other ways to use the FDR

The section above explained one approach: Choose a desired FDR and use that to decide which results count as a discovery. There is one FDR for the whole set of comparisons.

An alternative approach is to first decide on a threshold for defining "discovery". For example, in a gene-chip assay, you might choose the 5% of genes whose expression changed the most. Given that definition, you would then compute what the FDR must be. Again, there is one FDR for the entire set of comparisons.

A third alternative approach is to compute a FDR for each comparison. For each comparison, define "discovery" so that particular comparison just barely satisfies the definition. Using that definition, compute the overall FDR for all the comparisons. This value is called a q value. Repeat for each comparison. If you make 1,000 comparisons, you'll end up with 1,000 q values.

WHAT IS A FAMILY?

Both the traditional (Bonferroni) and the FDR approaches analyze a family of P values at once. But what is a family of comparisons? The answer is necessarily somewhat ambiguous. A family is a set of related comparisons. Usually, a family consists of the comparisons in one experiment or one major part of an experiment. When reading about results corrected for multiple comparisons, ask about how the investigators defined the family of comparisons.

THE BIG PICTURE

Coping with multiple comparisons is one of the biggest challenges in data analysis. If you calculate many P values, some are likely to be small just by random chance. It is easy to be fooled by these small P values.

This chapter explained three approaches to solve this problem. One approach is to analyze the data as usual, but to fully report the number of comparisons that were made, and then let the reader account for the number of comparisons. Another approach is to define the significance level to apply to the entire family of comparisons, rather than to each individual comparison. The third approach is to control or define the false discovery rate.

Looking ahead, Chapter 23 shows that the problem of multiple comparisons is pervasive, and Chapter 40 will explain special strategies for dealing with multiple comparisons after ANOVA.

CHAPTER 23

Multiple Comparison Traps

If the fishing expedition catches a boot, the fishermen should throw it back, and not claim that they were fishing for boots.

JAMES L. MILLS

Chapter 22 explained the problem of multiple comparisons. This chapter explains how pervasive this problem is. To interpret statistical analyses properly, you need to know how many comparisons were made. Thus, it is essential that all analyses be planned and that all planned analyses be conducted and reported. These simple guidelines are often violated.

ANALYZING DATA WITHOUT A PLAN

"Data torture" (Mills, 1993) occurs when investigators, without a clear plan, analyze their data in many ways, desperately seeking statistical significance.

Vickers (2006b) told this story:

STATISTICIAN: "Oh, so you have already calculated the P value?"
SURGEON: "Yes, I used multinomial logistic regression."
STATISTICIAN: "Really? How did you come up with that?"
SURGEON: "Well, I tried each analysis on the SPSS drop-down menus, and that was the one that gave the smallest P value."

Here is another example from the former Mayor of Washington, DC, Marion Barry:

If it weren't for the killings, Washington would have one of the lowest crime rates in the country.

Investigators have found many ways to wring statistical significance out of data: Change the definition of the outcome. Try different criteria for including or excluding a subject. Arbitrarily decide which points to remove as outliers. Try different ways to clump or separate subgroups. Try different algorithms for computing statistical tests. Try different statistical tests.

Fitting a multiple regression model (see Chapters 37 and 38) provides even more opportunities: Include or exclude possible confounding variables. Include

168

or exclude interactions. Change the definition of the outcome variable. Transform some of the variables.

If you try hard enough, eventually statistically significant findings will emerge from any reasonably complicated data set. Because the number of possible comparisons is not defined in advance and is almost unlimited, these results cannot be interpreted except perhaps as a method to generate hypotheses to be tested in future studies.

Does this kind of data abuse really happen? Chan, Hrobjartsson, Haahr, Gotzsche, and Altman (2004) showed that when studies have multiple outcomes, the outcomes with statistically significant improvement are far more likely to be reported than outcomes with no significant effect. Gotzsche (2006) used a clever approach to quantify this. He figured that if results were presented honestly, the number of P values between 0.04 and 0.05 would be about the same as the number of P values between 0.05 and 0.06. However, in 130 abstracts of papers published in 2003, he found five times more P values between 0.04 and 0.05 than between 0.05 and 0.06. He concluded that authors use tricks to push the marginal P values below 0.05. It is also possible that editors rejected the papers with the higher P values.

PUBLICATION BIAS

Editors prefer to publish papers that report results that are statistically significant. Interpreting published results becomes problematic when studies with not significant conclusions are abandoned, whereas the ones with statistically significant results get published. This means that the chance of observing a significant result in a published study can be much greater than 5% even if the null hypotheses are all true.

Turner, Matthews, Linardatos, Tell, and Rosenthal (2008) demonstrated this kind of selectivity—called *publication bias*—in industry-sponsored investigations of the efficacy of antidepressant drugs. Between 1987 and 2004, the FDA reviewed 74 such studies and categorized them as positive, negative, or questionable. The FDA reviewers found that 38 studies showed a positive result (the antidepressant worked). All but one of these studies was published. The FDA reviewers found that the remaining 36 studies had negative or questionable results. Of these, 22 were not published, 11 were published with a "spin" that made the results seem somewhat positive, and only 3 of the negative studies were published with clear negative findings.

Studies that show positive results are far more likely to be published than ones that reach negative or ambiguous conclusions. Selective publication makes it impossible to properly interpret the published literature.

MULTIPLE TIME POINTS—SEQUENTIAL ANALYSES

To properly interpret a P value, the experimental protocol must be set in advance. Usually this means choosing a sample size, collecting data, and then analyzing them.

But what if the results aren't quite statistically significant? The experimenter will be tempted to run the experiment a few more times (or add a few more subjects) and then analyze the data again, with the larger sample size. If the results still aren't significant, then do the experiment a few more times (or add more subjects) and reanalyze once again.

When data are analyzed in this way, it is impossible to interpret the results. This informal sequential approach should not be used.

If the null hypothesis of no difference is in fact true, the chance of obtaining a statistically significant result using that informal sequential approach is far higher than 5%. In fact, if you carry on that approach long enough, then every single experiment will eventually reach a significant conclusion, even if the null hypothesis is true. Of course, "long enough" might be very long indeed and exceed your budget or even your life span.

The problem is that the experiment continues when the result is not significant, but stops when the result is significant. If the experiment was continued after reaching significance, adding more data might then result in a not significant conclusion. But you'd never know this, because the experiment would have been terminated once significance was reached. If you keep running the experiment when you don't like the results but stop the experiment when you like the results, the results are impossible to interpret.

Statisticians have developed rigorous ways to handle sequential data analysis. These methods use much more stringent criteria to define significance to make up for the multiple comparisons. Without these special methods, you can't interpret the results unless the sample size is set in advance.

MULTIPLE SUBGROUPS

Analyzing multiple subgroups of data is a form of multiple comparisons. When a treatment works in some subgroups but not in others, analyses of subgroups becomes a form of multiple comparisons and it is easy to be fooled.

A simulated study by Lee (1980) and coworkers points out the problem. They pretended to compare survival following two "treatments" for coronary artery disease. They studied a group of real patients with coronary artery disease whom they randomly divided into two groups. In a real study, they would give the two groups different treatments and compare survival. In this simulated study, they treated the subjects identically but analyzed the data as if the two random groups actually represented two distinct treatments. As expected, the survival of the two groups was indistinguishable.

They then divided the patients into six groups depending on whether they had disease in one, two, or three coronary arteries and depending on whether the heart ventricle contracted normally. Because these are variables that are expected to affect survival of the patients, it made sense to evaluate the response to "treatment" separately in each of the six subgroups. Whereas they found no substantial difference in five of the subgroups, they found a striking result among the sickest patients. The patients with three-vessel disease who also had impaired ventric-ular contraction had much better survival under treatment B than treatment A. The difference between the two survival curves was statistically significant with a P value less than 0.025.

If this were an actual study, it would be tempting to conclude that treat-ment B is superior for the sickest patients, and to recommend treatment B to those patients in the future. But this was not a real study, and the two treatments reflected only random assignment of patients. The two treatments were identical, so the observed difference was absolutely, positively caused by chance.

It is not surprising that the authors found one low P value out of six compari-sons. Figure 22.1 shows that there is a 26% chance that one of six independent com-parisons will have a P value less than 0.05, even if all null hypotheses are true.

If all the subgroup comparisons are defined in advance, it is possible to correct for many comparisons—either as part of the analysis or informally while interpret-ing the results. But when this kind of subgroup analysis is not defined in advance, the results are impossible to interpret rigorously even if all the results are published and are misleading if only the statistically significant results are published.

COINCIDENCES

In 1991, President H. W. Bush and his wife, Barbara, both developed hyperthy-roidism caused by Graves' disease. Could it be a coincidence, or did something cause Graves' disease in both individuals? What is the chance that the President and his wife would both develop Graves' disease just by chance? It's hard to calculate that probability exactly, but it is less than 1 in a million. Because this would have been such a rare coincidence, there were extensive efforts to find a cause in the food, water, or air. No cause was ever found.

Was it really a 1 in a million coincidence? The problem with this "probabil-ity" is that the event had already happened before anyone thought to calculate the probability. A more appropriate question might be "What is the probability that a prominent person and his or her spouse would both develop the same disease this year?" But how prominent? Which diseases? Which time span?

Implicitly, many comparisons were made, so the coincidence no longer seems so strange. Because the question was prompted by the data, it really is impossible to calculate how rare (or common) the association is.

DISEASE CLUSTERS

Five children in a particular school developed leukemia last year. Is that a coinci-dence? Or does the clustering of cases suggest the presence of an environmental toxin that caused the disease? That's a very difficult question to answer (Thun & Sinks, 2004). It is tempting to estimate the answer to the question "What is the probability that five children in this particular school would all get leukemia this particular year?" You could calculate (or at least estimate) the answer to that question if you knew the overall incidence rates of leukemia among children and the number of children enrolled in the school. The answer will be tiny. Everyone intuitively knows that and so is alarmed by the cluster of cases.

But you've asked the wrong question once you've already observed the cluster of cases. The school only came to your attention because of the cluster of cases, so you must consider all other schools and other diseases. The right question is "What is the probability that five children in any school would develop the same severe disease in the same year?" This is a harder question to answer, because you must define the population of schools (this city or this state?), the time span you care about (1 year or 1 decade?), and the severity of diseases to include (does asthma count?). Clearly the answer to this question is much higher than the answer to the previous one.

About 1,000 cancer clusters are reported to U.S. health officials each year. About three quarters of these are not really clusters of similar kinds of cancers, but that leaves several hundred cancer clusters each year. These are fully investigated to look for known toxins and to be alert to other findings that might suggest a real problem. But virtually all disease clusters turn out to be simply a coincidence. It is surprising to find a cluster of one particular disease in one particular place at any one particular time. But chance alone will cause many clusters of various diseases in various places at various times.

MULTIPLE PREDICTIONS

In 2000, the Intergovernmental Panel on Climate Change made predictions about future climate. Pielke (2008) asked what seemed like a straightforward question: How accurate were those predictions over the next 7 years? That's not long enough to seriously assess predictions of global warming, but it is a necessary first step. Answering this question proved impossible (Tierney, 2008). The problems are that the report contained numerous predictions and didn't specify which sources of climate data should be used. Did the predictions come true? The answer depends on the choice of which prediction to test and which data set you test it against—"a feast for cherry pickers" (Pielke).

You can only evaluate the accuracy of a prediction or diagnosis when it is defined precisely, including the timing, methodology and data source. Otherwise, there are too many possible ways to assess the prediction, and you can get any answer you want.

COMBINING GROUPS

When comparing two groups, the groups must be defined as part of the study design. If the groups are defined by the data, many comparisons are being made implicitly and the results cannot be interpreted.

Austin and Goldwasser (2008) demonstrated this problem. They looked at the incidence of hospitalization for heart failure in Ontario, Canada, in 12 groups of patients defined by their astrological sign (based on their birthday). People born under the sign of Pisces happened to have the highest incidence of heart failure. They then did a simple statistics test to compare the incidence of heart failure among people born under Pisces with the incidence of heart failure among all others (born under all other 11 signs combined into one group). Taken at face value, this comparison showed that the difference in incidence rates is very unlikely to be the result of chance (the P value was 0.026). Pisces have a statistically significant higher incidence of heart failure than do people born under the other 11 signs.

The problem is that the investigators didn't test really one hypothesis; they tested 12. They only focused on Pisces after looking at the incidence of heart failure for people born under all 12 astrological signs. So it isn't fair to compare that one group against the others without considering the other 11 implicit comparisons. After correcting for those multiple comparisons, there was no significant association between astrological sign and heart failure.

MULTIPLE COMPARISONS IN MULTIPLE REGRESSION

Multiple regression (as well as logistic and proportional hazards regression) fit a model that predicts an outcome as a function of multiple independent (input) variables. Some programs offer automated methods to choose which independent variables are included, and which are omitted, from the model. Chapters 37 and 38 will discuss these techniques.

Freedman (1983) did simulations to show how these methods can lead to misleading results. His paper is reprinted within a text by Good and Hardin (2006). He simulated a study with 100 subjects, with data from 50 independent variables recorded from each subject. The simulations were performed so all the variation was random. The simulated outcome had no relationship at all to any of the simulated inputs. In other words, the data were all noise and no signal.

Multiple regression (Chapter 37) was used to find the equation that best predicted the outcome from all the inputs, and a P value was computed for each input variable. Each P values tested a null hypothesis that a particular input variable had no impact on predicting the outcome. The results were no surprise, with the P values randomly spread between 0 and 1. An overall P value, testing the null hypothesis that the overall model was not helpful in predicting the outcome, was high (0.53).

No surprises so far. Random variables went in, and a random assortment of P values came out. Anyone looking at the conclusion (and not knowing the data were randomly generated) would conclude that the 50 input variables have no ability to predict the outcome.

But wait, there's more!

He then selected the 15 input variables with the lowest P values (less than 0.25) and reran the multiple regression program using only those 15 input variables, rather than all 50 as before. Now the overall P value was tiny (0.0005). Of the 15 variables now in the model, 6 had an associated P value smaller than 0.05.

Anyone who saw only this analysis and didn't know the 15 input variables were selected from a larger group of 50 would conclude that the outcome variable is predicted reasonably well from the 15 input variables and that 6 input variables had a statistically significant ability to help predict the outcome. Because these are simulated data, it is clear that this conclusion would be wrong.

By including so many variables and selecting a subset that happened to be predictive, the investigators were performing multiple comparisons. Freedman (1983) knew this, and that is the entire point of this paper. But this kind of multiple comparison in variable selection happens often in analyzing large studies. When multiple regression analyses include lots of opportunity for variable selection, it is easy to be misled by the results.

OVERVIEW OF MULTIPLE COMPARISON TRAPS

Berry (2007, p 155) highlighted the importance and ubiquity of multiple comparisons:

> Most scientists are oblivious to the problems of multiplicities. Yet they are everywhere. In one or more of its forms, multiplicities are present in every statistical application. They may be out in the open or hidden. And even if they are out in the open, recognizing them is but the first step in a difficult process of inference. Problems of multiplicities are the most difficult that we statisticians face. They threaten the validity of every statistical conclusion.

CHAPTER 24

Gaussian or Not?

You need the subjunctive to explain statistics.
DAVID COLQUHOUN

Chapter 10 explained the origins and usefulness of the Gaussian distribution. This chapter explains how to test whether a data distribution is consistent with the assumption that the data were sampled from a Gaussian population.

THE GAUSSIAN DISTRIBUTION IS AN UNREACHABLE IDEAL

Many statistical tests (including t tests, ANOVA, and regression) assume that the data were sampled from a Gaussian distribution (Chapter 10). Is this assumption reasonable? This sounds like a simple question, but it really isn't.

In almost all cases, we can be 100% sure that the data were not sampled from an ideal Gaussian distribution. That is because an ideal Gaussian distribution includes some very low negative numbers and some superhigh positive values. Those values may comprise a tiny fraction of all the values in the population, but they are part of every ideal Gaussian distribution. In most scientific situations, there are constraints on the possible values. Blood pressures, concentrations, weights, and many other variables cannot have negative values, so cannot be sampled from perfect Gaussian distributions. Other variables can be negative, but have physical or physiological limits that don't allow super large values (or have extremely low negative values). These variables also cannot follow a perfect Gaussian distribution. Micceri (1989) looked at 440 different variables that psychologists measure and concluded that all deviated substantially from a Gaussian distribution. I suspect the same is true for most scientific fields.

Because almost no variables you measure follow an ideal Gaussian distribution, why use tests that rely on the Gaussian assumption? Plenty of studies with simulated data have shown that the statistical tests based on the Gaussian distribution are useful when data are sampled from a distribution that only approximates a Gaussian distribution. These tests are fairly robust to violations of the Gaussian assumption, especially if the sample sizes are equal. So the question that matters is not whether the data were sampled from an ideal Gaussian population, but rather whether the they were sampled from is close enough to Gaussian so that the results of the statistical tests are useful. Normality tests do not answer this question.

WHAT A GAUSSIAN DISTRIBUTION REALLY LOOKS LIKE

The ideal Gaussian frequency distribution was shown in Figure 10.1. With huge data sets, this is what you expect a Gaussian distribution to look like. But what about smaller data sets?

Figures 24.1 shows simulated data. Each of the eight frequency distributions shows the distribution of values randomly chosen from a Gaussian distribution. The top four distributions are four different samples with 12 values in each sample, and the bottom four graphs show samples with 130 values. Because of random sampling variation, none of these frequency distributions really looks completely bell shaped and symmetrical.

The bell-shape Gaussian distribution is an ideal distribution of the population. Unless the samples are huge, actual frequency distributions tend to be less symmetrical and more jagged. This is just the nature of random sampling.

Figure 24.2 makes the same point by showing individual values, rather than frequency distributions. Each sample was drawn from a Gaussian distribution. To many people, however, some of those distributions don't look Gaussian.

TESTING FOR NORMALITY

Statistical tests can be used to quantify how much a data set deviates from the expectations of a Gaussian distribution. Such tests are called *normality tests.*

The first step is to quantify how far a set of values differs from the predictions of a Gaussian distribution. One of the more popular normality tests is the *D'Agostino–Pearson omnibus K2 normality test.* It first computes two values that quantify how far the distribution deviates from the Gaussian ideal:

- Skewness quantifies symmetry. A distribution that is completely symmetrical has a skewness of 0. An ideal Gaussian distribution is symmetrical, so it would have a skewness of 0. When the distribution is asymmetric with the right tail heavier than the left tail, the skewness is positive. When the asymmetry goes the other way, with a heavy left tail, the skewness is negative.
- Kurtosis quantifies how peaked the distribution is. A Gaussian distribution is the ideal and has a kurtosis of 0.0. Distributions with a sharper peak and thinner tails have a positive kurtosis. Distributions with a rounded peak and wide shoulders have a negative kurtosis.

The D'Agostino–Pearson omnibus K2 normality test combines the skewness and kurtosis to a single value that describes how far a distribution is from Gaussian. Other normality tests (such as the Shapiro–Wilk test, the Kolmogorov–Smirnov

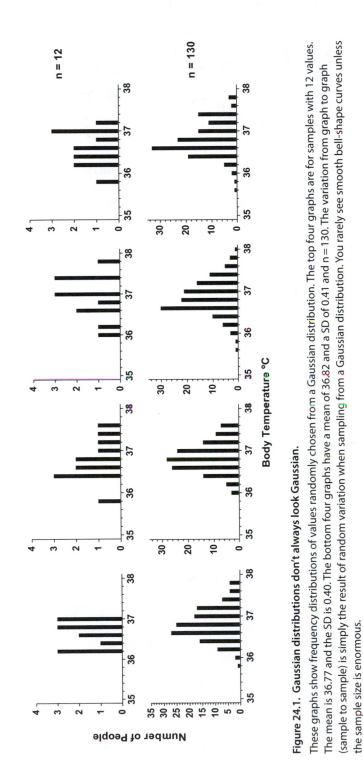

Figure 24.1. Gaussian distributions don't always look Gaussian.

These graphs show frequency distributions of values randomly chosen from a Gaussian distribution. The top four graphs are for samples with 12 values. The mean is 36.77 and the SD is 0.40. The bottom four graphs have a mean of 36.82 and a SD of 0.41 and n = 130. The variation from graph to graph (sample to sample) is simply the result of random variation when sampling from a Gaussian distribution. You rarely see smooth bell-shape curves unless the sample size is enormous.

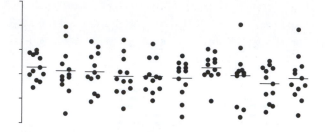

Figure 24.2. Samples from Gaussian distributions don't always look Gaussian.

All 10 samples were randomly sampled from Gaussian distributions. It is too easy to be fooled by random variation and think that the data are far from Gaussian.

test, and the Darling–Anderson test) use other approaches to quantify the discrepancy between the observed distribution and the Gaussian distribution.

INTERPRETING THE RESULTS OF A NORMALITY TEST

The meaning of a P value from a normality test

All normality tests then compute a P value that answers the following question:

> If you randomly sample from a Gaussian population, what is the probability of obtaining a sample that deviates from a Gaussian distribution as much (or more so) as this sample does?

High P value

If the P value from a normality test is large, all you can say is that the data are not inconsistent with a Gaussian distribution. Ugh! Statistics requires the use of double negatives.

A normality test cannot prove the data were sampled from a Gaussian distribution.

All the normality test can do is demonstrate that the deviation from the Gaussian ideal is not more than you'd expect to see with chance alone. With large data sets, this is reassuring. With smaller data sets, the normality tests don't have much power to detect modest deviations from the Gaussian ideal. How small is small? It depends on how far the distribution is from Gaussian.

Small P value

The null hypothesis is that the data are sampled from a Gaussian distribution. If the P value is small enough, you reject that null hypothesis and so accept the alternative hypothesis that the data are not sampled from a Gaussian population. If the data were sampled from a Gaussian distribution, it would be rare to find a sample that is as far from Gaussian as yours. With large data sets, a normality test can report a small P value even though the distribution only mildly deviates from a Gaussian distribution.

WHAT TO DO WHEN DATA FAIL
A NORMALITY TEST

If a normality test reports a small P value, you have several choices:

- The data may come from another identifiable distribution. If so, you may be able to transform your values to create a Gaussian distribution. Most commonly, if the data come from a lognormal distribution (Chapter 11), transform all values to their logarithms.
- The presence of one or a few outliers might be causing the normality test to fail. Run an outlier test (see Chapter 25).
- If the departure from normality is small, you may choose to do nothing. Statistical tests tend to be quite robust to mild violations of the Gaussian assumption.
- A final choice is to switch to nonparametric tests that don't assume a Gaussian distribution. Chapter 41 will explain the advantages and disadvantages of nonparametric tests.

Don't make the mistake of jumping directly to the fourth option, using a nonparametric test. It is very hard to decide when to use a statistical test based on a Gaussian distribution and when to use a nonparametric test. It really *is* difficult, requiring thinking and perspective and consistency.

This decision about how to handle data that fail a normality test should not be automated for these reasons:

- When analyzing a series of experiments, all should be analyzed the same way. Therefore, results from normality tests should not be used to choose a test for each particular experiment. Instead, your overall experience with a particular assay should dictate your choice of which statistical test to use for all experiments.
- In some cases, transforming the data (perhaps logarithms) can create a Gaussian distribution. In other cases, a single outlier (Chapter 25) may explain the low P value from a normality test.
- The decision of whether to use a parametric or nonparametric test is most important with small data sets (because the power of nonparametric tests is so low). But with small data sets, normality tests have little power. The concept of power was explained in Chapter 20.

Q & A: Normality Tests

Does it make sense to ask whether a particular data set is Gaussian?	No. A common misconception is to think that the normality test asks whether a particular set of data is Gaussian. But the term Gaussian
	refers to an entire population. In only makes sense to ask about the population your data were sampled from. Normality tests ask whether the data are consistent with the assumption of sampling from a Gaussian distribution.
Should a normality test be run as part of every experiment?	Not necessarily. You want to know whether a certain kind of data are consistent with sampling from a Gaussian distribution. The best way to find out is to run a special experiment just to ask about the distribution of data collected using a particular method. This experiment would need to generate plenty of data points, but would not have to make any comparisons or ask any scientific questions. If analysis of many data points convinces you that a particular experimental protocol generates data that are consistent with a Gaussian distribution, there is no point in testing smaller data sets from individual runs of that experiment.

CHAPTER 25

Outliers

There are liars, outliers, and out-and-out liars.
ROBERT DAWSON

A n outlier is a value that is so far from the others that it appears to have come from a different population. More informally, an outlier is a data point that is too extreme to fit your preconceptions. The presence of outliers can invalidate many statistical analyses. This chapter explains the challenges of identifying outliers.

HOW DO OUTLIERS ARISE?

Outliers—also called anomalous, spurious, rogue, wild, or contaminated observations—can occur for several reasons.

- Invalid data entry. The outlier may simply be the result of transposed digits or a shifted decimal point. If you suspect an outlier, the first thing to do is make sure the data were entered correctly and that any calculations (changing units, normalizing, etc.) were done accurately.
- Biological diversity. If each value comes from a different person or animal, the outlier may be a correct value. It is an outlier because that individual may truly be different from the others. This may be the most exciting finding in your data!
- Random chance. In any distribution, some values by chance are far from the others.
- Experimental mistakes. Most experiments have many steps, and it is possible that a mistake was made.
- Wrong assumption. If you assume data are sampled from a Gaussian distribution, you may conclude that a large value is an outlier. But if the distribution is, in fact, lognormal, then large values are common and are not outliers. See Chapter 11.

THE NEED FOR OUTLIER TESTS

The presence of an outlier can spoil many analyses, either creating the appearance of differences (associations, correlations…) or blocking discovery of real differences (etc.).

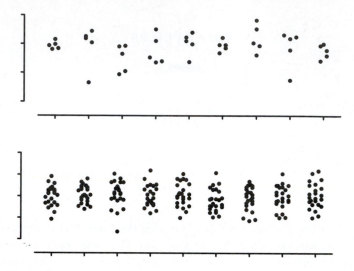

Figure 25.1. No outliers here.

All of these data sets were computer generated and sampled from a Gaussian distribution. But when you look at them, some points just seem too far from the rest to be part of the same distribution. They seem like real outliers, but are not. The human brain is too good at seeing patterns and exceptions from patterns, but is poor at recognizing random scatter.

It would seem that the presence of outliers would be obvious. If this were the case, outliers could be dealt with informally. But identifying outliers is harder than it seems.

Figure 25.1 shows the problem with attempting to identify outliers informally. It shows 18 data sets all sampled from a Gaussian distribution. Half of the samples have 5 values and half have 24. When you look at the graph, some points just seem to be too far from the rest. It seems obvious they are outliers. But in fact, all of these values were sampled from the same Gaussian distribution.

One problem with *ad hoc* removal of outliers is our tendency to see too many outliers. Another problem is that the experimenter is almost always biased. Even if you try to be fair and objective, your decision about which outliers to remove will probably be influenced by the results you want to see.

QUESTIONS TO ASK BEFORE USING
AN OUTLIER TEST

Before using an outlier test, ask yourself the following questions:

- Was there a mistake in data entry? If so, fix it. An outlier may simply be the result of transposed digits or a shifted decimal point.

- Is the outlier really a code for missing values? In some programs, one simply leaves a blank spot when a value is missing. With other programs, you might enter a value like 999. If you entered the wrong code for a missing value (or configured the program incorrectly), your analyses might give invalid results.
- Was a problem noticed during the experiment? Don't bother with outlier tests. Eliminate values if a problem with a value was noticed during the experiment.
- Could the extreme values be a result of biological variability? If so, this might be interesting. Don't even think about eliminating the extreme value without considering whether it could be real. You may have discovered a new polymorphism or mutation. You may have discovered that the disease you are studying is actually two distinct diseases.
- Is it possible the distribution is not Gaussian? If so, it may be possible to transform the values to make them Gaussian. Most outlier tests assume that the data (except the potential outliers) come from a Gaussian distribution.

OUTLIER TESTS

The question an outlier test answers

Having answered no to all the questions above, two possibilities remain:

- The extreme value came from the same distribution as the other values and just happened to be larger (or smaller) than the rest. In this case, the value should not be treated specially.
- The extreme value was the result of a mistake. This could be something like bad pipetting, voltage spike, or holes in filters. Or it could be a mistake in recording a value. These kinds of mistakes can happen, and are not always noticed during the collection of data. Because including an erroneous value in your analyses will give invalid results, you should remove it. In other words, the value comes from a different population than the other values and is misleading.

The problem, of course, is that you can never be sure which of these possibilities is correct. Mistake or chance? No mathematical calculation can tell you for sure whether the outlier came from the same, or a different, population than the others. An outlier test, however, can answer this question:

If the values really were all sampled from a Gaussian distribution, what is the chance that you would find one value as far from the others as you observed?

Interpreting a low P value

If this P value is small, then you will conclude that the outlier is not from the same distribution as the other values. Assuming you answered no to all five questions asked before using an outlier test, you have justification to exclude it from your analyses.

Interpreting a high P value

If the P value is high, you have no evidence that the extreme value came from a different distribution than the rest. This does not prove that the value in fact came from the same distribution as the others. All you can say is that there is no strong evidence that the value came from a different distribution.

How do outlier tests work?

Statisticians have devised several methods for detecting outliers. All of the methods first quantify how far the outlier is from the other values. This can be the difference between the extreme value and the mean of all values, the difference between the extreme value and the mean of the remaining values, or the difference between the extreme value and the next closest value. Next, this value is normalized by dividing by some measure of variability, such as the SD of all values, the SD of the remaining values, the distance to the closest value, or the range of the data. Finally, this ratio is compared with a table of critical values. If the ratio is too high, then the value is a statistically significant outlier. If all the values were really sampled from a Gaussian population, the chance of randomly finding a value that far from the other values is less than 5% (or whatever significance level you choose).

Detecting multiple outliers is much harder than identifying a single outlier. The presence of the second outlier can mask the first one, so neither is identified.

BEWARE OF LOGNORMAL DISTRIBUTIONS

Most outlier tests are based on the assumption that the data, except the potential outlier(s), are sampled from a Gaussian distribution. The results are misleading if the data were sampled from some other distribution.

Figure 25.2 shows that lognormal distributions can be especially misleading. These simulated values were all generated from a lognormal distribution. An outlier test, based on the assumption that most of the values were sampled from a Gaussian distribution, identified an outlier in three of the four data sets. But these values are not outliers. Extremely large values are common in a lognormal distribution.

If you don't realize that the data came from a lognormal distribution, an outlier test would be very misleading. Excluding these high values as outliers would be a mistake and lead to incorrect results. If you recognize that the data are lognormal, it is easy to analyze the data properly. Transform all the values to their logarithms (Figure 25.2, right) and the apparent outliers are gone.

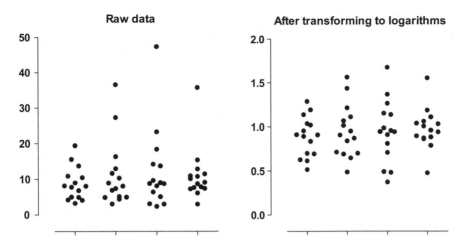

Figure 25.2. No outliers here.

(Left) The four data sets were randomly sampled by computer from a lognormal distribution. Grubbs's outlier test found a significant (P < 0.05) outlier in three of the four data sets. (Right) Graph of the same values after being transformed to their logarithms. No outliers were found. Most outlier tests are simply inappropriate when values are not sampled from a Gaussian distribution.

Q & A: Outliers

Is it legitimate to remove outliers?

Some people feel that removing outliers is "cheating." It can be viewed that way when outliers are removed in an *ad hoc* manner, especially when you remove only outliers that get in the way of obtaining results you like. But leaving outliers in the data you analyze is also cheating, because it can lead to invalid results.

It is not cheating when the decision of whether to remove an outlier is based on rules and methods established before the data were collected and these rules (and the number of outliers removed) are reported when the data are published.

When your experiment has a value flagged as an outlier, there are two possibilities. One possibility is that a coincidence occurred, the kind of coincidence that happens in 5% (or whatever level you pick) of experiments even if the entire scatter is Gaussian. The other possibility is that a "bad" point got included in your data.

Continued

	Which possibility is more likely? It depends on your experimental system. • If your experimental system generates one or more bad points in a few percent of experiments, eliminate the value as an outlier. It is more likely to be the result of an experimental mistake than to come from the same distribution as the other points. • If your system is very pure and controlled so bad values almost never occur, keep the value. It is more likely that the value comes from the same distribution as the other values than it is that it represents an experimental mistake.
What does it mean to remove or eliminate an outlier?	When an outlier is eliminated, the analyses are performed as if that value were never collected. If the outliers are graphed, they are clearly marked. Removing an outlier from an analysis does not mean the outlier should be erased from the lab notebook. Instead, the value of the outlier and the reason it was excluded should be recorded.
Can outlier tests be used with linear or nonlinear regression?	Yes. In fact, I published a method for doing so (Motulsky & Brown, 2006).
How should outlier removal be reported?	A scientific paper should state how many values were removed as outliers, the criteria used to identify the outliers, and whether those criteria were chosen as part of the experimental design. It can also make sense to report the results computed in two ways, with the outliers included and excluded.
Can reasonable scientists disagree about how to deal with outliers?	Yes!

ROBUST STATISTICS

Rather than eliminate outliers, an alternative strategy is to use statistical methods that are designed so outliers have little effect on the result. Methods of data analysis that are not much affected by the presence of outliers are called *robust*. You don't need to decide when to eliminate an outlier, because the method is designed to accommodate them. Outliers just automatically fade away.

The simplest robust statistic is the median. If one value is very high or very low, the value of the median won't change, whereas the value of the mean will change a lot. The median is robust; the mean is not.

To learn more about robust statistics, start with the book by Huber (2003).

N	CRITICAL G	N	CRITICAL G
3	1.15	27	2.86
4	1.48	28	2.88
5	1.71	29	2.89
6	1.89	30	2.91
7	2.02	31	2.92
8	2.13	32	2.94
9	2.21	33	2.95
10	2.29	34	2.97
11	2.34	35	2.98
12	2.41	36	2.99
13	2.46	37	3.00
14	2.51	38	3.01
15	2.55	39	3.03
16	2.59	40	3.04
17	2.62	50	3.13
18	2.65	60	3.20
19	2.68	70	3.26
20	2.71	80	3.31
21	2.73	90	3.35
22	2.76	100	3.38
23	2.78	110	3.42
24	2.80	120	3.44
25	2.82	130	3.47
26	2.84	140	3.49

Table 25.1. Critical values for Grubbs's outlier test ($\alpha = 0.05$).

HOW IT WORKS: GRUBBS'S OUTLIER TEST

Grubbs's method for assessing outliers is particularly easy to understand. This method is also called the *extreme studentized deviate* (ESD). It questions whether the most extreme value in a set of values is a significant outlier. It cannot detect more than one value.

1. Compute the mean and standard deviation of all values, including the suspected outlier.
2. Calculate the difference between each value and the mean and divide that difference by the standard deviation. Call the absolute value of this ratio G (not a standard abbreviation).
3. Find the largest value of G.
4. If the computed value of G is greater than the critical value from Table 25.1 (for the number of observations in your data set), then conclude that the extreme value is a significant outlier ($P < 0.05$).

Because 5% of the values in a Gaussian population are more than 1.96 SDs from the mean, your first thought might be to conclude that the outlier comes from a different population if G is greater than 1.96. But because any outlier would also increase the value of SD and so decrease the value of G, that rule doesn't work. With small samples, G can never get as high as 1.96. Consider a data set with these values: 1, 2, 3, 4, 999999. That last value is clearly an outlier, but G only equals 1.79.

For the example in the previous paragraph, n = 5, so the critical value of G is 1.71. The calculated value of G is higher (1.79), so the largest value (999999) is a significant outlier.

PART F

Statistical Tests

CHAPTER 26

Comparing Observed and Expected Distributions

It is a capital mistake to theorize before one has data.
Insensibly one begins to twist facts to suit theories, instead of
theories to fit facts.

SHERLOCK HOLMES

The chi-square test compares a discrete distribution of results to a distribution predicted by theory.

DO DATA FOLLOW AN EXPECTED DISTRIBUTION?

Kales and colleagues (2007) investigated why heart disease is the most frequent cause of on-duty death among firefighters. They wanted to find out whether those deaths resulting from heart disease primarily occurred while the firefighters actually fought fires.

For each death resulting from heart disease, they determined what duty the firefighter was performing at the time, as tabulated in the left column of Table 26.1 (which I simplified a bit from the original publication). About a third of those deaths happened while the firefighters were actively suppressing fires.

The null hypothesis is that deaths occur randomly throughout the work week and are not related to activity. The investigators compared the actual distribution of time of death with the prediction of that null hypothesis.

DUTY	NO. OBSERVED	NO. EXPECTED	% EXPECTED
Fire suppression	144	9.0	2.0
Alarm response and return	138	71.8	16.0
Physical training	56	35.9	8.0
Other duties	111	332.3	74.0
Total	449	449.0	100

Table 26.1. **Deaths resulting from coronary heart disease among firefighters.**
From Kale (2007). To simplify, I use only the data for municipal fire departments and pooled several categories to reduce the number of rows. The number of deaths that occurred while actually suppressing fires vastly exceeds the number expected (based on allocation of time).

In this example, there is no theory about the expected distribution. Instead, the investigators used data about how firefighters spend their time. For example, about 2% of a firefighter's time is spent suppressing fires. Under the null hypothesis, therefore, the number of deaths expected while fighting fires would be 2% of the total number of deaths (449), or 9. In fact, there were 144 coronary deaths while fighting fires. Table 26.1 compares the actual and predicted distributions. The discrepancy between the observed and expected distribution seems huge. The chi-square goodness-of-fit test does the calculations.

THE CHI-SQUARE GOODNESS-OF-FIT TEST

The chi-square test compares the observed and expected numbers of subjects in each category.

The observed values must be the actual numbers of subjects in each category. Don't try to run the chi-square test with percentages or any kind of normalized value. Each observed value must be a positive integer.

The expected values are the number of subjects you expect to see in each category. These values do not need to be integers. Each expected value is the average number you'd expect in that category if the experiment were repeated many times. In any one experiment, the observed value must be an integer. But the expected value, averaged over many experiments, can be a fraction.

The sum of all the observed values must equal the sum of all the expected values.

In this example, the categories have no intrinsic order. In other cases, the categories might be ordered.

The test is based on some approximations, which are only reasonably accurate when all the expected values are fairly large. If any expected value is less than 5, the results are dubious. This matters less when there are lots of categories (rows) and matters the most when there are only two categories (in which case the expected values should be 10 or higher).

The chi-square test combines the discrepancies between observed and expected counts to calculate a P value answering the following question:

> If the null hypothesis was true, what is the chance of randomly selecting subjects with this large a discrepancy between observed and expected distribution?

For the example, the P value is tiny, less than 0.0001. The data significantly depart from the predictions of the null hypothesis. Some factor beyond chance must account for the large number of coronary deaths while the firefighters actually fight fires.

If the P value is large, that means the observed distribution does not deviate from the theoretical distribution by more than you'd expect by random chance. This does not prove that the theory is correct, only that the deviations from that theory are small and consistent with random variation.

PHENOTYPE	OBSERVED NUMBER OF SEEDS IN THIS EXPERIMENT	EXPECTED PROPORTION	EXPECTED NUMBER IN THIS EXPERIMENT
Round and yellow	315	9/16	312.75
Round and green	108	3/16	104.25
Angular and yellow	101	3/16	104.25
Angular and green	32	1/16	34.75
Total	556	16/16	556.00

Table 26.2. Mendel's peas.
This shows one of Mendel's experiments (adapted from Cramer, 1999). The first column shows the actual distribution of traits in the seeds he collected. The last column shows the distribution expected by genetic theory.

CHI-SQUARE AND MENDELIAN GENETICS

Mendel pioneered the field of genetics. The chi-square test (developed after he died) can be used to compare actual data with the predictions of Mendel's model. Table 26.2 shows one of his experiments (from Cramer, 1999). In one of Mendel's experiments, he looked simultaneously at whether peas were round or angular and whether they were yellow or green. The yellow and round traits were dominant. Table 26.2 shows the expected proportions of the four phenotypes and the expected number in an experiment with 556 peas. These expected numbers are not integers, but that is OK because these are the average expectations if you did many experiments.

A chi-square test can compare the observed distribution with the expected distribution and compute a P value that answers the following question:

> If the theory that generated the expected distribution is correct, what is the chance that random sampling would lead to a deviation from expected as large or larger as observed in this experiment?

The P value is 0.93 (computed from a chi-square value of 0.470 with 3 df). With such a high P value, there is no reason to doubt that the data follow the expected distribution. (Many of Mendel's P values were high, which makes some wonder whether the data were fudged, as briefly discussed in Chapter 19.)

HOW IT WORKS: CHI-SQUARE GOODNESS-OF-FIT TEST

The observed and expected counts are combined into a single value as follows:

1. For each category, compute the difference between the observed and expected values. Square that difference. Divide that square by the expected value.
2. Add up the result of Step 1 for all categories. The result is a chi-square value, pronounced kī (rhymes with eye) square. For the firefighter example, $\chi^2 = 2245$. For the Mendel example, $\chi^2 = 0.470$.

3.   Define the number of df to equal the number of categories minus 1. Both examples have four categories and so have 3 df. This makes sense. Once you know the total number of firefighters and the number who died in three of the categories, you automatically know the number who died in the fourth category. Once you know the total number of peas and the number in three of the phenotype categories, you can figure out the number of peas in the remaining category.

4.   If the null hypothesis is true, the distribution of χ^2 (for a specified number of df) is known. Use a program or table to find (or approximate) the P value that corresponds to the calculated value of chi square and df.

Here it is as an equation:

$$\chi^2 = \sum \frac{(\text{Observed} - \text{Expected})^2}{\text{Expected}}$$

DON'T CONFUSE TWO DISTINCT CHI-SQUARE TESTS

The chi-square test is used in two distinct ways, and it is easy to mix them up.

This chapter explains how the chi-square test compares an observed distribution with one group of subjects with an expected distribution. For each category or outcome, you must enter both an observed and an expected count. The expected counts must come from theory or external data, and cannot be derived from the data being analyzed. In the example, the expected values were computed by calculating the total number of deaths times the fraction of the time firefighters (on average) spend doing various tasks. The chi-square test compares the observed and expected distributions.

Chapters 27 and 28 explain uses of the chi-square test of independence, which is used to analyze a contingency table. You enter data into the contingency table, which tabulates the number of subjects given (or exposed to) various treatments with alternative outcomes. A contingency table requires two or more alternative treatments or exposures, as well as two or more alternative outcomes. Table 26.1 is not a contingency table, because it shows various outcomes for one group of subjects.

Both tests are based on the same chi-square distribution, but the computations are done somewhat differently. When you analyze a contingency table, the expected values are computed from the experimental data and not from theory.

BINOMIAL TEST

The chi-square test described above is an approximation. When there are only two categories, the *binomial test* computes the exact P value, without any approximation or worry about sample size.

The coin-flipping example of Chapter 15 used the binomial test. To compute the binomial test, you must enter the number of observations, the fraction that had one of the two outcomes, and the fraction expected (under the null hypothesis) of having that outcome. In the coin-flipping example, the expected proportion was 50%, but this is not always the case.

CHAPTER 27

Comparing Proportions: Prospective and Experimental Studies

No one believes an hypothesis except its originator, but everyone believes an experiment except the experimenter.
W. I. B. BEVERIDGE

*This chapter and the next one explain how to interpret results that
compare two proportions. This chapter explains analyses of cross-
sectional, prospective, and experimental studies where the results are
summarized as the difference or ratio of two incidence or prevalence
rates.*

LINGO: CROSS-SECTIONAL, PROSPECTIVE, EXPERIMENTAL, AND RETROSPECTIVE STUDIES

This chapter and the next show how to answer a simple question. Does exposure to a risk factor cause disease? Before answering this question, you first must learn some terminology.

Incidence is the rate of new cases of disease.

Prevalence is the fraction of the group that has the disease.

In a *cross-sectional study*, the investigator selects a single sample of subjects, without regard to either the disease or the risk factor. The subjects are then divided into two groups based on previous exposure to the risk factor. The investigators then compare the prevalence of the disease in the two groups.

In a *prospective* study, also called a *longitudinal* study, the investigators select two groups of subjects. One group has been exposed to a possible risk factor. The other group hasn't. The investigator then waits while the natural history of the disease progresses and compares the incidence rates in the two groups.

In an *experimental* study, the investigator selects a single sample of subjects, which are randomly divided into two groups. Each of the groups gets a different treatment (or no treatment) and the investigators compare the incidence of the disease. The example in this chapter is an experimental study.

In a *case–control* study, the investigators select two groups of subjects. One group has the disease or condition being studied. These are the cases. The other

	DISEASE	NO DISEASE	TOTAL
Exposed or treated	A	B	A+B
Not exposed or placebo	C	D	C+D
Total	A+C	B+D	A+B+C+D

Table 27.1. Generic contingency table.
Each of the four values (A, B, C, and D) must be the actual count of number of subjects. Contingency tables must show the actual number of subjects rather than percentages, rates, averages, etc.

group is selected to be similar in many ways, but not to have the condition. These are the controls. The investigators then look back in time to compare the exposure of the two groups to a possible risk factor. Chapter 28 explains how to interpret data from case–control studies.

CONTINGENCY TABLES

The data from all four of these studies can be presented on a *contingency table*, as shown in Table 27.1. These tables show how the outcome is contingent on the treatment or exposure.

The rows represent exposure (or lack of exposure) to alternative treatments or possible risk factors. Each subject belongs to one row based on exposure or treatment. Columns denote alternative outcomes. Each subject belongs to one column based on outcome. Therefore, each "cell" in the table (the variables A, B, C, and D) is the number of subjects that were in one particular exposure (or treatment) group and had one particular outcome.

Not all tables are contingency tables. Contingency tables always show the actual number of subjects (or some other experimental unit) in various categories. Thus, each number must be a nonnegative integer. Tables of fractions, proportions, percentages, averages, changes, or durations are not contingency tables. Nor are tables of rates, such as number of cases per 1,000 population. Table 26.1, which compares observed and expected counts, is not a contingency table.

Applying methods appropriate for contingency tables to other kinds of data will generate meaningless results.

EXAMPLE OF AN EXPERIMENTAL STUDY: A CLINICAL TRIAL

Cooper et al. (1993) studied the effectiveness of zidovudine (also known as AZT) in treating asymptomatic people infected with human immunodeficiency virus (HIV). AZT benefits patients with the acquired immunodeficiency syndrome (AIDS) or asymptomatic patients infected with HIV who have low numbers of T-helper (CD4⁺) cells. Patients can be infected with HIV for many years before

TREATMENT	DISEASE PROGRESSED	NO PROGRESSION	TOTAL
AZT	76	399	475
Placebo	129	332	461
Total	205	731	936

Table 27.2. Results of the Cooper AZT study.

they develop any symptoms of AIDS and before their CD4$^+$ cells counts drop. Does AZT help these HIV$^+$ patients?

The investigators selected adults who were infected with HIV but had no symptoms and randomly assigned them to receive AZT or placebo. The subjects were followed for 3 years. The authors analyzed the data in several ways and looked at several outcomes. We'll just look at one outcome—whether the disease progressed in 3 years, yes or no. The authors defined disease progression to be when a patient developed symptoms of AIDS or when the number of CD4$^+$ cells dropped substantially. They questioned whether treatment with AZT reduces progression of the disease.

The investigators measured other outcomes and analyzed these results too. They also looked at drug-induced side effects. Before you reach an overall conclusion from this study, you must look at all the data. Although statistical tests focus on one result at a time, you must integrate various results before reaching an overall conclusion.

This study is called a randomized, double-blind prospective study.

It is a *randomized* study because the assignment of subjects to receive AZT or placebo was determined randomly. Patients or physicians could not request one treatment or the other.

It is *double blind* because neither patient nor investigator knew who was getting AZT and who was getting placebo. This is sometimes called a *double-masked* study. Until the study was complete, the information about which patient got which drug was coded, and the code was not available to any of the participating subjects or investigators (except in a medical emergency).

It is *prospective* because the subjects were followed forward over time. Chapter 28 explains retrospective case–control studies, which look back in time.

The results are shown in Table 27.2. The disease progressed in 28% of the patients receiving placebo (129/461) and in only 16% of the patients receiving AZT (76/475).

The goal is to generalize about the general population of patients infected with HIV. You already know one way to make inferences from the data by calculating the 95% CI for each of the two proportions using the methods introduced in Chapter 4. Disease progressed in 16% of the patients receiving AZT, and the 95% CI ranges from 13 to 20%. Disease progressed in 28% of the subjects receiving placebo, and the 95% CI ranges from 24 and 32%.

THE ATTRIBUTABLE RISK

One way to summarize the results is to calculate the difference between the two proportions. Disease progressed in 28% of placebo-treated subjects and in 16% of AZT-treated subjects. In our sample, the difference is 28–16%, or 12%. This difference between two incidence rates is called *attributable risk*.

The 95% CI of the difference ranges from 6.7 to 17.3%. These calculations are done by many computer programs, so are not detailed in this book. If we assume our subjects are representative of the larger population of adults infected with HIV but not yet symptomatic, we are 95% confident that treatment with AZT will reduce the incidence of disease progression by somewhere between 6.7 and 17.3%. Note that these calculations deal with the actual difference in incidence rates (subtraction), not the relative change (division).

NUMBER NEEDED TO TREAT (NNT)

Laupacis and colleagues (1988) have suggested reporting the reciprocal of the difference and term the reciprocal the *number needed to treat* (NNT). This value tells you how many patients would require treatment with a form of medication to reduce the expected number of cases of a defined endpoint by 1. In this example, the reciprocal of 0.12 is 8.3. For every eight patients who receive the treatment, you'd expect disease progression to be prevented in one. The CI of the NNT is obtained by taking the reciprocal of each end of the CI of the attributable risk, so it extends from 5.7 to 14.9. In other words, you'd expect somewhere between 1 of 6 to 1 of 15 patients to benefit from the treatment. Of course, you don't know before treating a patient whether he or she will benefit.

There are two advantages to reporting results as the NNT. One advantage is that it avoids the need to think about small fractions. The other advantage is that it puts the results in a clinically relevant context.

When the treatment or exposure causes harm, the term NNT doesn't fit, so this value is renamed the *number needed to harm*.

THE RELATIVE RISK

It is often more intuitive to think of the ratio of two proportions rather than the difference. This ratio is termed the *relative risk*. Disease progressed in 28% of placebo-treated subjects and in 16% of AZT-treated subjects. The ratio is 16/28%, or 0.57. In other words, subjects treated with AZT were 57% as likely as placebo-treated subjects to have disease progression. A relative risk between 0.0 and 1.0 means that the risk decreases with treatment (or exposure to risk factor). A relative risk greater than 1.0 means that the risk increases. A relative risk = 1.0 means that the risk is identical in the two groups.

We could also have calculated the ratio the other way, as 28/16%, which is 1.75. This means that subjects receiving the placebo were 1.75 times more likely to have disease progression than subjects receiving AZT. When interpreting relative risks, make sure you know which group has the higher risk.

The 95% CI of the relative risk extends from 0.44 to 0.74. These calculations are done by many computer programs, so they are not explained here. The interpretation is now familiar. If we assume our subjects are representative of the larger population of adults infected with HIV but not yet symptomatic, we are 95% sure that treatment with AZT will reduce the relative incidence of disease progression by somewhere between 44 and 74%.

Don't get confused by the two uses of percentages. When computing the difference between proportions, the percentages are percentage of subjects. When computing a relative risk, the percentages quantify a relative change.

In this example, the term *risk* is appropriate because it refers to disease progression. In other contexts, one alternative outcome may not be worse than the other, and the *relative risk* is more appropriately termed the *relative probability* or *relative rate*.

RELATIVE RISK OR DIFFERENCE
BETWEEN PROPORTIONS?

The relative risk and the difference between proportions both summarize the data as one value. Chapter 28 will explain a third summary value: the odds ratio. But any simplification can also be misleading, because one number is not really sufficient to summarize the data.

Consider a vaccine that halves the risk of a particular infection. In other words, the vaccinated subjects have a relative risk of 0.5 of getting that infection compared with unvaccinated subjects. How important are these results? The answer depends on the prevalence of the disease that the vaccine prevents. If the risk in unexposed people is 2 in 10 million, then halving the risk to 1 in 10 million isn't so important. If the risk in unexposed people is 20%, then halving the risk to 10% would have immense public health consequences. The relative risk alone does not differentiate between the two cases.

Expressing the data as the difference in risks (rather than the ratio) is more helpful in this example. In the first example, the difference is 0.0000001; in the second case it is 0.1. The NNT is the reciprocal of the difference. In our example, NNT = 10,000,000 for the first example and 10 in the second. In other words, to prevent 1 case of disease you have to vaccinate 10 million people in the first case and only 10 people in the second.

CALCULATING A P VALUE

The CIs can be (but don't need to be) supplemented with a P value. All P values start with a null hypothesis, which in this case is that AZT does not alter the probability of disease progression. The P value answers the following question:

> If the null hypothesis was true, what is the chance that random sampling of subjects would result in incidence rates as different (or more so) from what we observed?

The P value depends on sample size and on how far the relative risk is from 1.0. Computer programs can compute the P value, and this book will not explain the calculations. The best test to use is *Fisher's exact test*. With large sample sizes (larger than used here), Fisher's test is mathematically unwieldy, so a *chi-square test* is used instead.

The P value (calculated with either test) is tiny, less than 0.0001. Interpreting the P value is straightforward: If the null hypothesis is true, there is less than a 0.01% chance of randomly picking subjects with such a large (or larger) difference in incidence rates.

ASSUMPTIONS

Interpreting the results of a prospective or experimental study depends on the following assumptions:

Assumption: Random (or representative) sample

The 95% CI is based on the assumption that your sample was randomly selected from the population. In many cases, this assumption is not true. You can still interpret the CI as long as you assume that your sample is representative of the population.

The patients in the example were certainly not randomly selected, but it is reasonable to think that they are representative of adult asymptomatic people infected with HIV.

Beware of the two uses of the term *random*. Each subject was randomly assigned to receive drug or placebo. However, the subjects in the study were not randomly selected from the population of all people with asymptomatic HIV infection.

Assumption: Independent observations

The 95% CI is only valid when all subjects are sampled from the same population and each has been selected independently of the others. Selecting one member of the population should not change the chance of selecting anyone else.

This assumption would be violated if the study included several people from one family or clusters of individuals who are likely to have the same strain of HIV.

Assumption: Accurate data

The 95% CI is only valid when the number of subjects in each category is tabulated correctly. This assumption would be violated in our first example if one of the patients had taken a different drug or if one of the "drug side effects" was actually caused by something else. The assumption would be violated in the election example if the pollster recorded some of the opinions incorrectly.

Assumption: Assessing an event you really care about

The 95% CI allows you to extrapolate from the sample to the population for the event that you tabulated. But sometimes you really care about a different event.

This study can tell you about disease progression as defined by symptoms and CD4$^+$ cell counts. It cannot tell you about the variable you really care about. What you really want to know is whether the drugs will reduce suffering and prolong life. It's easy to forget this point and to generalize results too far.

Assumption: No difference between the two groups except treatment

In this study, subjects were randomly assigned to receive drug or placebo, so there is no reason to think that the two groups differ. But it is possible that, just by chance, the two groups differ in important ways. The authors presented data showing that the two groups were indistinguishable in terms of age, T-cell counts, sex, and HIV risk factors.

Q & A: Comparing Proportions

How is the chi-square test mentioned in this chapter related to the chi-square mentioned in Chapter 26?	The chi-square test in Chapter 26 compares an observed distribution with a distribution expected by theory. The chi-square test mentioned here compares the observed distribution of a contingency table with an expected distribution that is computed right from the data assuming the null hypothesis.
What if there are more than three groups or more than three outcomes?	The chi-square test can handle more than two rows or columns. It won't be possible to compute an attributable or relative risk, but it is possible to compute a P value.
If there are more than three rows or columns, does it matter in what order they are placed?	The usual chi-square test pays no attention to the order of rows or columns. If your table has two columns and three or more rows where the order matters (for example, doses or ages), *the chi-square test for trend* questions whether there is a significant trend between row number and the distribution of the outcomes.
What is Yates's correction?	When you use a program to analyze contingency tables, you might be asked about Yates's correction. The chi-square test used to analyze a contingency table can be computed in two ways. Yates's correction increases the resulting P value to adjust for a bias in the usual chi-square test, but it overcorrects. With small samples, Fisher's test is better and avoids the need to think about Yates's correction. With large samples, the Yates's correction makes very little difference.
Are special analyses available for paired data where each subject is measured before and after an intervention?	Yes. McNemar's test is explained in Chapter 31.

CHAPTER 28

Comparing Proportions: Case–Control Studies

It is now proven beyond doubt that smoking is one of the leading causes of statistics.

FLETCHER KNEBEL

*T*his chapter explains how to interpret results from a case–control study (also called retrospective studies). In these studies, the investigators select two groups of subjects: cases with the disease or condition being studied and controls selected to be similar in many ways, but not to have the condition. The investigators then look back in time to compare the exposure of the two groups to a possible risk factor (or treatment).

EXAMPLE: DOES A CHOLERA VACCINE WORK?

Cholera kills many people in Africa. Although vaccines were not very effective against cholera in the past, newer vaccines hold great promise for preventing this awful disease.

Lucas and coauthors (2005) investigated whether a cholera vaccine was effective. An ideal approach would be to recruit people who are vaccinated and those who are not and follow both groups for many years to compare the incidence of cholera. Such a study would take many years to conduct, would require a huge number of subjects, and would require withholding vaccine from many. Instead, the investigators performed a case–control study to compare whether people with cholera are less likely to have been vaccinated than those who did not get cholera.

This kind of study is called a *case–control study* because the investigators pick cases and controls to study. It is also called a retrospective study, because the investigators start with the disease and look back in time to try to learn about the cause.

Table 28.1 shows the results. Note the difference between this contingency table and the one from the example in Chapter 27 (AZT). In the AZT example, the investigators set the row totals by choosing how many subjects got each treatment

	CASES (CHOLERA)	CONTROLS
Received vaccine	10	94
No vaccine	33	78
Total	43	172

Table 28.1. Case–control study to investigate association of cholera with lack of vaccination.

From Lucas et al. (2005).

and observed the outcome tabulated in the two columns. In this example, the investigators set the column totals by choosing how many cases and controls to study and then determined whether each group had been vaccinated.

COMPUTING THE RELATIVE RISK FROM CASE–CONTROL DATA IS MEANINGLESS

Don't try to calculate the relative risk from a case–control study. It would be a mistake to look at Table 28.1 and divide 10 (number of people with cholera who were vaccinated) by 104 (the total number of vaccinated people in the study) to calculate "there is a 10% risk that vaccinated people get cholera." This is not a helpful calculation or a true statement. The authors chose to have four times as many controls as cases. If they had chosen to use only twice as many controls as cases, that same calculation would have divided 10 into 52 and concluded that "there is a 20% risk that vaccinated people get cholera." Computing a relative risk directly from a case–control study is invalid.

THE ODDS RATIO

Case–control studies are best summarized with the odds ratio.

Probabilities Versus Odds

Chance can be expressed either as a probability or as odds. In most contexts, there is no particular advantage to thinking about odds rather than probabilities. Most scientists (except maybe those who spend too much time at the race track) tend to feel more comfortable thinking about probabilities than odds.

- The *probability* that an event will occur is the fraction of times you expect to see that event in many trials.
- The *odds* are defined as the probability that the event will occur divided by the probability that the event will not occur.

Probabilities always range between 0 and 1. Odds may be any positive number (or zero). A probability of 0 is the same as odds of 0. A probability of 0.5 is the same as odds of 1.0. The probability of flipping a coin to heads is 50%.

The odds are "fifty:fifty," which equals 1.0. As the probability goes from 0.5 to 1.0, the odds increase from 1.0 to approach infinity. For example, if the probability is 0.75, then the odds are 75:25, three to one, or 3.0.

To convert from a probability to odds, divide the probability by one minus that probability. So if the probability is 10% or 0.10, then the odds are 0.1/0.9, one to nine, or 0.111.

To convert from odds to a probability, divide the odds by 1 plus the odds. So to convert odds of 1/9 to a probability, divide 1/9 by 10/9 to obtain the probability of 0.10.

The Odds Ratio

Results from a case–control study are summarized as an odds ratio. Among the cases, the odds of being vaccinated are 10:33, or 0.303. Among the controls, the odds of being vaccinated are 94:78, or 1.205. The odds ratio is 0.303/1.205 = 0.25. A computer program can compute the 95% CI, which extends from 0.12 to 0.54.

It isn't obvious, but if the disease is fairly rare (affects less than about 10% of the population studied), then the odds ratio calculated from a case–control study will be approximately equal to the true relative risk. If you are curious, an informal proof is at the end of the chapter. For this example, the odds ratio is 0.25. If we assume that cholera is rare, we can conclude that vaccinated individuals are 25% as likely to get cholera as unvaccinated people.

In the case of vaccination studies, it makes sense to subtract the odds ratio from 1.0. Here that difference is 0.75, which means the vaccine is 75% effective in preventing cholera. The CI for this is obtained by subtracting each end of the odds ratio CI from 1.0. The 95% CI for vaccine effectiveness extends from 46 to 88%. (The numbers reported in the original paper are slightly different than these, because they analyzed the data in a fancier method called conditional logistic regression to account for the matching of controls with each case).

INTERPRETING A P VALUE

The odds ratio and its CI are usually accompanied by a P value. The null hypothesis is that there is no association between the vaccination rate in the cases and controls. The P value for the example is 0.0003 (computed by Fisher's exact test).

The P value is easy to interpret. If the vaccination rates were really the same among patients and controls, there is only a 0.03% chance that an experiment of this size would show such a strong association between disease and vaccination. This is a two-tail P value, so it includes the possibilities of seeing either less disease or more disease with vaccines.

When using a computer program, Fisher's exact test is preferred. An alternative is to use a chi-square test (much easier if you are doing the calculations manually, but why would you?). The P value is 0.0002 or 0.0004 depending on exactly how the chi-square calculations are done.

THE CHALLENGE OF CASE-CONTROL STUDIES

The advantage of case–control studies is that they can be done relatively quickly with a relatively small sample size, from previously recorded data. The alternative method of assessing the effectiveness of the vaccine would be to follow thousands of vaccinated and unvaccinated people for a year or two. Cholera is a disease with rapid onset, so a prospective study could be done in one year. Many diseases have a much slower natural history, thus requiring prospective studies that last many years or decades. For these diseases, case–control studies are particularly advantageous.

The challenge with case–control studies is to pick the right controls. The idea is to control for extraneous factors that might confuse the results, but not control away the effects you are looking for.

In the cholera example, the authors picked controls by visiting homes near the patient. There are some problems with this approach:

- The controls were picked because they were the same gender as the subject (with a few exceptions). Therefore, the study could not determine whether the vaccine reduces the incidence of cholera differently in men and women.
- The controls were picked to have the same age as the subjects. Therefore, the study could not determine anything about whether the vaccine reduces the incidence of cholera more in people of one age group than another.
- The subjects obviously knew they had cholera and so may recall their vaccination more vividly than the controls.
- The interviewers knew whether they were talking to a control subject or to a case (someone who had cholera). Although they tried to ask the questions consistently, they may have inadvertently used different emphasis with the cases.
- The subjects had suffered from cholera and may be motivated to help the researchers learn more about the disease. The controls may be more focused on ending the interview as quickly as possible. Thus, cases and controls may not give equally detailed or accurate information.
- The only way patients became part of the study was coming to the Cholera Treatment Center. Thus, the study did not include people who had mild cases of the disease and did not seek medical attention. Not everyone who is sick seeks medical attention, and this study selects for people who go to doctors when ill. This selection criterion was not applied to the controls.
- The only way that controls became part of the study was to be home when the investigators visited. This method selects for people who stay home a lot. This selection criterion was not applied to the cases.

These kinds of problems are inherent in all case–control studies. The investigators in this study were very aware of these potential problems. To test whether these biases affected their results, they ran a second case–control study. Here, the cases were patients with bloody diarrhea that turned out to not be caused by cholera.

The controls were selected in the same way as in the first study. The second study, which would have almost the same set of biases as the first, did not detect an association between diarrhea and cholera vaccination. The odds ratio was 0.64, with a 95% CI extending from 0.34 to 1.18 (I computed these values from their data; they reported slightly different results caused by use of a logistic regression analysis; see Chapter 37). Because the CI spans 1.0, the study shows no association between cholera vaccination and bloody diarrhea not caused by cholera. The negative results of the second study suggest that the association reported in the main study really was caused by vaccination, rather than by any of the biases listed above.

Because of these problems, some statisticians suggest being very skeptical unless the odds ratio is greater than 3 or 4 (or less than 0.33 or 0.25), even if the P value is tiny and the CI narrow (Taubes, 1995). There are too many ways for subtle biases to affect the results. How do you know when to accept the results? Results are more likely to be true when the odds ratio is large, when the results are repeated, and when the results make sense biologically.

ASSUMPTIONS IN CASE–CONTROL STUDIES

Assumption: Random (or representative) sample

The 95% CI is based on the assumption that your cases and controls were randomly selected from the populations. In many cases, this assumption is not true. You can still interpret the CI as long as you assume that your sample is representative of the population you are generalizing about.

The patients in the example were certainly not a random selection of all those with cholera, but it is reasonable to think that they are representative of adults with cholera in that particular city and perhaps all of Africa.

Assumption: Independent observations

The 95% CI is only valid when all subjects are sampled from the same population and each has been selected independently of the others. Selecting one member of the population should not change the chance of selecting anyone else.

This assumption would be violated if the study included several people from one family or if there were several unique strains of cholera.

Assumption: Accurate data

The 95% CI is only valid when the number of subjects in each category is tabulated correctly. This assumption would be violated in the example if some of the patients actually didn't have cholera or if some of the controls did.

Assumption: Assessing an event you really care about

The 95% CI allows you to extrapolate from the sample to the population for the event that you tabulated. In many cases, the event measured in the study is a few steps removed from the event you really care about. This is not a problem here, because this study looked at exactly the event you cared about—getting cholera.

	CASES (CHOLERA)	CONTROLS
Received vaccine	A	B
No vaccine	C	D
Total	A+C	B+D

Table 28.2. Hypothetical data if the entire population were studied.

Assumption: No difference between the two groups except disease

The validity of a case–control study depends on the assumption that the controls do not differ systematically from the cases in any way except for the absence of disease. As discussed above, it can be very difficult to be sure a case–control study has complied with this assumption.

WHY ODDS RATIOS APPROXIMATE THE RELATIVE RISK

Earlier I stated (but did not prove) an important point: If the disease is fairly rare, then the odds ratio calculated from a case–control study will approximately equal the true relative risk. Because that conclusion is not obvious, this section presents an informal proof.

The odds ratio from a cross-sectional study has a value very close to the relative risk when the disease is rare

Imagine what the data would look like if the investigators could have done a cross-sectional study. They would have collected information about cholera vaccine and cholera from a huge number of people in the area at risk. The data would look like Table 28.2. This is called a cross-sectional study. Note that subjects are picked at random from the entire population, regardless of whether they have cholera or were vaccinated.

If we had all these data, the relative risk of cholera among those vaccinated (compared with those who were not) is

$$\text{Relative Risk} = \frac{\dfrac{A}{A+B}}{\dfrac{C}{C+D}}$$

If we assume that cholera is rare, then A must be much smaller than B, and C must be much smaller than D, and the equation can be simplified (as an approximation) to

$$\text{Relative Risk} = \frac{\dfrac{A}{A+B}}{\dfrac{C}{C+D}} \approx \frac{A/B}{C/D} = \text{Odds Ratio}$$

	CASES (CHOLERA)	CONTROLS
Received vaccine	A*M	B*K
No vaccine	C*M	D*K
Total	(A+C)*M	(B+D)*K

Table 28.3. In a case–control study, you select cases and controls.

In this hypothetical table, extended from Table 28.2, we have selected a fraction M of the cases to study and a fraction K of the controls.

The odds ratio from a case–control study has a value very close to the relative risk from a cross-sectional study

When performing a case–control study, the investigators choose the relative number of cases and controls (Table 28.3). Of all the cases, they chose some fraction (we'll call it M) to study. Of all the people without cholera, the investigators studied some fraction (we'll call it K) for the study.

Note that the investigators don't know any of the six variables in Table 28.3! The only way to know A through D would be to perform a full cross-sectional study. And the investigators don't know what fraction of all cases and controls in the population they have surveyed, so they don't know K and M.

The values of K and M drop out of the equation when computing the odds ratio.

$$\text{Odds Ratio} = \frac{\dfrac{A \cdot M}{B \cdot K}}{\dfrac{C \cdot M}{D \cdot K}} \approx \frac{A/B}{C/D}$$

The odds ratio calculated from the case–control study is expected to be identical to the odds ratio you would have calculated from a cross-sectional study.

The odds ratio from a case–control study approximate the relative risk

The first part of this informal proof showed that with a cross-sectional study of a rare disease, the odds ratio and relative risk are almost the same. The second part showed that the odds ratio from a case–control study is about the same as the odds ratio you would have calculated from a cross-sectional study. Combine those two ideas, and the odds ratio from a case–control study of a rare disease approximates the relative risk.

CHAPTER 29

Comparing Survival Curves

A statistician is a person who draws a mathematically
precise line from an unwarranted assumption to a foregone
conclusion.

Unknown author

*C*hapter 5 *explained how survival curves were generated and how to
interpret the confidence interval of survival curves. This chapter
explains how to compare two survival curves.*

EXAMPLE SURVIVAL DATA

Patients with chronic active hepatitis were treated with prednisolone or placebo,
and their survival was compared (Kirk, Jain, Pocock, Thomas, & Sherlock, 1980;
raw data from Altman & Bland, 1998). Some patients were still alive at the time
the data were collected, and these are shown in Table 29.1 with an asterisk. The
information from these patients (that they lived at least up to the time of data collection) is an essential part of the data collected from the study. These values are
entered into a computer program as censored values. Additionally, one patient
taking prednisolone was lost to follow-up at 56 months. His data are also said
to be censored and are entered into a survival analysis program the same as the
other censored values. He lived at least 56 months, but we don't know what happened after that.

Figure 29.1 shows the Kaplan–Meier graph of the survival data, as previously
explained in Chapter 5.

ASSUMPTIONS WHEN COMPARING SURVIVAL CURVES

This list summarizes the assumptions, explained in detail in Chapter 5, that must
be accepted to interpret survival analyses.

- Random (or representative) sample
- Independent subjects
- Consistent entry criteria
- Consistent definition of the end point
- Clear definition of the starting point

PREDNISOLONE	CONTROL
2	2
6	3
12	4
54	7
56 (left study)	10
68	22
89	28
96	29
96	32
125*	37
128*	40
131*	41
140*	54
141*	61
143	63
145*	71
146	127*
148*	140*
162*	146*
168	158*
173*	167*
181*	182*

Table 29.1. Sample survival data from Kirk et al. (1980) with raw data from Altman and Brand (1998).

Patients with chronic active hepatitis were treated with prednisolone or placebo, and their survival was compared. The values are survival time in months. The asterisks denote patients still alive at the time the data were analyzed. These values are said to be censored.

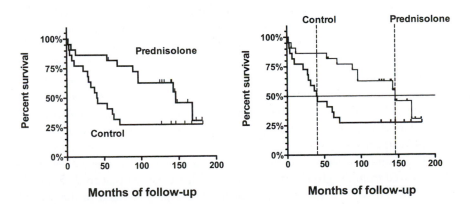

Figure 29.1. Kaplan–Meier survival curves created from the data in Table 29.1.

Each drop in the survival curve shows the time of one (or more) patient's death. The blips show the time of censoring. One subject was censored when he left the study. The data for the others are censored because they were alive when the data collection ended. The graph on the right shows how median survival times are determined.

- Time of censoring is unrelated to survival
- Average survival doesn't change during the study

When comparing curves, there are additional assumptions, as follows.

Assumption: Treatment groups were defined before data collection began

When you compare groups, the groups must be defined before data collection begins. It is not valid to divide a single group of patients (all treated the same way) into two groups based on whether they responded to treatment. It can be tempting, for example, to compare survival of subjects whose tumor got smaller with treatment with those whose tumors stayed the same size, or to compare those whose lab tests improved with those whose lab tests didn't. Comparing survival of responders with nonresponders is invalid for two reasons.

The first reason is that a patient cannot be defined to be a "responder" unless he or she survived long enough for you to measure the tumor. Any patient who died early in the study would certainly be defined into the nonresponder group. In other words, survival influenced which group the patient was assigned to. Therefore, you can't learn anything by comparing survival in the two groups.

The second reason is that the disease may be heterogeneous. The patients who responded may have a different form of the disease than those who didn't respond. In this case, the responders may have survived longer even if they hadn't been treated.

You must define the groups you are comparing before starting the experimental phase of the study. Be very wary of studies that use data collected during the experimental phase of the study to divide patients into groups or to adjust the data.

Assumption: Groups are defined consistently as data are accrued

Some survival studies accrue patients over several years. In these studies, it is essential that the diagnostic groups are defined consistently.

Here is an example where that assumption might be violated. You are comparing the survival of patients whose cancer has metastasized to the survival of patients whose cancer remains localized. Average survival is longer for the patients without metastases. Now a fancier scanner becomes available, making it possible to detect metastases earlier. What happens to the survival of patients in the two groups?

The group of patients without metastases will be smaller. The patients who are removed from the group are those with small metastases that could not have been detected without the new technology. These patients tend to die sooner than the patients without detectable metastases. By taking away these patients, the average survival of the patients remaining in the "no metastases" group will probably improve.

What about the other group? The group of patients with metastases is now larger. The additional patients, however, are those with small metastases. These patients tend to live longer than patients with larger metastases. Thus, the average survival of all patients in the "with metastases" group will probably also improve.

Changing the diagnostic method paradoxically increased the average survival of both groups! Feinstein, Sosin, and Wells (1985) termed this paradox the *Will Rogers phenomenon* from a quote attributed to the humorist Will Rogers: "When the Okies left Oklahoma and moved to California, they raised the average intelligence in both states."

Assumption: Subjects actually received the assigned treatment

When comparing the survival of people randomly assigned to receive different treatments, one must assume that they actually got their assigned treatment—including all the doses of a drug or all boosters of a vaccine. Unfortunately, this assumption is often violated, and handling the resulting data is problematic. It seems sensible to just exclude from analysis all data from people who didn't receive the full assigned treatment. This is called the *per protocol approach*, because you only compare survival of subjects who got the full treatment according to the study protocol. But this approach would lead to biased results if the noncompliance has any association with disease progression and treatment. The preferred approach is called *intention to treat* (Hollis & Campbell, 1999). With this approach, the data are analyzed based on the assigned treatment, even if it was not given or was incomplete.

Some studies analyze the data both with the per protocol and with the intention-to-treat approaches. If the results are similar, then you know that the subjects who didn't get the assigned treatment (or didn't get a complete treatment) didn't affect the results much. If the two analysis approaches lead to substantially different conclusions, then the results are simply ambiguous.

Assumption: Proportional hazards

Hazard is defined as the slope of the survival curve—a measure of how rapidly subjects are dying. The hazard ratio compares two treatments. If the hazard ratio is 2.0, then the rate of deaths in one treatment group is twice the rate in the other group. Figure 29.2 shows ideal curves with a consistent hazard ratio. Both curves start, of course, with 100% and end at 0%. At any time along the curve, the slope of one curve is twice the other. The hazards are proportional.

The assumption of *proportional hazards* is required for most comparisons of survival curves. This means that the relative hazards are consistent over time and that any differences are caused by random sampling. This assumption would be true if, at all times, patients from one treatment group die at about half the rate of patients from the other group. It would not be true if the death rate in one group is much higher at early times, but lower at late times. This situation is common when comparing surgery (high initial risk, lower later risk) with medical therapy (less initial risk, higher later risk).

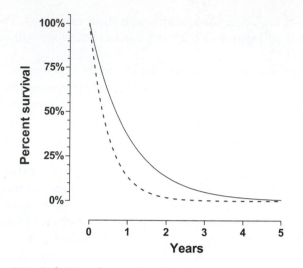

Figure 29.2. Definition of proportional hazards.
At every time point, the dotted curve is twice as steep as the solid curve. The hazard ratio is 2.0 (or 0.5, depending on how you compute it) at all time points.

If two survival curves cross, the assumption of proportional hazards is unlikely to be true. The exception would be when the curves only cross at late time points when there are few patients still being followed.

COMPARING TWO SURVIVAL CURVES USING CIs

Survival curves can be compared with P values (next section) and CIs.

Viewing the confidence bands

Chapter 5 showed confidence bands of a survival curve. Figure 29.3 shows the example survival curves with their 95% confidence bands. The curves overlap a bit, so plotting both curves together creates a very cluttered graph. Instead, the two are placed side by side. Both curves start at 100% of course, so they overlap somewhat. But they don't overlap at all for many months. This graph is enough to convince you that the prednisolone worked.

Hazard ratio

If the assumption of proportional hazards is accepted (which does not seem unreasonable with the sample data), the two survival curves can be summarized with the hazard ratio, which is essentially the same as a relative risk (see Chapter 27). For the example data, the hazard ratio is 0.42, with a 95% CI ranging from 0.19 to 0.92. In other words, the treated patients are dying at 42% of the rate of control patients, and we have 95% confidence that the true ratio is between 19 and 92%.

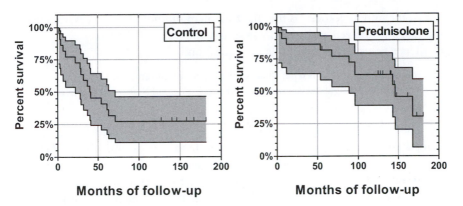

Figure 29.3. Survival curves showing the 95% confidence bands.

More specifically, this means in any particular day or week, a treated patient has 42% of the chance of dying as a control patient.

If the two survival curves were identical, the hazard ratio would equal 1.0. Because the 95% CI does not include 1.0, we can be at least 95% certain that the two populations have different survival experiences.

Ratio of median survival times

Median survival time is defined as the time it takes until half the subjects have died. The right panel of Figure 29.1 shows the median survival of the sample data. The horizontal line is at 50% survival. The time at which each survival curve crosses that line is the median survival. The median survival of the control patients is 40.5 months, whereas the median survival of the patients treated with prednisolone is 146 months, 3.61 times longer.

It is possible to compute a 95% CI for that ratio of median survivals. This calculation is based not only on the assumption of proportional hazards (see prior section), but also on an additional assumption: that the chance of dying in a small time interval is the same early in the study and late in the study. In other words, the survival curve follows the same pattern as an exponential decay curve. This assumption does not seem unreasonable for the sample data. For the sample data, the ratio of median survivals is 3.61, with a 95% CI ranging from 3.14 to 4.07. In other words, we are 95% sure that treatment with prednisolone triples to quadruples the median survival time.

COMPARING SURVIVAL CURVES USING A P VALUE

The comparison of two survival curves can be supplemented with a P value.

All P values test a null hypothesis. When comparing two survival curves, the null hypothesis is that the survival curves of the two populations are identical and any observed discrepancy is the result of random sampling error. In other words, the null hypothesis is that the treatment did not change survival overall and that any difference observed was simply the result of chance.

The P value answers the following question:

> If the null hypothesis is true, what is the probability of randomly selecting subjects whose survival curves are as different (or more so) than what was actually observed?

The calculation of the P value is best left to computer programs. The *log-rank method*, also known as the *Mantel–Cox method* (and nearly identical to the *Mantel–Haenszel method*), is used most frequently. The assumption of proportional hazards (explained earlier in this chapter) is required to interpret this P value.

For the sample data, the two-tail P value is 0.031. If the treatment was really ineffective, it is possible that the patients who were randomly selected to be given one treatment just happened to live longer (or shorter) than the patients given the other treatment. The P value tells us that the chance of this happening is only 3%. Because that is less than the traditional significance cutoff of 5%, we can say that the increase in survival with treatment by prednisolone is statistically significant.

An alternative method to compute the P value is known as the *Gehan–Breslow–Wilcoxon method*. Although the log-rank test gives equal weight to all time points, the Gehan–Breslow–Wilcoxon method gives more weight to deaths at early time points. This often makes lots of sense, but the results can be misleading when a large fraction of patients are censored at early time points. The Gehan–Wilcoxon test does not require a consistent hazard ratio, but does require that one group consistently have a higher risk than the other.

For the sample data, the P value computed by the Gehan–Breslow–Wilcoxon method is 0.011.

Q & A: Comparing Survival Curves

Is the log-rank test the same as the Mantel–Haenszel test?	Almost. The two differ only in how they deal with multiple deaths at exactly the same time point. The results will be very similar.
Is the Gehan–Wilcoxon test also the same?	No. The Gehan–Wilcoxon method (also attributed to Breslow) gives more weight to deaths at early time points, which makes lots of sense. But the results can be misleading when a large fraction of patients are censored at early time points. In contrast, the log-rank test gives equal weight to all time points. The Gehan–Wilcoxon test does not require a consistent hazard ratio, but does require that one group consistently has a higher risk than the other. Of course, you should choose the test as part of the experimental design.

Continued

Q&A Continued

What if the two survival curves cross?	If two survival curves truly cross, then one group has a higher risk at early time points and the other group has a higher risk at late time points. If the two curves are based on plenty of data and the crossing point is near the middle of the time span, then the data violate the assumptions of both the log-rank and the Wilcoxon–Gehan test and you'd need to use more specialized methods (beyond this book). When survival curves overlap only at later time points, it may be a matter of chance and mean nothing. At those late time points, fewer patients are followed, and the two curves may cross as the result of chance.
Why compare entire survival curves? Why not just compare the mean age of death?	There are three reasons why it is rarely helpful to compare mean age of death: • You usually will want to tabulate the data before every subject has died. If some people are still alive, it would not be helpful to compute the average age of death of only those who died. • If the data for any subject were censored, it would be impossible to calculate a meaningful average age of death. • Even if every subject died (and none were censored), the mean age of death may not be meaningful. It is likely that the distribution of ages is not Gaussian. If so, summarizing the data with the mean may not be informative. And calculations like the 95% CI of the mean wouldn't be helpful if the distribution is far from Gaussian.

Continued

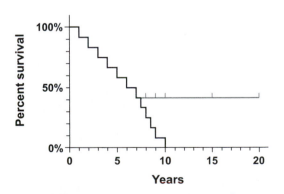

Figure 29.4. Two curves with identical five-year survivals and identical median survival times. Yet the curves are very different.

Q&A Continued

Why compare entire survival curves? Why not just compare the median age of death?	Figure 29.4 shows two simulated survival curves. The first parts of the curves are identical, so they appear superimposed. They have the same median survival (6.5 years) and the same 5-year survival rate (58%). But after year 7, the two curves diverge drastically. If you had a choice between the two treatments, you'd choose the one whose survival curve levels off with 40% of the patients still living after 20 years, rather than the treatment where all subjects had died by year 10.

CHAPTER 30

Comparing Two Means: Unpaired t Test

Researchers often want Bioinformaticians to be Biomagicians, people who can make significant results out of non-significant data, or Biomorticians, people who can bury data that disagree with the researcher's prior hypothesis.

DAN MASYS

The unpaired t test compares the means of two groups, assuming the data were sampled from a Gaussian population.

EXAMPLE: MAXIMUM RELAXATION OF BLADDER MUSCLES

Frazier et al. (2006) measured how well the neurotransmitter norepinephrine relaxes bladder muscle. Chapter 11 looked at the concentrations required to get half-maximal relaxation as an example of lognormal data. Here we will compare the maximal relaxation that can be achieved by large doses of norepinephrine and compare old with young rats.

The raw data are listed in Table 30.1 and plotted in Figure 30.1. The two means are fairly far apart, but there is a lot of variation and the two sets of data overlap considerably. Do young and old rats differ? Or is the difference observed here just a matter of chance? Statistical calculations can help you answer that question by calculating the following:

- A CI for the difference between two means or
- A P value that tests the null hypothesis that the two population means are identical.

An unpaired t test does these analyses.

INTERPRETING RESULTS FROM AN UNPAIRED t TEST

Table 30.2 shows the results of an unpaired t test.

OLD	YOUNG
20.8	45.5
2.8	55.0
50.0	60.7
33.3	61.5
29.4	61.1
38.9	65.5
29.4	42.9
52.6	37.5
14.3	

Table 30.1. Maximal relaxation of muscle strips of old and young rat bladders stimulated with high concentrations of norepinephrine (Frazier et al., 2006).

Larger values reflect more muscle relaxation. These values are graphed in Figure 30.1.

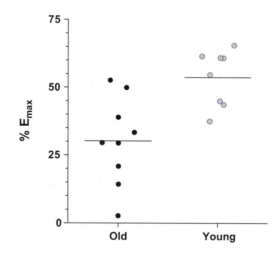

Figure 30.1. Maximal relaxation of muscle strips of old and young rat bladders stimulated with high concentrations of norepinephrine.

More relaxation is shown as larger numbers. Each symbol represents a measurement from one rat. The horizontal lines represent the means.

CI

A t test compares two means. The mean maximum response in old rats is 23.5 lower than in young rats. The 95% CI for the difference ranges from 9.3 to 37.8 (Figure 30.2).

Is this difference large? It depends on the scientific context of the work. Because the maximum conceivable difference in this example would be 100%,

UNPAIRED t TEST

P value	0.0030
P value summary	**
Are means significantly different? (P < 0.05)	Yes
One- or two-tail P value?	Two tailed
t, df	$t = 3.531$, $df = 15$

HOW BIG IS THE DIFFERENCE?

Mean ± SEM of column A	53.71 ± 3.664, $n = 8$
Mean ± SEM of column B	30.17 ± 5.365, $n = 9$

DIFFERENCE BETWEEN MEANS **23.55 ± 6.667**

95% CI	9.338 to 37.75
R^2	0.4540

F TEST TO COMPARE VARIANCES

F, DFn, Dfd	2.412, 8, 7
P value	0.2631
P value summary	ns
Are variances significantly different?	No

Table 30.2. Results of unpaired t test from GraphPad Prism 5.0.

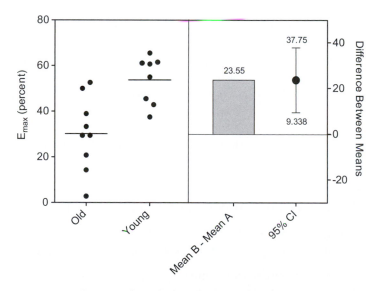

Figure 30.2. The CI for the difference between two means.

The first two columns show the actual data. The third column shows the difference between the two means and the fourth column shows the 95% CI for that difference (plotted on the right axis).

the difference seems reasonably large. The two sets of data overlap, and there are only 8 or 9 values per group, so the CI is wide. Because the CI does not include zero, we are 95% sure that the mean response in old animals is less than the mean response in young ones.

P value

The null hypothesis is that both sets of data are randomly sampled from populations with identical means. The P value answers the following question:

> If the null hypothesis was true, what is the chance of randomly observing a difference as larger or larger than observed in this experiment?

The P value is 0.0030. Random sampling is unlikely to have created the difference. The difference between the two means is statistically significant.

As explained in Chapter 15, the P value can be one or two sided. Here, the P value is two sided (two tailed). If the null hypothesis was true, the probability of observing a difference as large as that observed here with the young rats having the larger mean is 0.0015, and the chance of observing a difference as large as observed here with the old rats having the larger mean is also 0.0015. The sum of those two probabilities equals the two-side P value (0.0030).

R^2

Not all programs report R^2 with t test results, so you can ignore this value if it seems confusing. Chapter 35 will explain this in more detail. The idea of R^2 is to quantify the fraction of all the variation among the values that is explained by a difference between the group means. The rest of the variation is within the two groups. For these data, $R^2 = 0.45$. In other words, a bit less than half the variation among all the values is due to differences between the group means and a bit more than half of the variation is due to differences within the groups.

t ratio

The P value is calculated from the t ratio and sample size. The t ratio is explained later in this chapter.

ASSUMPTIONS: UNPAIRED t TEST

When assessing any statistical results, it is essential to review the list of assumptions. The t test is based on a familiar list of assumptions (see Chapter 12).

- Random (or representative) samples
- Independent observations
- Accurate data
- The values in the population are distributed in a Gaussian manner, at least approximately

The t test makes one additional assumption, that two populations have the same standard deviation, even if their means are distinct. More about this assumption below.

THE ASSUMPTION OF EQUAL VARIANCE

The unpaired t test depends on the assumption that the two data sets are sampled from populations that have identical standard deviations (and thus identical variances).

Testing the assumption

In the sample of data collected in this experiment, you can see that there is more variability among the old animals than the young. The standard deviations are 16.09 and 10.36. The old animals have a SD 1.55 times larger than the young animals. The square of that ratio (2.41) is called an F ratio.

The t test assumes that both groups are sampled from populations with equal variances. Are the data consistent with that assumption? To find out, let's compute another P value.

If that assumption were true, the distribution of the F ratio is known, so a P value can be computed. This P value equals 0.26. If the assumption of equal variances were true, there would be a 26% chance that random sampling would result in as large a discrepancy between the two SD values as observed here (or larger still). The P value is large, so the data are consistent with the assumption.

Don't mix up this P value, which tests the null hypothesis that the two populations have the same SD, with the P value that tests the null hypothesis that the two populations have the same mean.

What if the assumption is violated?

What should you do if the P value (from the F test) is small, indicating that the assumption of equal variances is unlikely to be true? This is a difficult question, and there is no real consensus among statisticians. There are seven possible answers.

- Ignore the result. The t test is fairly robust to violations of the assumption of equal variances, so long as the sample size isn't tiny and the two samples have equal, or nearly equal, number of observations. This is probably the approach that most biologists use.
- Emphasize the result and conclude that the populations are different. If the standard deviations truly differ, then the populations are not the same. That conclusion is solid, whether the two means are close together or far apart.
- Transform the data (often to logarithms) in an attempt to equalize the variances, and then run the t test on the transformed results.

- Instead of running the ordinary unpaired t test, run a modified t test that allows for unequal variance (the Welch modification to allow for different variances). If you always use this modified test, you don't have to think about the assumption of equal variances. The drawback is that this modified t test has less power to detect differences.
- Use the result of the test to compare variances to decide whether to run the usual unpaired t test or the modified t test that allows for unequal variance. Although this approach sounds sensible, it should not be used because the results will be misleading (Moser & Stevens, 1992).
- Analyze the data using linear regression (as explained in Chapter 33) and weight by the reciprocal of each group's variability (as explained in Chapter 36).
- Use the result of the test that compares variances to decide whether to run a t test or the nonparametric Mann–Whitney test. This approach also sounds very reasonable, but is not recommended. Chapter 41 will explain why.

OVERLAPPING ERROR BARS AND THE t TEST

Figure 30.1 showed the individual data points of the t test example. More often (for no good reason), you'll see data plotted as a bar graph showing mean and error bars. These error bars can show the SD or the SEM. Chapter 13 explains the difference.

It is tempting to look at whether two error bars overlap and try to reach a conclusion about whether the difference between means is statistically significant. Resist that temptation, because you really don't learn much by asking whether two error bars overlap (Lanzante, 2005).

SD error bars

Figure 30.3 graphs the mean and SD. The graph on the left is typical of graphs you'll see in journals, with the error bar only sticking up. But of course, the scatter goes in both directions. The graph on the right shows this.

The two error bars overlap. The upper error bar for the data from the old rats is higher than the lower error bar for the young rats. What can you conclude from that overlap?

The SD error bars quantify the scatter among the values. Looking at whether the error bars overlap lets you compare the difference between the mean with the amount of scatter within the groups. But the t test also takes into account sample size (in this example, the number of rats studied). If the samples were larger (more rats), with the same means and same SDs, the P value would be much smaller. If the samples were smaller (fewer rats), with the same means and same SDs, the P value would be larger.

When the difference between two means is statistically significant ($P < 0.05$), the two SD error bars may or may not overlap. Likewise, when the difference between two means is not statistically significant ($P > 0.05$), the two SD error bars

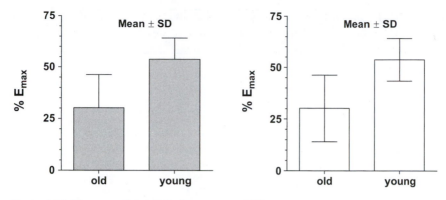

Figure 30.3. The same data plotted as mean and SD.
The left graph is similar to ones you'll often see in publications. The right graph shows the error bars going both up and down to emphasize that of course the scatter goes in both directions. The two error bars overlap. However, the fact that two SD error bars overlap tells you nothing about whether the difference between the two means is or is not statistically significant.

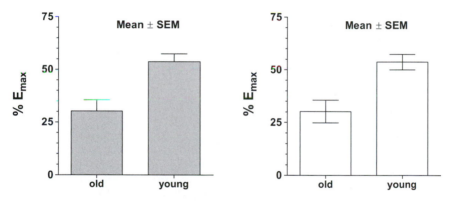

Figure 30.4. The same data plotted as mean and SEM.
Compare this with Figure 30.3. SEM error bars are always shorter than SD error bars. The left graph is similar to ones that you'll often see in publications. The right graph shows the error bars going both up and down to emphasize that of course the uncertainty goes in both directions. The two error bars do not overlap. However, the fact that two SEM error bars do not overlap tells you nothing about whether the difference between the two means is or is not statistically significant.

may or may not overlap. Knowing whether SD error bars overlap, therefore, does not let you conclude whether the difference between the means is statistically significant.

SEM error bars

Figure 30.4 is similar to Figure 30.3 but plots the mean and SEM instead of the SD.

Q & A: Unpaired t Test

Can a t test be computed from the mean, SD, and sample size of each group?	Yes. You don't need the raw data to compute an unpaired t test. It is enough to know the mean, SD or SEM, and sample size of each group.
Why is it called an unpaired test?	As its name suggests, it is used when the values in the two groups are not matched. It is not used when you compare two measurements in each subject (perhaps before and after an intervention) or if each measurement in one group is matched to a particular value in the other group. These kinds of data are analyzed by the paired t test, which will be explained
	in Chapter 31. If the pairing is effective in controlling for experimental variability, the paired t test will be more powerful than the unpaired test.
Is it sometimes called Student's t test because it is the first statistical test inflicted on students of statistics?	No. W. S. Gossett developed the t test when he was employed by a brewery that did not allow employees to publish. To submit the paper anonymously, he signed the paper "Student." Gossett is no longer anonymous, but the name Student is still attached to the test.
How is the z test different than the t test?	Some statistics texts compare the t and z tests. The t test compares the difference between the two sample means with the standard error of that difference, which is computed from the two sample standard deviations and sample sizes. The z test assumes that you know the standard deviation of the populations precisely. With large samples, this doesn't help much. With small samples, this extra information is quite useful and gives the z test more power than the t test. This is great if the SD of the population is actually known precisely. That is rare, so the z test is rarely useful.
Does it matter whether the two groups have different numbers of observations?	No. The t test does not require equal n. However, the t test is more robust to violations of the Gaussian assumption when the sample sizes are equal or nearly equal.
Why is the t ratio sometimes positive and sometimes negative?	The sign (positive or negative) of t depends on which group had the larger mean and in which order they were entered into the statistical program. Because the order you enter the groups into a program is arbitrary, the sign of the t ratio is irrelevant. In the example data, the t ratio might be reported as 3.53 or −3.53. It doesn't matter, because the CI and P value will be the same either way.

The two error bars do not overlap—the upper error bar for the data from the old rats is lower than the lower error bar for the young rats. What can you conclude from the lack of overlap?

The SEM error bars quantify how precisely you know the mean, taking into account both the SD and the sample size. Looking at whether the error bars overlap, therefore, lets you compare the difference between the mean with the precision of those means. This sounds promising. But in fact, you don't learn much by looking at whether SEM error bars overlap. By taking into account sample size and considering how far apart two error bars are, Cumming, Fidler, and Vaux (2007) came up with some rules for deciding when a difference is significant. But these rules are hard to remember and apply.

Here is a conclusion that is easy to remember. If two SEM error bars overlap, the P value is (much) greater than 0.05, so the difference is not statistically significant. The opposite rule does not apply. If two SEM error bars do not overlap, the P value could be less than, or greater than, 0.05.

CI error bars
The error bars in Figure 30.5 show the 95% CI of each mean. Because the two 95% CI error bars do not overlap, the P value must be less than 0.05—a lot less (Payton, Greenstone, & Schenker, 2003). But it would be a mistake to look at overlapping 95% CI error bars and conclude that the P value is greater than 0.05. That relationship, although commonly believed, is just not true. When two 95% CIs overlap, the P value might be greater than 0.05 and it also might be less than 0.05.

Summary
Table 30.3 summarizes the rules of thumb.

COMMON MISTAKES: UNPAIRED t TEST

Mistake: If the result is almost statistically significant, collect more data to increase the sample size and then recalculate the t test.
You can only really interpret the results of any statistical calculation when the sample size was chosen in advance or you use special methods designed to handle sequential accumulation of data.

What's wrong with collecting more data when the P value is higher than 0.05? The problem is that it biases you toward getting small P values, even if the null hypothesis is true. If you stop when you get a P value you like, but otherwise keep collecting more data, you can no longer interpret the P values. With this sequential approach, the chance of eventually reaching a conclusion that the result is statistically significant with $P < 0.05$ is much higher than 5%, even if the null hypothesis is true.

Mistake: If your experiment has three or more treatment groups, use the unpaired t test to compare two groups at a time.

If you perform multiple t tests this way, it is too easy to reach misleading conclusions. Use one-way ANOVA, followed by multiple comparisons posttests as explained in Chapters 39 and 40.

Mistake: If your experiment has three or more treatment groups, compare the largest mean with the smallest mean with a single unpaired t test.

You didn't know which group would have the largest mean and which would have the smallest mean until after you collected the data. So although you are formally just doing one t test to compare two groups, you are really comparing all the groups. Use one-way ANOVA.

Mistake: If the P value is larger than 0.05, try other tests to see whether they give a lower P value?

It's so tempting. If the P value is "too high" with one test, try another. If you don't like the results from an unpaired t test, switch to a nonparametric test to see whether the P value is smaller. If that doesn't give you a low enough P value, run a test for outliers, remove the outliers, and run the t test again. If the P value still isn't low enough, try running the t test on log-transformed data.

If you try multiple tests and choose to only report the results you like the most, those results will be misleading. You can't interpret the P value at face value when it was chosen from a menu of P values computed using different methods. You should pick one test before collecting data and use it.

HOW IT WORKS: UNPAIRED t TEST

Standard error of the difference between two means

Chapter 12 explained the SEM. The unpaired t test compares two means, so the calculations are based on the standard error of the difference between the two means. This is calculated by combining the two SEMs using a messy equation that accounts for any difference in sample size. The standard error of the difference between two means will always be larger than either SEM, but smaller than their sum. For the example, the standard error of the difference between the two means equals 6.67.

CI

The CI for the difference between the two population means is centered on the difference between the means of the two samples. The CI extends in each direction by a distance computed by multiplying the standard error of the difference (previous section) by a critical value from the t distribution (see Appendix D). For the sample data, the margin of error equals 6.67 (previous section) times 2.1314 (critical value from t distribution for 95% CI and 15 df), or 14.22. The observed

TYPE OF ERROR BAR	CONCLUSION IF THEY OVERLAP	CONCLUSION IF THEY DON'T OVERLAP
SD	No conclusion	No conclusion
SEM	P > 0.05	No conclusion
95% CI	No conclusion	P << 0.05

Table 30.3. Conclusions you can reach when two error bars do or do not overlap. This applies to comparing two means with an unpaired t test.

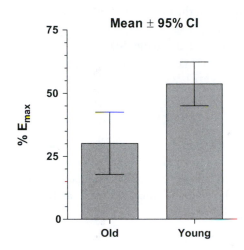

Figure 30.5. The same data plotted as means with 95% CIs.
Compare this with Figure 30.4. The 95% error bars are always longer than SEM error bars. The two error bars do not overlap, which means the P value must be less than 0.005.

difference between means was 23.55, so the 95% CI extends from 23.55 – 14.22 to 23.55 + 14.22, or from 9.33 to 37.76.

Thus, the width of the CI depends on three values:

- Variability. If the data are widely scattered (large SD), then the CI will be wider. If the data are very consistent (low SD), the CI will be narrower.
- Sample size. Everything else being equal, larger samples generate narrower CIs and smaller samples generate wider CIs.
- Degree of confidence. If you wish to have more confidence (i.e., 99% rather than 95%), the interval will be wider. If you are willing to accept less confidence (i.e., 90% confidence), the interval will be narrower.

t ratio

The P value is calculated from the t ratio. The t ratio is computed by dividing the difference between the two sample means (23.5) by the standard error of that difference (6.67). The numerator and denominator have the same units, so the t ratio has no units. In the example, t = 3.53. This tells you that difference between the two sample means is about three and a half times larger than the standard error of the difference between the two means.

P value

The P value is computed from the t ratio and the number of df, which equals the total number of values minus 2. Its value depends on the following:

- Difference between the means. Everything else being equal, the P value will be smaller when the means are further apart;
- The SDs. Everything else being equal, the P value will be smaller when the data are more consistent (smaller SD);
- The sample size. Everything else being equal, the P value will be smaller when the samples are larger.

LOOKING FORWARD

Chapter 31 explains the paired t test. Chapter 39 will explain the nonparametric Mann–Whitney test (and computer-intensive bootstrapping methods). Chapter 39 will explain one-way ANOVA to compare three or more means.

Chapter 35 will show how an unpaired t test can be viewed as a comparison of the fit of two models.

Comparing Two Paired Groups

To call in the statistician after the experiment is done may be no more than asking him to perform a postmortem examination: he may be able to say what the experiment died of.

R. A. FISHER

The paired t test compares two matched or paired groups when the outcome is continuous. McNemar's test compares two matched or paired groups when the outcome is binomial.

WHEN TO USE SPECIAL TESTS FOR PAIRED DATA

Often, experiments are designed so that the same patients or experimental preparations are measured before and after an intervention. These data should not be analyzed with an unpaired t test or the nonparametric Mann–Whitney test. Unpaired tests do not distinguish variability among subjects from differences caused by treatment.

When subjects are matched or paired, you should use a special paired test instead. Paired analyses are appropriate in these types of protocols:

- A variable is measured in each subject before and after an intervention.
- Subjects are recruited as pairs and matched for variables such as age, postal code, or diagnosis. One of each pair receives one intervention, whereas the other receives an alternative treatment.
- Twins or siblings are recruited as pairs. Each receives a different treatment.
- Each run of a laboratory experiment has a control and treated preparation handled in parallel.
- A part of the body on one side is treated with a control treatment and the corresponding part of the body on the other side is treated with the experimental treatment (e.g., right and left eyes).

CROSS FERTILIZED	SELF-FERTILIZED	DIFFERENCE
23.500	17.375	6.125
12.000	20.375	−8.375
21.000	20.000	1.000
22.000	20.000	2.000
19.125	18.375	0.750
21.500	18.625	2.875
22.125	18.625	3.500
20.375	15.250	5.125
18.250	16.500	1.750
21.625	18.000	3.625
23.250	16.250	7.000
21.000	18.000	3.000
22.125	12.750	9.375
23.000	15.500	7.500
12.000	18.000	−6.000

Table 31.1. Sample data for paired t test.

These data were collected by Charles Darwin, who compared the growth of cross-fertilized and self-fertilized plants. The values are the height of the plants in inches (measured to the nearest eighth of an inch). Each row represents a matched pair of self- and cross-fertilized seeds, grown under the same conditions. The last column is the difference.

EXAMPLE OF PAIRED t TEST

Most of the examples in this book are from the fairly recent medical literature. For this example, however, we'll go back over a century to an example that was used by Ronald Fisher, one of the pioneers of statistics (Fisher, 1935). Charles Darwin compared the growth of plants from seeds that were self-fertilized with that of seeds that were cross-fertilized (Darwin, 1876).

Table 31.1 shows the data. Each row in the table represents one matched set, with the two kinds of seeds grown side by side. By designing the experiments this way, Darwin controlled for any changes in soil, temperature, or sunlight that would affect both kinds of seeds. Figure 31.1 graphs the data on a before–after plot. This kind of graph gets is name from its common use to where the same measurement is made in each subject before and after an experimental intervention. Here the lines don't connect before and after measurements, but rather each of the 15 lines connects measurements of plants grown from matched seeds.

Figure 31.2 shows the same data as a bar graph, plotting the mean and SEM of each group. This kind of graph is commonly used, but it shows much less information than Figure 31.1. It shows you nothing about the pairing, and only indirectly (via the SEM) gives you a sense of variation. When possible, avoid bar graphs and graph the actual data.

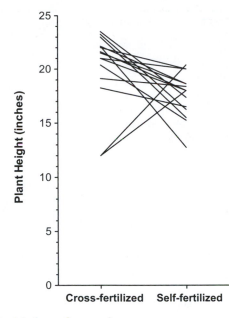

Figure 31.1. A before–after graph.

Usually, this kind of graph is used to plot values where the same measurement is made in each subject before and after an experimental intervention. Each of the 15 lines connects measurements from matched seeds.

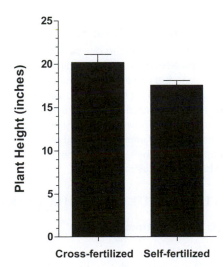

Figure 31.2. An alternative, but inferior approach.

This graph plots the same data as Figure 31.1, but showing only the mean and SEM of each group without accounting for pairing.

PAIRED t TEST	
P value	0.0497
P value summary	*
Are means significantly different? (P < 0.05)	Yes
One- or two-tail P value?	Two-tail
t, df	t = 2.148, df = 14
Number of pairs	15
HOW BIG IS THE DIFFERENCE?	
Mean of differences	2.617
95% CI	0.003639 to 5.230
HOW EFFECTIVE WAS THE PAIRING?	
Correlation coefficient (r)	−0.3348
P value (one tailed)	0.1113
P value summary	ns
Was the pairing significantly effective?	No

Table 31.2. Results of a paired t test as computed by GraphPad Prism.

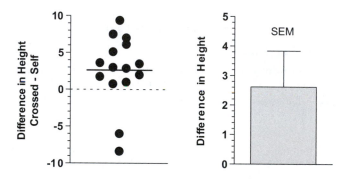

Figure 31.3. The difference between matched measurements.

Each of the circles on the left represents one paired experiment. The length of the self-fertilized plant was subtracted from the length of the cross-fertilized plant, and that difference is plotted. The cross-fertilized seed grew more than the self-fertilized seed in 13 of the 15 paired experiments, resulting in a positive difference. The other two experiments resulted in more growth in the cross-fertilized plant and so the difference is negative. The graph on the right plots only the mean and SEM. This graph takes up the same amount of space, but shows less information and isn't really easier to interpret.

INTERPRETING RESULTS FROM A PAIRED t TEST

Table 31.2 shows the results of a paired t test.

CI

A paired t test looks at the difference in measurements between two matched subjects (as in our example; see Figure 31.3) or a measurement made before and after an experimental intervention. For the sample data, the average difference in plant length between self- and cross-fertilized seeds is 2.62 inches. To put this in perspective, the self-fertilized plants have an average height of 17.6 inches, so this difference is approximately 15%.

The 95% CI for the difference ranges from 0.003639 inches to 5.230 inches. Because the CI does not include zero, we are 95% sure that the cross-fertilized seeds grow more than the self-fertilized seeds. But the CI extends from a tiny difference (especially considering that plant height was only measured to the nearest eighth of an inch) to a fairly large difference.

P value

The null hypothesis is there is no difference in the height of the two kinds of plants. In other words, the differences we measure are sampled from a population where the average difference is zero. The P value answers the following question:

> If the null hypothesis was true, what is the chance of randomly observing a difference as larger or larger than observed in this experiment?

The P value is 0.0497. If the null hypothesis was true, 5% of random samples of 15 pairs would have a difference this large or larger. Using the traditional definition, the difference is statistically significant because the P value is less than 0.05.

As explained in Chapter 15, the P value can be one or two sided. Here the P value is two sided (two tailed). Assuming the null hypothesis is true, the probability of observing a difference as large as that observed here with the self-fertilized plants growing more is 0.0248. The chance of observing a difference as large as observed here with the cross-fertilized plants growing more is also 0.0248. The sum of those two probabilities equals the two-side P value (0.0497).

t ratio

The P value is calculated from the t ratio and sample size. The t ratio is explained later in this chapter.

How effective was the pairing?

Darwin's experiment worked with pairs of seeds. Each pair of seeds was exposed to the same conditions. But different pairs were measured at different times, over several years. The idea of a paired t test is to account for that pairing. If the seeds were grown under great conditions, both seeds would grow tall. If grown under worse conditions, both seeds would grow less. In either case, the difference between the two kinds of seeds would be consistent.

Figure 31.4 shows that, in fact, there is no positive correlation among the data. Because the whole point of a paired t test is to use the internal controls to get more consistent data, the paired t test actually has a larger P value than an unpaired t test with these data (the P value from an unpaired t test is 0.02). This situation is rare. Usually, if you design an experiment with matched samples, you'll see a strong positive correlation.

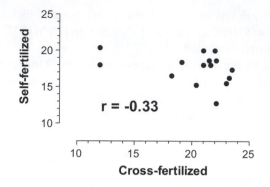

Figure 31.4. Testing the need for a paired t test.
The whole point of a paired t test is that you expect the paired values to be correlated—if one is higher, so is the other. This graph shows that sample data show a slight negative correlation. This negative trend is far from convincing and is almost certainly a coincidence. But it is clear that there is no strong positive correlation. Chapter 32 explains correlation coefficients.

With these data, is it fair to switch to an unpaired t test? It certainly is not fair to "shop around" for the P value you want. You'd need to establish the protocol for switching before collecting any data. Darwin didn't do that.

Assumptions

When assessing any statistical results, it is essential to review the list of assumption. The paired t test is based on a familiar list of assumptions (see Chapter 12).

- The paired values are randomly sampled from (or at least are representative of) a population or paired samples.
- In that population, the differences between the matched values follow a Gaussian distribution.
- Each pair is selected independently of the others.

Q & A: Paired t Test

Can I decide how the subjects are matched after collecting the data?	No. Pairing must be part of the experimental protocol decided before the data are collected. The decision about pairing is a question of experimental design and should be made long before the data are analyzed.
When computing the difference for each pair, in which order is the subtraction done?	It doesn't matter much. For each pair in the example, the length of the self-fertilized plant was subtracted from the length of the cross-fertilized plant. If the calculation were

Continued

Q&A Continued

	done the other way (if the length of the cross-fertilized plant was subtracted from the length of the self-fertilized plant), all the differences would have the opposite sign, as would the t ratio. The P value would be the same. It is very important, of course, that the subtraction be done the same way for every pair. It is also essential that the program doing the calculations doesn't lose track of which differences are positive and which are negative.
What if one of the values for a pair is missing?	The paired t test analyzes the differences between each set of pairs. If one value for a pair is missing, that pair can contribute no information at all, so it must be excluded from the analysis. A paired t test program will ignore pairs where you have only entered one of the two values.
Can a paired t test be computed from only the set of differences, without the original data?	Yes. All you need to compute a paired t test is the list of differences, where each difference is the value in one of the pairs minus the value in the other. It is essential that the difference be computed the same way for each pair.
Can a paired t test be computed if you know only the mean and SD of the two groups (or two time points) and the number of pairs?	No.
Can a paired t test be computed if you know only the mean and SD of the set of differences (as well as the number of pairs)? What about the mean and SEM?	Yes. All you need to compute a paired t test is the mean of the differences, the number of pairs, and the SD or SEM of the differences.
Does it matter whether the two groups are sampled from populations that are not Gaussian?	Not necessarily. The paired t test only analyses the set of paired differences, which it assumes is sampled from a Gaussian distribution. This doesn't mean that the two individual sets of values need to be Gaussian. If you are going to run a normality test on paired t test data, it only makes sense to test the list of differences (one value per pair). It does not make sense to test the two sets of data separately.
Will a paired t test always compute a lower P value than an unpaired test?	No. With the Darwin example, an unpaired test computes a lower P value than a paired test. When the pairing is effective (when the set of differences is more consistent than either set of values), the paired test will usually compute a lower P value.

THE RATIO PAIRED t TEST

Example data: Does a treatment change enzyme activity?

Table 31.3 shows example data that test whether treating cultured cells with a drug increases the activity of an enzyme. Five different clones of the cell were

CONTROL	TREATED
24	52
6	11
16	28
5	8
2	4

Table 31.3. Sample data for ratio t test.
These data (which are not real) test whether treating cultured cells with a drug increases the activity of an enzyme.

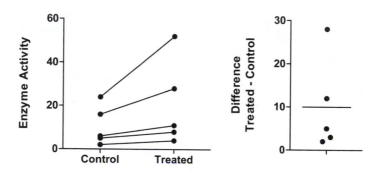

Figure 31.5. Enzyme activity in matched sets of control and treated cells.

tested. With each clone, control and treated cells were tested side by side. In all five clones, the treatment increased the activity of the enzyme. Figure 31.5 plots the data as a before–after graph and also as a graph of the differences.

The mean of the differences (treated-control) is 10.0. The 95% CI for the average differences ranges from –3.4 to 23.4. Because that CI includes zero, you can't be sure (with 95% confidence) whether the treatment has any effect on the activity. The P value (two tailed, from paired t test) is 0.107, which is not low enough to convince you that the difference between control and treated is real. It could easily just be the result of random sampling. With only five pairs and inconsistent data, the data only lead to a very fuzzy conclusion.

Relative differences versus absolute differences

But look more carefully at the left panel of Figure 31.5. The difference between control and treated depends on where you start. The clones with higher enzyme activity in the control condition had a larger increment with treatment. The treatment multiplies the enzyme activity by a certain factor, rather than adding a certain amount.

Figure 31.6 shows a simple way to align the multiplicative experimental model with the additive model used by the paired t test. That graph has a

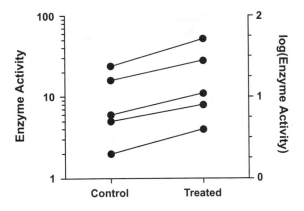

Figure 31.6. The same data as Figure 31.5 and Table 31.3 plotted on a logarithmic axis.

The right axis shows the logarithms. The left axis is labeled with the original values, logarithmically spaced. Both sets of data are plotted on both axes, which plot the same values but expressed differently.

logarithmic Y-axis. Now, all five of the increases are about the same size. The treatment increases the logarithm of the outcome (enzyme activity) by a constant amount, because the treatment multiplies the increases the activity by a constant factor, rather than adding a constant factor. On a log scale, multiplication becomes addition.

If you are not comfortable working with logarithms, this seems a bit mysterious. But read on to see how logarithms are used practically to analyze these kinds of data.

Results from a ratio paired t test

To analyze these data with a paired t test, first transform all values to their logarithms (base 10) and then perform the paired t test on those results (logarithms and antilogarithms are reviewed in Appendix E). The mean of the difference between logarithms is 0.26. Transform that back to its original ratio scale: $10^{0.26} = 1.82$. On average, the treatment multiplies the enzyme activity by a factor of 1.82. In other words, the treatment increases activity by 82%.

The 95% CI for the difference of logarithms is 0.21 to 0.33. Transform both those values to their antilogarithms to find the 95% CI for the ratio (treated/control), which is 1.62 to 2.14. This interval doesn't include 1.0 (a ratio of 1.0 means no change) and doesn't even come close to including 1.0. Thus, the increase in activity with treatment is very unlikely to be a coincidence. The P value is 0.0003, low enough to convince you that the treatment effect is very unlikely to be caused by chance. Analyzed this way, the conclusion is very crisp.

I call this procedure (paired t test of data transformed to logarithms) a *ratio t test*, but that term is not widely used. However, the idea of transforming values to make the differences more consistent is entirely standard. Of course, you really should pick the analysis method before collecting data. It is not fair to analyze the data lots of different ways and then pick the P value you like the best.

HOW A PAIRED t TEST WORKS

Because computer programs do the calculations, there is no need to learn the equation used to compute the paired t test. But it is important that you know what values enter the calculations.

Only the differences are analyzed
For each set of before–after measurements or each set of matched pairs, a paired t test first computes the differences between the two values for each pair. Only this set of differences is used to compute the CI and P value.

CI
The CI for the mean difference is calculated exactly as explained in Chapter 12, except that the values entering the calculations are the set of differences. The width of the CI depends on three values:

- Variability. If the observed differences are widely scattered, with some pairs having a large difference and some pairs a small difference (or a difference in the opposite direction), then the CI will be wider. If the data are very consistent, the CI will be narrower.
- Sample size. Everything else being equal, a sample with more pairs will generate narrower CIs, and a sample with fewer pairs will generate wider CIs.
- Degree of confidence. If you wish to have more confidence (i.e., 99% rather than 95%), the interval will be wider. If you are willing to accept less confidence (i.e., 90% confidence), the interval will be narrower.

t ratio
The t ratio is computed by dividing the average difference (2.62 inches) by the SEM of those differences (1.22 inches). The numerator and denominator have the same units, so the t ratio is unitless. In the example, t = 2.15.

P value
The P value is computed from the t ratio and the number of df, which equals the number of pairs minus 1. The size of the P value depends on the following:

- Mean difference. Everything else being equal, the P value will be smaller when the average of the differences is far from zero.
- Variability. If the observed differences are widely scattered, with some pairs having a large difference and some pairs a small difference, then the P value will be higher. If the data are very consistent, the P value will be smaller.

CONTROLS	CASES		
	RISK FACTOR +	RISK FACTOR −	TOTAL
Risk factor +	13	4	17
Risk factor −	25	92	117
Total	38	96	134

Table 31.4. A matched pairs case–control study.

Each value in the table represents a matched case and control. The total number of the four values is 134, because the study used 134 pairs of subjects (so 268 subjects in all). This is not a contingency table, and analysis by programs designed for contingency tables would be invalid.

	RISK FACTOR +	RISK FACTOR −	TOTAL
Case	38	96	134
Control	17	117	134
Total	55	213	268

Table 31.5. Data from Table 31.4 expressed as a contingency table.

Each value in the table represents 1 subject. The study had 134 patient–control pairs, so 268 subjects in total. This is a contingency table. This arrangement of the data obscures the fact that the study was designed with a matched control for each case. Table 31.4 is more informative.

- Sample size. Everything else being equal, the P value will be smaller when the sample has more data pairs.

MCNEMAR'S TEST FOR A PAIRED CASE-CONTROL STUDY

McNemar's test analyzes matched data when the outcome is binomial (two possible outcomes).

In a standard case–control study, the investigator compares a group of controls with a group of cases. As a group, the controls are chosen to be similar to the cases (except for the absence of disease and for exposure to the putative risk factor). An alternative way to design a case–control study is to match each case with a specific control based on age, gender, occupation, location, and other relevant variables.

An example is shown in Table 31.4. The investigators studied 134 cases and 134 matched controls. Each entry in the table represents one pair (a case and a control). This is not a contingency table, and entering this table into a program designed to analyze contingency tables would lead to invalid results. Table 31.5 shows these data as a contingency table.

The 13 pairs in which both cases and controls were exposed to the risk factor provide no information about the association between risk factor and disease. Similarly, the 92 pairs in which both cases and controls were not exposed to the risk factor provide no useful information. The association between risk factor and disease depends on the other two values in the table, and their ratio is the odds ratio.

For the example, the odds ratio is the number of pairs in which the case was exposed to the risk factor but the control was not (25) divided by the number of pairs where the control was exposed to the risk factor but the case was not (4), which equals 6.25.

McNemar's test computes the 95% CI of the odds ratio and a P value from the two discordant values (25 and 4 for this example). Not all statistics programs compute McNemar's test, but it can be computed using a free Web calculator in the QuickCalcs section of graphpad.com.

The 95% CI for the odds ratio ranges from 2.16 to 24.7. Assuming the disease is fairly rare, the odds ratio can be interpreted as a relative risk (Chapter 28). These data show that exposure to the risk factor increases one's risk 6.25-fold and that there is 95% confidence that the range from 2.16 to 23.7 contains the true population odds ratio.

McNemar's test also computes a P value, 0.0002. To interpret a P value, the first step is to define the null hypothesis, which is that there really is no association between risk factor and disease, so the population odds ratio is 1.0. If that null hypothesis was true, the chance of randomly selecting 134 pairs of cases and controls with an odds ratio so far from 1.0 is only 0.02%.

RELATED TESTS

Chapter 30 explained the unpaired t test.

Chapter 41 will explain the nonparametric Wilcoxon test (and computer-intensive bootstrapping methods). Chapter 39 will explain repeated-measures one-way ANOVA to compare three or more groups.

CHAPTER 32

Correlation

The invalid assumption that correlation implies cause is probably among the two or three most serious and common errors of human reasoning.

STEPHEN JAY GOULD

The association between two continuous variables can be quantified by the correlation coefficient, r.

INTRODUCING THE CORRELATION COEFFICIENT

Borkman and colleagues (1993) wanted to understand why insulin sensitivity varies so much among individuals. They hypothesized that the lipid composition of the cell membranes of skeletal muscle affected the sensitivity of the muscle for insulin.

They determined insulin sensitivity of 13 healthy men by infusing insulin at a standard rate (adjusting for size differences) and quantifying how much glucose they needed to infuse to maintain a constant blood glucose level. Insulin causes the muscles to take up glucose and thus causes the level of glucose in the blood to fall, so people with high insulin sensitivity will require a larger glucose infusion.

They also took a small muscle biopsy from each subject and measured its fatty acid composition. We'll focus on the fraction of polyunsaturated fatty acids that have between 20 and 22 carbon atoms (%C20–22).

Table 32.1 shows the data (interpolated from the author's published graph), which are graphed in Figure 32.1. Note that both variables are scattered. The mean of the insulin-sensitivity index is 284 and the SD is 114 mg/m^2/min. The CV is 114/284, which equals 40.1%. This is quite high. The authors knew that there would be a great deal of variability, and that is why they explored the causes of the variability. The fatty acid content is less variable, with a CV of 11.6%. If you don't look at the graph carefully, you could be misled. The X-axis does not start at 0, so you get the impression that the variability is greater than it actually is.

The graph shows a clear relationship between the two variables. Individuals whose muscles have more C20–22 polyunsaturated fatty acids tend to have greater sensitivity to insulin. The two variables vary together—statisticians say that there is a lot of *covariation* or a lot of *correlation*.

INSULIN SENSITIVITY (MG/M²/MIN)	% C20–22 POLYUNSATURATED FATTY ACIDS
250	17.9
220	18.3
145	18.3
115	18.4
230	18.4
200	20.2
330	20.3
400	21.8
370	21.9
260	22.1
270	23.1
530	24.2
375	24.4

Table 32.1. Correlation between %C20–22 and insulin sensitivity.

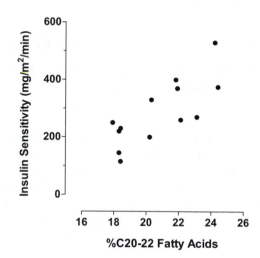

Figure 32.1. Correlation between %C20–22 and insulin sensitivity.

The direction and magnitude of the linear correlation can be quantified with a correlation coefficient, abbreviated r. Its value can range from –1 to 1. If the correlation coefficient is 0, then the two variables do not vary together at all. If the correlation coefficient is positive, the two variables tend to increase or decrease together. If the correlation coefficient is negative, the two variables are inversely related, that is, as one variable tends to decrease, the other one tends to increase. If the correlation coefficient is 1 or –1, the two variables vary together completely, that is, a graph of the data points forms a straight line.

In the example, the two variables increase together, so the correlation coefficient must be positive. But there is some scatter, so the correlation coefficient must be less than 1.0. In fact, the correlation coefficient equals 0.77.

CI OF THE CORRELATION COEFFICIENT

The 95% CI for the correlation coefficient ranges from 0.38 to 0.93. Assuming these data were randomly sampled from a larger population (and that other assumptions listed later in Chapter 32 are true), there is a 95% chance that this range includes the population correlation coefficient.

Note that the CI is not symmetrical. In this example, it extends much further below the correlation coefficient than it extends above it. This makes sense. The correlation coefficient can never be larger than 1.0 or smaller than –1.0, and so the CI is usually asymmetrical. The asymmetry is especially noticeable when r is far from zero and when the sample size is small.

INTERPRETING A P VALUE

The P value is 0.0021. To interpret any P value, define the null hypothesis. Here, the null hypothesis is that there is no correlation between insulin sensitivity and the lipid composition of membranes in the overall population. The two-tail P value answers this question: If the null hypothesis was true, what is the chance that 13 randomly picked subjects would have an r greater than 0.77 or less than –0.77?

Because the P value is so low, the data provide strong evidence to reject the null hypothesis.

CORRELATION AND CAUSATION

Why do the two variables correlate so well? There are five possible explanations:

- The lipid content of the membranes determines insulin sensitivity.
- The insulin sensitivity of the membranes somehow affects lipid content.
- Both insulin sensitivity and lipid content are under the control of some other factor, perhaps a hormone.
- Lipid content, insulin sensitivity, and other factors are all part of a complex molecular/biochemical/physiological network, perhaps with positive and/or negative feedback components. In this case, the observed correlation is just a peek at a much more complicated set of relationships.
- The two variables don't correlate in the population at all, and the observed correlation in our sample was a coincidence.

You can never rule out the last possibility, but the P value tells you how rare the coincidence would be. In this example, you would observe a correlation that strong (or stronger) in 0.21% of experiments if there is no correlation in the overall population.

You cannot decide among the first four possibilities by analyzing only these data. The only way to figure out which is true is to perform additional experiments where you manipulate the variables. Remember that this study simply measured both values in a set of subjects. Nothing was experimentally manipulated.

The authors, of course, want to believe the first possibility based on their knowledge of physiology. That does not mean they believe that the lipid composition is the *only* factor that determines insulin sensitivity, only that it is one factor.

Most people immediately think of the first two possibilities but ignore the rest. Correlation does not necessarily imply simple causality. Two variables can be correlated because both are influenced by the same third variable. Infant mortality in various countries is negatively correlated with the number of telephones per capita, but buying telephones will not make kids live longer. Instead, increased wealth (and thus increased purchases of telephones) relates to better plumbing, better nutrition, less crowded living conditions, more vaccinations, etc.

ASSUMPTIONS: CORRELATION

You can calculate the correlation coefficient from any set of data, and it may be a useful descriptor of the data. However, interpreting the CI and P value depends on the following assumptions.

Assumption: Random sample
Like all statistical analyses, you must assume that subjects are randomly selected from, or at least representative of, a larger population.

Assumption: Paired samples
Each subject (or each experimental unit) must have both X and Y values.

Assumption: Sampling from one population
Correlation assumes that all the points were randomly sampled from one population. If you sampled some subjects from one population and some from another, the correlation coefficient and P value will be misleading.

Assumption: Independent observations
Correlation assumes that any random factor affects only one subject and not others. The relationship between all the subjects should be the same. In this example, the assumption of independence would be violated if some of the subjects are related (i.e., siblings). It would also be violated if the investigator purposely chose some people with diabetes and some without or if the investigator measured each subject on two occasions and treated the values as two separate data points.

Assumption: X values were not used to compute Y values

The correlation calculations are not meaningful if the values of X and Y are not measured separately. For example, it would not be meaningful to calculate the correlation between a midterm exam score and the overall course score, because the midterm exam is one of the components of the course score.

Assumption: X values were not experimentally controlled

If you systematically controlled the X variable (i.e., concentration, dose, or time), you should calculate linear regression rather than correlation (see Chapter 33). You will get the same value for R^2 and the P value. However, the CI of r cannot be interpreted if the experimenter controlled the value of X.

Assumption: Both variables follow a Gaussian distribution

The X and Y values must each be sampled from populations that follow a Gaussian distribution, at least approximately.

Assumption: All covariation is linear

The correlation coefficient would not be meaningful, for example, if Y increases as X increases up to a certain point but then Y decreases as X increases further. Curved relationships are common, but are not quantified with a correlation coefficient.

Assumption: No outliers

Calculation of the correlation coefficient can be heavily influenced by one outlying point. Change or exclude that single point and the results may be quite different. Outliers can influence all statistical calculations, but especially in correlation. You should look at graphs of the data before reaching any conclusion from correlation coefficients. Don't instantly dismiss outliers as bad points that mess up the analysis. It is possible that the outliers are the most interesting observations in the study!

R^2

The square of the correlation coefficient is an easier value to interpret than r. For the example, $r = 0.77$, so $R^2 = 0.59$ (referred to as "r squared"). Because r is always between -1 and 1, R^2 is always between 0 and 1. Note that when you square a fraction, the result is a smaller fraction.

If you can accept the assumptions listed in the previous section, R^2 is the fraction of the variance shared between the two variables. In the example, 59% of the variability in insulin tolerance is associated with variability in lipid content. Knowing the lipid content of the membranes lets you explain 59% of the variance in the insulin sensitivity. That leaves 41% of the variance that is explained by other factors or by measurement error. X and Y are symmetrical in correlation analysis, so you can also say that 59% of the variability in lipid content is associated with variability in insulin tolerance.

BEWARE OF LARGE SAMPLES

Arden and colleagues (2008) asked whether there is a correlation between intelligence and sperm count. Really!

They obtained data from a study of U.S. Vietnam-era veterans, which measured both intelligence and the number and motility of sperm in ejaculate. The variation in sperm count (measured as sperm per milliliter, or sperm per ejaculate) among individuals was very skewed, so they transformed all the values to logarithms. This makes perfect sense, because the values approximated a lognormal distribution (Chapter 11).

With data from 425 men, they computed the correlation coefficient between a measure of intelligence and three assessments of sperm quality (logarithm of sperm count per volume and per ejaculate, and the percentage of those sperm that were motile). The results are shown in Table 32.2, which demonstrates three points:

- The r values are all positive. This tells you that the trend is positive, that increased intelligence was associated with increased sperm count and motility.
- The P values were all quite small. If there really were no relationship between sperm and intelligence, there is only a tiny chance of obtaining a correlation this strong.
- No corrections were made for multiple comparisons (Chapters 22 and 23). This is appropriate because the three variables that assess sperm are all sort of related. These aren't three independent measurements. It makes perfect sense to report all three P values without correction for multiple comparisons (but it wouldn't be fair to report only the lowest and not mention the other two). The fact that they all are tiny and all correlations go in the same direction helps make the data convincing.
- The r values are all small. It is easier to interpret the R^2 values, which show that only 2–3% of the variation in intelligence is associated with variation in sperm count and motility.

The last two points show a common situation. With large samples, data can show tiny effects (in this case R^2 values of 2–3%) and still have tiny P values. The fact that the P values are small tells you that the effect is unlikely to be a coincidence of random sampling. But the size of the P value does not tell you how large the effect is. With these data, r and R^2 measure the effect size, which is tiny.

Is an R^2 value of 2–3% large enough to be considered interesting and worth pursuing? That is a scientific question, not a statistical one. The investigators of this study seem to think so. Other investigators might conclude that such a tiny effect is not worthy of much attention. I doubt that many newspaper reporters who wrote about the link between sperm count and intelligence understood how weak the reported relationship really is.

	R	R²	P VALUE
Log(sperm count, per ml)	0.15	0.023	0.0019
Log(sperm count, per ejaculate)	0.19	0.036	<0.0001
Fraction of sperm that are motile (%)	0.14	0.020	0.0038

Table 32.2. Correlation between a measure of intelligence and three measures of sperm quality.

Data from Arden (2008) with $n = 425$.

HOW IT WORKS: CALCULATING
THE CORRELATION COEFFICIENT

The calculation of the correlation coefficient is built in to computer programs, so there is no reason to do the calculations manually. The explanation below is provided to give you a feel for what the correlation coefficient means.

1. Calculate the average of all X values. Also calculate the average of all Y values. These two averages define a point at "the center of gravity" of the data.

2. Compare the position of each point to that center. Subtract the average X from each X value. The result will be positive for points to the right of the center and negative for points to the left. Similarly, subtract the average Y from each Y value. The result will be positive for points above the center and negative for points below.

3. Standardize those X distances by dividing by the standard deviation of all the X values. Similarly, divide each Y distance by the standard deviation of all Y values. Dividing a distance by the SD cancels out the units, so these ratios are fractions without units.

4. Multiply the two standardized distances for each data point. The product will be positive for points that are northeast (product of two positive numbers) or southwest (product of two negative numbers) of the center. The product will be negative for points that are to the northwest or southeast (product of a negative and a positive number).

5. Add up all the products computed in Step 4.

6. Account for sample size by dividing the sum by n-1, where n is the number of XY pairs.

If X and Y are not correlated, then the positive products in Step 4 will approximately balance the negative ones, and the correlation coefficient will be close to 0. If X and Y are correlated, the positive and negative products will not balance, and the correlation coefficient will be far from 0.

Nonparametric Spearman correlation (Chapter 41) adds one step at the beginning. First, separately rank the X and Y values, with the smallest value getting a rank of 1. Then calculate the correlation coefficient between the X ranks and the Y ranks, as explained above.

Q & A: Correlation

Does it matter which variable is called X and which is called Y?	No. X and Y are totally symmetrical in correlation calculations. But note this is not true for linear regression (Chapter 33). When analyzing data with linear regression, you must carefully choose which variable is X and which is Y.
Do X and Y have to be measured in the same units to calculate a correlation coefficient? Can they be measured in the same units?	X and Y do not have to be measured in the same units, but they can be.
What units is r expressed in?	None. It is unitless.
Can r be negative?	Yes. It is negative when one variable tends to go down as the other goes up. When r is positive, one variable tends to go up as the other variable goes up.
Can correlation be calculated if all X values are the same? If all Y values are the same?	No. If all the X or Y values are the same, it makes no sense to calculate correlation.
Why no best-fit lines in the figures?	Correlation quantifies the relationship, but does not fit a line. Chapter 33 explains linear regression, which finds the best-fit line.
If all the X or Y values are transformed to new units, will r change?	No. Multiplying by a factor to change units (inches to centimeters, milligrams per milliliter to millimolar) will not change the correlation coefficient.
If all the X or Y values are transformed to their logarithm, will r change?	Yes. A logarithmic transform, or any that changes the relative values of the points, will change the value of r. However, the nonparametric Spearman correlation coefficient (Chapter 41), which depends only on the order of the values, will not change.
If you interchange X and Y, will r change?	No. X and Y are completely symmetrical in calculating and interpreting the correlation coefficient.
If you double the number of points, but r doesn't change, what happens to the CI and P value?	With more data points, the CI gets narrower. With more data points and the same value of r, the P value gets lower.
Why is it essential to view a graph as well as the correlation coefficient?	Figure 32.2 shows four data sets designed by Anscombe (1973). The correlation coefficients are identical (0.816), but the data are very different.
Can correlation be used to quantify how closely two alternative assay methods agree?	No. This is a common mistake. If you want to compare two different analysis methods, special methods are needed. Look up the Bland–Altman plot.
Is there a distinction between r^2 and R^2?	No. Upper and lower case mean the same thing. However, the correlation coefficient, r, is always written in lower case.

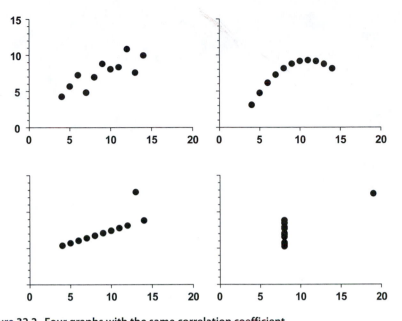

Figure 32.2. Four graphs with the same correlation coefficient.
In all four cases, the correlation coefficient (r) is 0.8164. Only the first graph seems to meet the assumptions of correlation.

LINGO: CORRELATION

Correlation
When you encounter the word "correlation," distinguish its strict statistical meaning (this chapter) from its more general usage (the rest of this book).

As used by statistics texts and programs, correlation quantifies the association between two continuous (interval or ratio) variables.

The word *correlation* is often used much more generally to describe the association of any two variables, but the term *correlation* is not strictly correct if either (or both) of the variables are not continuous variables. It is not possible to compute a correlation coefficient to help you figure out whether survival times are correlated with choice of drug, or whether antibody levels are correlated with gender.

Coefficient of determination
This is just a fancy term for R^2. Most scientists and statisticians just call it r square or r squared.

PART G

Fitting Models to Data

CHAPTER 33

Simple Linear Regression

In the space of 126 years, the Lower Mississippi has shortened
itself 242 miles. This is an average of a trifle over one mile and
a third per year. Therefore...any person can see that seven
hundred and forty-two years from now, the lower Mississippi
will be only a mile and three-quarter long...

MARK TWAIN *Life on the Mississippi*

*O*ne way to think about linear regression is that it fits the "best line"
through a graph of data points. Another way to look at it is that linear regression fits a simple model to the data to determine the most likely
values of the parameters that define that model (slope and intercept).
Chapter 34 will introduce the more general concepts of fitting a model to
data.

THE GOALS OF LINEAR REGRESSION

Recall the example of Chapter 32. The investigators were curious to understand
why insulin sensitivity varies so much between individuals. They measured insulin sensitivity in 13 men and also measured the lipid content of muscle obtained
at biopsy. You've already seen that the two variables (insulin sensitivity and
the fraction of the fatty acids that are unsaturated with 20–22 carbon atoms,
%C20–22) correlate substantially.

In this example, the authors concluded that differences in the lipid composition affect insulin sensitivity and proposed a simple model—that insulin sensitivity is a linear function of %C20–22. As %C20–22 goes up, so does insulin
sensitivity. Expressed as an equation,

Insulin Sensitivity = Intercept + Slope · %C20–22.

Let's define the insulin sensitivity to be Y, the %C20-22 to be X, the intercept
to be b, and the slope to be m. Now the model takes this standard form:

$Y = b + m \cdot X$.

That model is not complete, because it doesn't account for random variation.
The investigators used the standard assumption that random variability from the
predictions of the model follow a Gaussian distribution.

BEST-FIT VALUES

Slope	37.21 ± 9.296
Y intercept when X = 0.0	-486.5 ± 193.7
X intercept when Y = 0.0	13.08
1/slope	0.02688

95% CIS

Slope	16.75 to 57.67
Y intercept when X = 0.0	-912.9 to -60.17
X intercept when Y = 0.0	3.562 to 15.97

GOODNESS OF FIT

r^2	0.5929
Sy.x	75.90

IS SLOPE SIGNIFICANTLY NONZERO?

F	16.02
DFn, DFd	1.000, 11.00
P value	0.0021
Deviation from zero?	Significant

DATA

Number of X values	13
Maximum number of Y replicates	1
Total number of values	13
Number of missing values	0

Table 33.1. Linear regression results.

These results are from GraphPad Prism; other programs would format the results differently.

We can't possibly know the one true population value for the intercept or the one true population value for the slope. From the sample of data, our goal is to find values for the intercept and slope that are most likely to be correct and to quantify the imprecision with CIs. Table 33.1 shows the results of linear regression. The next section will review all of these results.

It helps to think of the model graphically (Figure 33.1). A simple way to view linear regression is that it finds the line straight that comes closest to the points. That's a bit too simple. More precisely, it finds the line that best predicts Y from X. To do so, linear regression only considers the vertical distances of the points from the line and, rather than minimizing the distances of the points from the line, it minimizes the sum of the square of those distances. Chapter 34 explains why.

LINEAR REGRESSION RESULTS

The slope

The best-fit value of the slope is 37.2. This means that when %C20–22 increases by 1.0, the average insulin sensitivity is expected to increase by 37.2 mg/m²/min.

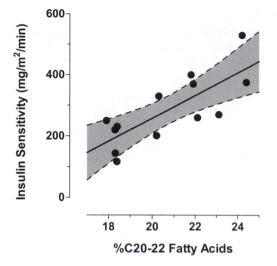

Figure 33.1. The best-fit linear regression line along with its 95% confidence band (shaded).

The CI is an essential (but often omitted) part of the analysis. The 95% CI of the slope ranges from 16.7 to 57.7 mg/m²/min. Although the CI is fairly wide, it does not include zero and doesn't even come close to zero. This is strong evidence that the observed relationship between lipid content of the muscles and insulin sensitivity is very unlikely to be a coincidence of random sampling.

The range of the CI is reasonably wide. The CI would be narrower if the sample size were larger.

Some programs report the standard errors of the slope instead of (or in addition to) the CIs. The standard error of the slope is 9.30 mg/m²/min. CIs are easier to interpret than standard errors, but the two are related. If you read a paper that reports the standard error of the slope but not its CI, compute the CI using these steps:

1. Look in Appendix D to find the critical value of the t distribution. The number of df equals the number data points minus 2. For this example, there were 13 data points, so there are 11 df, and the critical t ratio for a 95% CI is 2.201.
2. Multiply the value from Step 2 times the SE of the slope reported by the linear regression program. For the example, multiply 2.201 times 9.30. The margin of error of the CI equals 20.47.
3. Add and subtract the value computed in Step 3 from the best-fit value of the slope to obtain the CI. For the example, the interval begins at 37.2 − 20.5 = 16.7. It ends at 37.2 + 20.5 = 57.5.

The intercept

A line is defined both by its slope and its Y-intercept, the value of the insulin sensitivity when the %C20–22 equals zero.

For this example, the Y-intercept is not a scientifically relevant value. The range of %C20–22 in this example extends from about 18 to 24%. Extrapolating back to zero is not helpful. The best-fit value of the intercept is –486.5 with a 95% CI ranging from –912.9 to –60.17. Negative values are not biologically possible, because insulin sensitivity is assessed as the amount of glucose needed to maintain a constant blood level and so must be positive. These results tell us that the linear model cannot be correct when extrapolated way beyond the range of the data.

Graphical results

Figure 33.1 shows the best-fit regression line defined by values for slope and intercept determined by linear regression.

The shaded area in Figure 33.1 shows the 95% confidence bands of the regression line, which combine the CIs of the slope and intercept. The best-fit line determined from this particular sample of subjects (solid black line) is unlikely to really be the best-fit line for the entire (infinite) population. If the assumptions of linear regression are true (later Chapter 33), you can be 95% sure that the overall best-fit regression line lies somewhere within the shaded confidence bands.

The 95% confidence bands are curved, but do not allow for the possibility of a curved (nonlinear) relationship between X and Y. The confidence bands are computed as part of linear regression, so they are based on the same assumptions as linear regression. The curvature simply is a way to enclose possible straight lines, of which Figure 33.2 shows two.

The 95% confidence bands enclose a region that you can be 95% confident includes the true best-fit line (which you can't determine from a finite sample of data). But note that only 6 of the 13 data points in Figure 33.2 are included within the confidence bands. If the sample was much larger, the best-fit line would be determined more precisely, the confidence bands would be narrower, and a smaller fraction of data points would be included within the confidence bands. Note the similarity to the 95% CI for a mean, which does not include 95% of the values (Chapter 12).

R^2

The R^2 value (0.5929) means that 59% of all the variance in insulin sensitivity can be accounted for by the linear regression model, and the remaining 41% of the variance may be caused by other factors, measurement errors, biological variation, or a nonlinear relationship between insulin sensitivity and %C20–22. Chapter 35 will define R^2 more rigorously. The value of R^2 for linear regression ranges between 0.0 (no linear relationship between X and Y) and 1.0 (the graph of X vs. Y forms a perfect line).

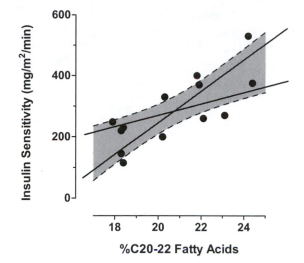

Figure 33.2. Although the confidence band is shaded, it is for linear regression and only considers the fits of straight lines.

Two lines that fit within the confidence band. Given the assumptions of the analysis, you can be 95% sure the true (population) line can be drawn within the shaded area.

P value

Linear regression programs report a P value, 0.0021. To interpret any P value, the null hypothesis must be stated. With linear regression, the null hypothesis is that there really is no linear relationship between insulin sensitivity and %C20–22. If the null hypothesis was true, the best-fit line in the overall population would be horizontal with a slope of zero. In this example, the 95% CI for slope does not include zero (and does not come close), so the P value must be less than 0.05. In fact, it is 0.0021. The P value answers the following question:

> If that null hypothesis were true, what is the chance that linear regression of data from a random sample of subjects would have a slope as far from zero (or further) than actually observed?

In this example, the P value is tiny, so we conclude that the null hypothesis is very unlikely to be true and that the observed relationship is unlikely to be caused by a coincidence of random sampling.

With this example, it made sense to analyze the data both with correlation (Chapter 32) and linear regression (Chapter 33). The two are related. The null hypothesis for correlation is that there is no correlation between X and Y. The null hypothesis for linear regression is that a horizontal line is correct. Those two null hypotheses are essentially equivalent, so the P values reported by correlation and linear regression are identical.

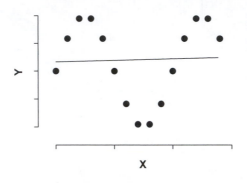

Figure 33.3. Linear regression only looks at linear relationships.
X and Y are definitely related here, just not in a linear fashion. The line is drawn by linear regression and misses the relationship entirely.

ASSUMPTIONS: LINEAR REGRESSION

Assumption: The model is correct

Not all relationships are linear (see Figure 33.3). In many experiments, the relationship between X and Y is curved, making simple linear regression inappropriate. Chapter 36 will explain nonlinear regression.

The linear regression equation defines a line that extends infinitely in both directions. For any value of X, no matter how high or how low, the equation can predict a Y value. Of course, it rarely makes sense to believe that a model can extend infinitely. But the model can be salvaged by using the predictions of the model only within a defined range of X values. Thus we only need to assume that the relationship between X and Y is linear within that range. In the example, we know that the model cannot be accurate over a broad range of X values. At some values of X, the model even predicts that Y would be negative, a biological impossibility. But the linear regression model is useful within the range of X values actually observed in the experiment.

Assumption: The scatter of data around the line is Gaussian

Linear regression analysis assumes that the scatter of data around the model (true best-fit line) is Gaussian. The CIs and P values cannot be interpreted if the distribution of scatter is far from Gaussian or if some of the values are outliers from another distribution.

Assumption: The variability is the same everywhere

Linear regression assumes that scatter of points around the best-fit line has the same standard deviation all along the curve. The assumption is violated if the points with high or low X values tend to be further from the best-fit line. The assumption that the standard deviation is the same everywhere is termed *homoscedasticity*.

Assumption: Data points are independent

Whether one point is above or below the line is a matter of chance and does not influence whether another point is above or below the line.

Assumption: X and Y values are not intertwined

If the value of X is used to calculate Y (or the value of Y is used to calculate X), then linear regression calculations will be misleading. One example is a Scatchard plot, used by pharmacologists to summarize binding data. The Y value (drug bound to receptors divided by drug free in solution) is calculated from the X value (free drug), so linear regression is not appropriate. Another example would be a graph of midterm exam scores (X) versus total course grades (Y). Because the midterm exam score is a component of the total course grade, linear regression is not valid for these data.

Assumption: The X values are known precisely

Regression assumes that the X values are known and all the variation is in the Y direction. If X is something you measure (rather than control) and the measurement is not precise, the linear regression calculations might be misleading.

COMPARISON OF LINEAR REGRESSION AND CORRELATION

The example data have now been analyzed twice, using correlation (Chapter 32) and linear regression. The two analyses are similar, yet distinct.

Correlation quantifies the degree to which two variables are related, but does not fit a line. The correlation coefficient tells you the extent (and direction) that one variable tends to change when the other one does. The CI of the correlation coefficient can only be interpreted when both X and Y are measured and both are assumed to follow Gaussian distributions. In the example, the experimenters measured both insulin sensitivity and %C20–22. You cannot interpret the CI of the correlation coefficient if the experimenters manipulated (rather than measured) X.

With correlation, you don't have to think about cause and effect. You simply quantify how well two variables relate to each other. It doesn't matter which variable you call X and which you call Y. If you reversed the definition, all of the results would be identical. With regression, you do need to think about cause and effect. Regression finds the best line that predicts Y from X, and that line is not the same as the line that best predicts X from Y.

It made sense to interpret the linear regression line only because the investigators hypothesized that the lipid content of the membranes influenced insulin sensitivity and so defined %C20–22 to be X and insulin sensitivity to be Y. The results of linear regression (but not correlation) would be different if the definitions of X and Y were swapped (so changes in insulin sensitivity somehow changed the lipid content of the membranes).

With most data sets, it makes sense to calculate either linear regression or correlation but not both. The example here (lipids and insulin sensitivity) is one where both correlation and regression make sense. The R^2 is the same whether computed by a correlation or linear regression program.

LINGO: LINEAR REGRESSION

Regression

The term regression is used to fit a model to data. Why the strange term? In the 19th century, Sir Francis Galton studied the relationship between parents and children. Children of tall parents tended to be shorter than their parents. Children of short parents tended to be taller than their parents. In each case, the height of the children reverted, or "regressed," toward the mean height of all children. Somehow, the term "regression" has taken on a much more general meaning.

Residuals

The vertical distances of the points from the regression line are called residuals. A residual is the discrepancy between the actual Y value and the Y value predicted by the regression model.

Least squares

Linear regression finds the value of slope and intercept that minimizes the sum of the squares of the vertical distances of the points from the line. This goal gives linear regression the alternative name *linear least squares*.

Linear

The word linear has a special meaning to mathematical statisticians. It can be used to describe the mathematical relationship between model parameters and the outcome. Thus, it is possible for the relationship between X and Y to be curved, but for the mathematical model to be considered linear.

Simple versus multiple linear regression

This chapter explained simple linear regression. The term simple is used because there is only one X variable. Chapter 37 will explain multiple linear regression. The term multiple is used because there are two or more X variables.

COMMON MISTAKES: LINEAR REGRESSION

Mistake: Concluding there is no relationship between X and Y when R^2 is low

A low R^2 value from linear regression means there is little linear relationship between X and Y. But not all relationships are linear. Linear regression in Figure 33.3 has a R^2 of 0.001, but X and Y are clearly related (just not linearly).

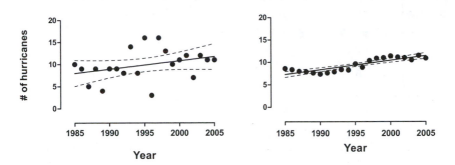

Figure 33.4. Don't smooth.
Smoothing, or computing a rolling average (which is a form of smoothing), appears to reduce the scatter of data and so gives misleading results.

Mistake: Fitting rolling averages or smoothed data

Figure 33.4 shows a synthetic example to demonstrate the problem of fitting smoothed data. The graph plots the number of hurricanes over time. The graph on the left shows actual "data," which jump around a lot. In fact, these are random values (from a Poisson distribution with a mean of 10), and each was chosen without regard to the others. There is no true underlying trend.

The graph on the right of Figure 33.4 shows a *rolling average* (adapted from Briggs, 2008). This is also called *smoothing* the data. There are many ways to smooth. For this graph, each value plotted is the average of the number of hurricanes for that year plus the prior 8 years (a rolling average). The idea of smoothing is to reduce the noise so you can see underlying trends. Indeed, the smoothed graph shows a clear upward trend. The R^2 is much higher, and the P value is very low. But this trend is entirely an artifact of smoothing. Calculating the running average makes any random swing to a high or low value look more consistent than it really is, because neighboring values also become low or high.

One of the assumptions of linear regression is that each point contributes independent information. When the data are smoothed, the values are not independent. Accordingly, the regression line is misleading, and the P value and R^2 are meaningless.

Mistake: Fitting data where X and Y are intertwined

When interpreting the results of linear regression, make sure that the X and Y axes represent separate measurements. If the X and Y values are intertwined, the results will be misleading. Here is an example.

Figure 33.5 shows computer-generated data simulating an experiment where blood pressure was measured before and after an experimental intervention.

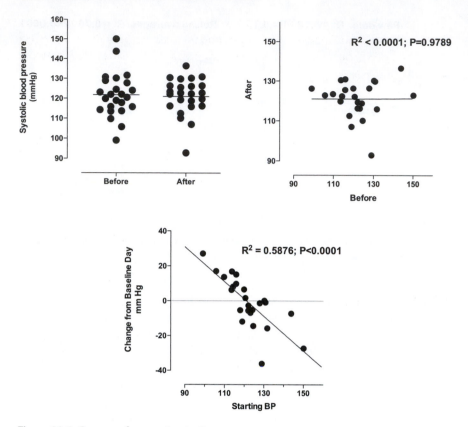

Figure 33.5. Beware of regression to the mean.

(Left) Actual data (which are simulated). The before and after values are indistinguishable. (Middle) Graph of one set of measurements versus the others. There is no trend at all. (Right) Graph of the starting (before) blood pressure versus the change (after–before). The apparent trend is an illusion. All it tells you is that if your blood pressure happens to be very high on one reading, it is likely to be lower on the next. And when it is low on one reading, it is likely to be high on the next. Regressions where X and Y are intertwined like this are not useful.

The graph on the left shows the data. Each point represents an individual whose blood pressure was measured before (X-axis) and after (Y-axis) an intervention. Each value was sampled from a Gaussian distribution with mean = 120 and SD = 10. The data are entirely random, and the two data sets (Figure 33.5, left) look about the same. Therefore, a best-fit regression line (Figure 33.5, middle) is horizontal. Although blood pressure levels varied between measurements, there was no systematic effect of the treatment. The graph on the right shows the same data. But now the vertical axis shows the change in blood pressure (after–before). Note the striking linear relationship. Individuals who initially had low pressures tended to increase; individuals with high pressures tended to decrease. This is entirely an artifact of data analysis and tells you nothing about the effect of the treatment, only about the stability of the blood pressure levels between treatments.

Graphing a change in a variable versus the initial value of the variable is quite misleading. Attributing a significant correlation on such a graph to an experimental intervention is termed the *regression fallacy*. Such a plot should not be analyzed by linear regression because these data (so presented) violate one of the assumptions of linear regression, that the X and Y values were determined independently.

Mistake: Not thinking about which variable is X and which is Y

Unlike correlation, linear regression calculations are not symmetrical with respect to X and Y. Switching the labels X and Y will produce a different regression line (unless the data are perfect, with all points lying directly on the line). This makes sense, because the whole point is to find the line that best predicts Y from X, which is not the same as the line that best predicts X from Y.

Consider the extreme case, when X and Y are not correlated at all. The linear regression line that best predicts Y from X is a horizontal line through the mean Y value. In contrast, the best line to predict X from Y is a vertical line through the mean of all X values, 90° different. With most data, the two lines are far closer than that, but are not the same.

Mistake: Looking at numerical results of regression without viewing a graph

Figure 33.6 shows four linear regressions designed by Anscombe (1973). The best-fit values of the slopes are identical for all four data sets. The best-fit values of the Y intercept are also identical. Even the R^2 values are identical. But a glance at the graph shows you that the data are very different!

Mistake: Using standard unweighted linear regression when scatter increases as Y increases

It is common for biological data to violate the assumption that variability is the same for all values of Y. Instead, it is common for variability to be proportional to Y. Few linear regression programs can handle this situation, but most nonlinear regressions can. If you want to fit a linear model to data where scatter increases with Y, use a nonlinear regression program to fit a straight line model and choose to weight the data points to account for unequal variation (see Chapter 36).

Mistake: Extrapolating beyond the data

The best-fit values of slope and intercept define a linear equation that defines Y for any value of X. So, for the example, it is easy enough to plug numbers in to

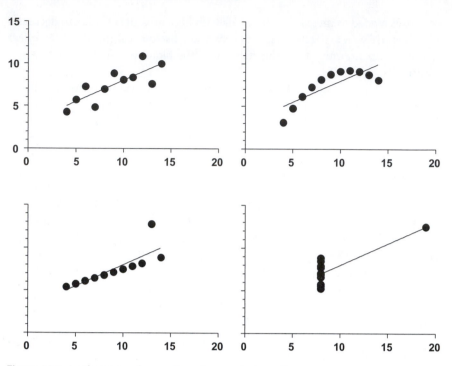

Figure 33.6. Look at a graph as well as at numerical results.
The linear regressions of these four data sets all have identical best-fit values for slope, best-fit value for the Y intercept, and R^2. Yet the data are far from identical.

the equation and predict what Y (glucose sensitivity) would be if X (lipid composition as %C20–22) were 100%. But the data were only collected with X values between 18 and 24, and there is no reason to think that the linear relationship would continue much beyond the range of the data. Predictions substantially beyond that range are likely to be very wrong.

Figure 33.7 shows why you must beware predictions that go beyond the range of the data. The top graph shows data that are fit by a linear regression model very well. The data range from X = 1 to X = 15.

The bottom graphs predict will happen at later times. The left graph on the bottom shows the prediction of linear regression. The other two graphs show predictions of two other models. Each of these models actually fit the data slightly better than does linear regression, so the R^2 values are slightly higher. The three models make very different predictions at late time points. Which prediction is most likely to be correct? It is impossible to answer that question without more data or at least information and theory about the scientific context. The predictions of linear regression, far beyond the data, may be very wrong.

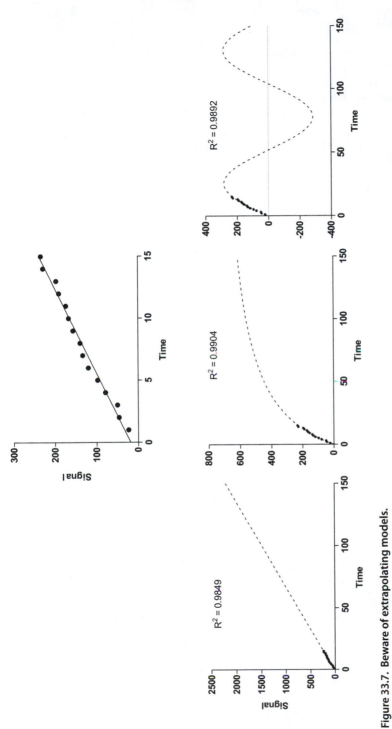

Figure 33.7. Beware of extrapolating models.

(Top) Data that fit a linear regression model very well. What happens at later time points? The three graphs on the bottom show three alternative predictions. (Left) The prediction of linear regression. (Middle and right) Predictions of two other models that actually fit the data slightly better than a straight line does. The predictions of linear regression, far beyond the data, may be very wrong.

Q & A: Linear Regression

Do the X and Y values have to have the same units to perform linear regression?	No, but they can. In the example, X and Y are in different units.
Can linear regression work when all X values are the same? When all Y values are the same?	No. The whole point of linear regression is to predict Y based on X. If all X values are the same, they won't help predict Y. If all Y values are the same, there is nothing to predict.
Can linear regression be used when the X values are actually categories?	If you are comparing two groups, you can assign the groups to $X = 1$ and $X = 0$ and use linear regression. This is identical to performing an unpaired t test, as will be explained in Chapter 35. If there are more than two groups, using simple linear regression only makes sense when the groups are ordered and equally spaced, so they can be assigned sensible numbers. If you need to use a categorical variable with more than two possible values, read about indicator variables (also called dummy variables) in a text about multiple linear regression.
Is the standard error of the slope the same as the SEM?	No. The standard error is a way to express the precision of a computed value (parameter). The first standard error encountered in this book happened to be the standard error of the mean (Chapter 14). The standard error of a slope is quite different. Standard errors can also be computed for almost any other parameter.
What does the variable $\hat{Y}$ (used in other statistics books) mean?	More mathematical books distinguish between the Y values of the data you collected from the Y values predicted by the model. The actual Y values are called Y_i, where i indicates which value you are referring to. For example, Y_3 is the actual Y value of the third subject or data point. The Y values predicted by the model are called $\hat{Y}$, pronounced "Y hat." So $\hat{Y}_3$ is the value the model predicts for the third subject or data point. That value is predicted from the X value for the third data point, but doesn't take into account the actual value of Y.
Will the regression line be the same if you exchange X and Y?	Linear regression fits a model that best predicts Y from X. If you swap the definitions of X and Y, the regression line will be different unless the data points line up perfectly, so every point is on the line. However, swapping X and Y will not change the value of R^2.

Continued

Q&A Continued

Can R^2 ever be 0? Negative?	It will equal 0 if there is no trend whatsoever between X and Y, so the best-fit line is exactly horizontal. R^2 cannot be negative with linear regression, but Chapter 36 explains that R^2 can be negative with nonlinear regression.
Do you need more than one Y value for each X value to calculate linear regression? Does it help?	Linear regression does not require more than one Y value for each X value. If you have collected replicate Y values at each X, additional calculations (not explained in this book) can test whether the data are best fit by a straight line. This test compares the variation among replicates with the distances of the points from the regression line. If your points are "too far" from the line (given the consistency of the replicates) then the P value will be small, which is evidence that the relationship between X and Y is not linear.

CHAPTER 34

Introducing Models

A mathematical model is neither a hypothesis nor a theory.
Unlike scientific hypotheses, a model is not verifiable directly
by an experiment. For all models are both true and false.... The
validation of a model is not that it is "true" but that it generates
good testable hypotheses relevant to important problems.

R. LEVINS (1966)

*Chapter 33 explained how linear regression fits a simple model to
data. This chapter generalizes the concept of fitting a model to data.
The goal in fitting a model is to find the best-fit values of the parameters
that define the model. It is essential to understand these basic ideas of
fitting models, before reading about the various kinds of regression in
Chapters 35–39.*

LINGO: MODELS, PARAMETERS, AND VARIABLES

Model

In general, a model is a representation of something else. We study models
because they are less expensive and more accessible than the real thing, and easier to manipulate (perhaps with fewer ethical issues).

A *mathematical model* is an equation or set of equations that describe, represent, or approximate a physical, chemical, or biological state or process. Using a
model can help you think about chemical and physiological processes or mecha-
nisms, so you can design better experiments and comprehend the results.

Your goal in using a model is not necessarily to describe your system perfectly. A perfect model may have too many parameters and variables to be useful. Rather, your goal is to find as simple a model as possible that comes close to
describing your system for your intended purpose. You want a model to be simple
enough so it is easy to collect enough data to fit the model to, yet complicated
enough to do a good job of explaining the data. It is common for new fields of
science to begin with simple models and then gradually use more and more complicated models as the systems are better understood.

Creating new useful models from general principles is very difficult. In contrast, fitting models to data (a major theme of this book) and

simulating data from models (a minor theme of this book) are much easier tasks.

When you fit a model to your data, you obtain best-fit values (parameter estimates) that you can interpret in the context of the model.

Random component

A mathematical model must specify both the ideal predictions and how the data will be randomly scattered around those predictions. The following two equivalent, crude equations point out that a full model must specify a random component (noise) as well as the ideal component (signal).

Data = Ideal + Random
Response = Signal + Noise

Parameters, statistics, and variables

A model is defined by an equation, or a set of equations. The equation defines the outcome, called the *dependent variable*, as a function of one or more *independent variables*, one or more *parameters*, and often one or more true constants. The model in Chapter 33 defined insulin sensitivity (the independent variable) as a function of %C20–22 (the independent variable) and the slope and intercepts (the parameters). It had no true constants.

When fitting a model, you provide the computer program with a set of dependent and independent values, and then the program finds the values of the parameters that make the model do the best possible job of predicting the dependent variable. The true constants, such as 1, 2, 0.693, π, etc., just come along for the ride and provide structure to the mathematical model.

Note that each data point has its own values for the independent and dependent variables. The population has one set of true parameters, which are unknown. Fitting the model to sample data generates an estimated value for each parameter in the model, along with a CI for each parameter.

The values of each parameter are given several interchangeable names: parameter estimates, best-fit values of parameters, and sample statistics (distinct from population parameters).

Estimate

When regression is used to fit a model to data, it reports values for each parameter in the model. These can be called best-fit values or "estimated" values. Note that this use of the term *estimate* is very different than the word's conventional use to mean an informed guess. The estimates provided by regression are the results of calculations. The best-fit value is called a *point estimate*. The CI for each parameter is called an *interval estimate*.

Fitting a model to data

Regression fits a model to data. It does this by adjusting the values of the parameters in the model to make the predictions of the model come as close as possible to the actual data, taking into account the mathematical model for random error (a Gaussian distribution in the case of linear regression).

Note that regression does not fit data to a model, a phrase that implies fudging the data to make it comply with the predictions of the model. The model is fit to the data.

Think of models as shoes in a shoe store and data as the pair of feet that you bring into the store. The shoe salesman fits a set of shoes of varying styles, lengths, and widths (parameter estimates) to your feet to find a good, comfortable fit. The salesman does not bring over one pair of universal shoes along with surgical tools to fit your feet to the shoes.

THE SIMPLEST MODEL

To compute an average, add up all the values and then divide by the number of values. That average, also called a mean, is a way to describe a stack of numbers with a single value. But what makes an average special?

When you sample values from a population that follows a Gaussian distribution, each value can be defined by this simple model:

$$Y = \mu + \varepsilon.$$

Y is the dependent variable, which is different for each value (data point).

μ (the population mean) is a parameter with a single value (which you are trying to find out). It is traditional to use Greek letters to denote population parameters and regular letters to denote sample statistics.

ε (random error) is different for each data point, randomly drawn from a Gaussian distribution centered at zero. Thus, ε is equally likely to be positive or negative, so each Y is equally likely to be higher or lower than μ. The random variable is often referred to as "error". As used in this statistical context, the term *error* refers to any random variability, whether caused by experimental imprecision or by biological variation.

This kind of model is often written like this:

$$Y_i = \mu + \varepsilon_i.$$

The subscript i tells you that each Y and ε has a different value, but the population parameter μ has only a single value.

Note that the right side of this model equation has two parts. The first part computes the *expected* value of Y. In this case, it is always equal to the parameter μ, the population mean. More complicated models would have more complicated calculations here, involving more than one parameter. The second part of the model takes into account the random error. In this model, the random scatter follows a Gaussian distribution and is centered at zero. This is a pretty standard assumption, but is not the only model of scatter.

Now you have a set of values, and you are willing to assume that this model is correct. You don't know the population value of μ, but you want to determine its value from the sample of data. What value of the parameter μ is most likely to be correct? Mathematicians have proven that if the random scatter follows a Gaussian distribution, then the value of μ that is most likely to be correct is the sample mean or average. To use some mathematical lingo, the mean is the *maximum likelihood estimate* of μ.

What I've done so far is to take the simple idea of computing the average and turn it into a complicated process using statistical jargon and Greek letters. This doesn't help you understand the idea of a sample mean, but it warms you up for understanding more complicated models, where the jargon really is helpful.

THE LINEAR REGRESSION MODEL

Recall the linear regression example of Chapter 33. The investigators were curious to understand why insulin sensitivity varies so much among individuals. They measured insulin sensitivity in 13 men, and also measured the lipid content of muscle obtained at biopsy. To find out how much insulin sensitivity increases for every percentage point increase in C20–22, linear regression was used to fit this model to the data:

Y = intercept + slope $\times$ X + scatter.

This equation describes a straight line. It defines the dependent variable Y (insulin sensitivity) as a function of the independent variable X (%C20–22), two parameters (the slope and Y intercept), and scatter (a random factor). It can be rewritten in a more standard mathematical form:

$$Y_i = \beta_0 + \beta_1 \times X_i + \varepsilon_i$$

The intercept (β_0) and slope (β_1) are parameters that each have a single true underlying population value. In contrast, the random component of the model takes on a different value for each data point. These random values are assumed to follow a Gaussian distribution with a mean of 0. Any point is just as likely to be above the line as below it, but more likely to be close to the line than far from it. Remember that the term *error* refers to any random variability, whether caused by experimental imprecision or biological variation.

Note that this model is very simple and certainly not 100% correct. Although data were only collected with X values ranging from 18 to 24, the model predicts Y values for any value of X. Predictions beyond the range of the data are unlikely to be accurate or useful. This model even predicts Y values when X has values outside the range 0–100, although X quantifies the percentage of lipid that is C20–22, so values outside the range of 0 to 100% make no sense at all. Furthermore, the model assumes Gaussian random scatter. As discussed earlier in Chapter 10, this assumption is never 100% true.

It's OK that the model is simple and cannot possibly be 100% accurate. That is the nature of scientific models. If a model is too simple, it won't provide useful results. If a model is too complicated, it won't be possible to collect enough data to fit all the parameters. Useful models are simple, but not too simple.

WHY LEAST SQUARES?

Linear regression finds the "best" values of the slope and intercept by minimizing the sum of the squares of the vertical distances of the points from the line. Why minimize the sum of the squared distances rather than the sum of the absolute values of the distances?

This question can't really be answered without delving into math, but the answer is related to the assumption that the random scatter follows a Gaussian distribution.

If the goal were to minimize the sum of the distances, the regression would be indifferent to fitting a model where the distances of two points from the line are each 5.0, versus a model where the distances are 1.0 and 9.0. The sum of the distances equals 10.0 in both cases. But if the scatter is Gaussian, the first model is far more likely, so the model that places the line equidistant from both points should be preferred. Minimizing the sum of squares accomplishes this. The sums of squares from the two models are 50 and 82, so minimizing the sum of squares makes the first model preferable.

A more rigorous answer is that the regression line determined by the least-squares method is identical to the line determined by maximum likelihood calculations. What does that mean? Given any hypothetical set of parameter values, it is possible to compute the chance of observing our particular data. Maximum likelihood methods find the set of parameter values for which the observed data are most probable.

Given the assumption that scatter follows a Gaussian distribution (with a uniform standard deviation), it can be proven that the maximum likelihood approach leads to identical results as does minimizing the sum of the squares. More simply (perhaps a bit too simple), minimizing the sum of squares finds values for the parameters that are most likely to be correct.

OTHER MODELS AND OTHER KINDS OF REGRESSION

Regression includes a large family of techniques beyond linear regression:

- Nonlinear regression (Chapter 36). Like linear regression, Y is a measured variable, and there is a single X variable. But, a graph of X versus Y is curved, and the model has a nonlinear relationship between the parameters and Y.
- Multiple linear regression (Chapter 37). "Multiple" means there are two or more independent X variables.
- Multiple nonlinear regression.
- Logistic regression (Chapter 37). Here, Y is a binary variable (or proportion) such as infected/not infected or cancer/no cancer. There may be only

one X variable, but logistic regression is more commonly used with several X values.

- Proportional hazards regression. Here, the outcome is survival time. There may be only one X variable, but proportional hazards regression is more commonly used with several X variables.
- Poisson regression. The outcomes are counts that follow a Poisson distribution (Chapter 6).

CHAPTER 35

—✦—

Comparing Models

Beware of geeks bearing formulas.
WARREN BUFFETT

A t first glance, comparing the fit of two models seems simple. Just choose the model whose predictions come closer to the data. In fact, choosing a model is more complicated than that, and requires accounting for both the number of parameters and the goodness of fit. The concept of comparing models provides an alternative perspective for understanding much of statistics.

COMPARING MODELS IS A MAJOR PART OF STATISTICS

So far, this book has explained the concepts of P values and hypothesis testing in the context of comparing two groups. Statistics is used in many other situations, and many of these can be thought of as comparing the fits of two models. Chapter 36 will briefly explain how to compare the fits of two different nonlinear models. Chapters 37–39 explain multiple regression models (including logistic and proportional hazards regression) and a major part of these analyses involves comparing alternative models. One-way ANOVA, explained in Chapter 40, can also be thought of as comparing models.

To set the stage for these later chapters, this chapter looks back at linear regression (Chapter 33) and the unpaired t test (Chapter 30), and presents them as a comparison of models.

What's so hard about comparing models? It seems as though the answer is simple: Pick the one that comes closest to the data. In fact, that approach is not useful, because models with more parameters almost always fit the sample data better, but don't reflect what is actually going on in the population. A useful comparison must also take into account the number of parameters fit by each model.

A model with too few parameters won't fit the sample data well. A model with too many parameters will fit the sample data well, but the CIs of the parameters will be wide. If the goal of the model is to predict future values, a model with too many parameters won't make precise predictions. If the goal of the model is

276

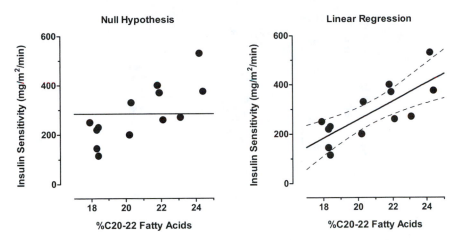

Figure 35.1. Fitting the sample data with two alternative models.

to obtain parameter values that can be interpreted scientifically, fitting a model with too many parameters leads to estimated parameter values that are very uncertain (wide CIs).

LINEAR REGRESSION AS COMPARISON OF MODELS

Chapter 33 explained how to informally interpret the P value and R^2 from linear regression. Here we use the same example (insulin sensitivity), but switch the focus to comparing two models:

- The linear regression model is shown (again) on the right of Figure 35.1. The right side of Figure 35.2 shows the variability of points around the linear regression line. Each point in the graph shows the vertical distance of a point from the regression line. Points above the horizontal line at zero represent points that are above the regression line, whereas points below that line represent points that are below the regression line.
- The alternative, null hypothesis model is a horizontal line. The left side of Figure 35.1 shows the horizontal line fit through the data. The left side of Figure 35.2 shows how well the null hypothesis model fits the data. Each point in the graph shows the difference between a Y value and the mean of all Y values. Points above the horizontal line at zero represent Y values that are greater than the mean, and points below that horizontal line represent Y values that are less than the mean.

The meaning of R^2

The linear regression model fits the data better. The variability of points around the regression line (right side of Figure 35.1) is less than the variability of points around the null hypothesis horizontal line (left side of Figure 35.1).

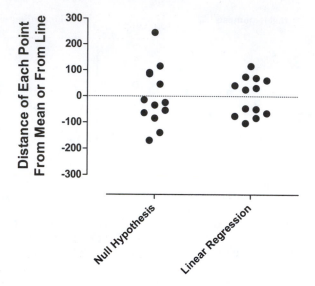

Figure 35.2. Residuals (distance from line) of each point from both models. The Y-axis has the same units as the Y-axis of Figure 35.1.

HYPOTHESIS	SCATTER FROM	SUM OF SQUARES	PERCENTAGE OF VARIATION	
Null	Horizontal line	155,642	100.0	
Alternative	Regression line	63,361	40.7	
Difference	Improvement	92,281	59.3	$R^2 = 0.593$

Table 35.1. Comparing the fit of a horizontal line versus the best-fit linear regression line.

The points are closer to the regression line, so the sum of squares is lower.

How much less?

Table 35.1 compares the sum of squares. The first row shows the sum of the squared distances of points from the horizontal line that is the null hypothesis. The second row shows the sum of the squared distances of points from the linear regression line.

The regression line fits the data better than a horizontal line, so the sum of squares is lower. The bottom row in Table 35.1 shows the difference between the fit of the two models. It shows how much better the linear regression model fits.

The fourth column shows the two sums of squares as a percentage of the total. Scatter around the regression line accounts for 40.7% of the variation. Therefore, the linear regression line model itself accounts for 100%−40.7% = 59.3% of the variation. This is the definition of R^2, which equals 0.593.

SOURCE OF VARIATION	SUM OF SQUARES	DF	MS	F RATIO
Regression	92,281	1	92281.0	16.0
Random	63,361	11	5760.1	
Total	155,642	12		

Table 35.2. Comparing the fit of a horizontal line versus the best-fit linear regression line.

The points are closer to the regression line, so the F ratio is high. Table 35.2 uses the format of ANOVA, which will be explained in Chapter 39.

P value

Table 35.2 is labeled to match other statistics books and programs. Note that the order of the rows is also changed. The focus is no longer on comparing the fit of two models, but on dividing the total sum of squares into its components. The first row quantifies how well the linear regression model explains the data. The second row quantifies the scatter of data around the predictions of the model. The third row quantifies the scatter of the data from the predictions (horizontal line) of the null hypothesis.

The important point is that overall variation among data points is quantified with the sum of the squared distances between the point and a prediction of a model and that the sum of squares can be divided into various sources of variation.

The third column of Table 35.2 shows the number of degrees of freedom (df). The bottom row shows the sum of squares of the distances from the fit of the null hypothesis model. There are 13 data points and only 1 parameter is fit (the mean), which leaves 12 df. The next row up shows the sum of squares from the linear regression line. Two parameters are fit (slope and intercept), so there are 11 degrees of freedom (13 data points minus 2 parameters). The top row shows the difference. The linear regression model has one more parameter than the null hypothesis model, so there is only 1 df in this row. The df, like the sums of squares, can be partitioned so the bottom row is the sum of values in the rows above.

The fourth column of Table 35.2 divides the sums of squares by the number of df to compute the mean square (MS), which could also be called variances. Note that it is not possible to add the MS in the top two rows to obtain the MS in the bottom row.

Even if the null hypothesis were correct, you'd expect the sum of squares around the regression line to be a bit smaller than the sum of squares around the horizontal null hypothesis line. Dividing by the number of df accounts for this difference. If the null hypothesis were true, the ratio of the two MS values would be expected to have similar values, so their ratio would be close to 1.0. In fact, for this example the ratio equals 16.0.

This ratio of the two MS values is called the F ratio, named after the pioneering statistician, Ronald Fisher. The distribution of F ratios is known when the null hypothesis is true. So for any value of F, and for particular values of the two df values, a P value can be computed. When using a program to find the P value from F, be sure to distinguish the df of the numerator (1 in this example) and the df for the denominator (11 in this example). If you mix up those two df values, you'll get the wrong P.

The P value, which you already saw in Chapter 30, is 0.0021. From the point of view of probability distributions, this P value answers the following question:

> If the null hypothesis were true, and given an experimental design with 1 and
> 11 df, what is the chance that random sampling would result in data with such
> a strong linear trend that the F ratio would be 16.0 or higher?

UNPAIRED t TEST RECAST AS COMPARING
THE FIT OF TWO MODELS

Chapter 30 explained how to compare the means of two unpaired groups with an unpaired t test. Here we present that same example (bladder relaxation in young and old rats), with a different mindset—comparing the fit of the data to two models.

Unpaired t test as linear regression

To view the unpaired t test as a comparison of the fits of two models, consider it a special case of linear regression.

The example compares two groups, old and young. Lets call the variable that defines age X, and assign X = 0 to the old group and X = 1 to the young group (those values are arbitrary). Figure 35.3 shows the data analyzed by linear regression.

The slope of the regression line is the increase in Y when the X value increases by 1 unit. The X values denoting old and young groups are 1 unit apart, so the slope of the best-fit regression line equals the difference between means. The best-fit value of the slope is 23.5%, with a 95% CI ranging from 9.338% to 37.75%. These values match the results reported by the unpaired t test.

The P value from linear regression tests the null hypothesis that the slope is horizontal. This is another way to state the null hypothesis of the unpaired t test (that the two populations share the same mean). Because the two null hypotheses are equivalent, the P value determined by linear regression (0.0030) is identical to the P value reported by the t test.

Goodness of fit and R^2

The top row of the Table 35.3 and the left side of Figure 35.4 quantify how well the null hypothesis model (a horizontal line) fits the data. Goodness of fit is quantified by the sum of squares of the difference between each value and the grand mean (totally ignoring any distinction between the two groups). Figure 35.4 plots the distance of each value from the grand mean, and Table 35.3 shows the sum of squares.

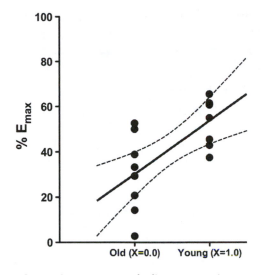

Figure 35.3. Comparing two groups by linear regression.

The data are maximal bladder relaxation in percent, as explained in Chapter 30. The two groups were assigned arbitrary X values, and the data were fit by linear regression. The best-fit slope of the regression line equals the difference between the two group means, and the CI of the slope equals the CI for the difference between two means. Linear regression reports a two-tail P value, testing the null hypothesis that the true slope is 0.

	HYPOTHESIS	SCATTER FROM	SUM OF SQUARES	PERCENTAGE OF VARIATION	
	Null	Grand mean	5,172	100.0	
−	Alternative	Group means	2,824	54.6	
=	Difference	Improvement	2,348	45.4	$R^2 = 0.454$

Table 35.3. The t test example of Chapter 30 recast as a comparison of models.

Values are closer to their group means than the grand mean, so the sum of squares of the alternative hypothesis is lower.

The second row of Table 35.3 and the right side of Figure 35.4 show how well the alternative hypothesis fits the data. Figure 35.4 plots the distance of each value from its own group mean, and Table 35.3 reports the sum of squares of the difference between each value and the mean of the group that value came from.

The third row shows the difference in variation. Of all the variation (sum of squares from the null hypothesis grand mean), 54.6% is caused by scatter within the groups, and 45.5% of the total variation is caused by a difference between the two group means. Therefore, $R^2 = 0.454$.

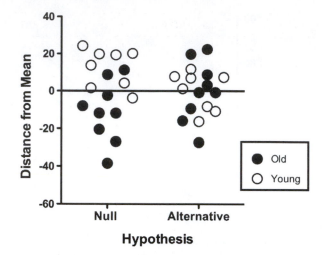

Figure 35.4. How well the t test example data fit the two models.
(Left) The fit of the model defined by the null hypothesis that both
groups share the same population mean showing the difference
between each value and the grand mean. (Right) How well the data fit
the alternative model that the groups have different population means.
This part of the graph shows the difference between each value and the
mean of its group.

P value

Determining the P value requires more than partitioning the variance into its
components. It also requires accounting for the number of values and the number of parameters fit by each model.

The third column of Table 35.4 shows the number of df. The bottom row
shows the fit of the null hypothesis model. There are 17 data points and only 1
parameter is fit (the grand mean), which leaves 16 df. The next row up quantifies
the fit of the alternative model. Two parameters are fit (the mean of each group),
so there are 15 df (17 data points minus 2 parameters). The top row shows the
difference. The alternative model (two distinct means) has one more parameter
than the null hypothesis model (one mean for both groups), so there is only 1 df
in this row. The df, like the sum of squares, can be partitioned so the bottom row
is the sum of values in the two rows above. The fourth column divides the sum
of squares by the number of df to compute the MS, which could also be called
variance. Note that it is not possible to add the MS in the top two rows to obtain
the MS in the bottom row.

If the null hypothesis were correct, you'd expect the sum of squares around
the individual means to be a bit smaller than the sum of squares around the grand
mean. But after dividing by df, the MS values would be expected to be about the
same if the null hypothesis is in fact true. Therefore, if the null hypothesis were

SOURCE OF VARIATION	SUM OF SQUARES	DF	MS	F RATIO	P VALUE
Between groups	2,348	1	2348.0	12.47	0.0030
Within groups	2,824	15	188.3		
Total	5,172	16			

Table 35.4. The t test example of Chapter 30 recast as a comparison of models.

Values are closer to their group means than the grand mean, so the F ratio is high and the P value is low.

true, the ratio of the two MS values would be expected to be close to 1.0. If fact, for this example, the ratio (called the F ratio) equals 12.47.

The F distribution under the null hypothesis is known, and so the P value can be computed. The P value is 0.0030. It is the answer to the following question:

> If the simpler (null hypothesis) model were correct, what is the chance that randomly chosen values would have group means far enough apart to yield a F ratio of 12.47 or higher.

Summary

The t test data can be viewed as comparing how well the data are fit by two models. One model is the null hypothesis—that the two groups of data are sampled from two populations with the same mean. Viewed in terms of linear regression, this model is a horizontal line with a slope equal to 0.0. The alternative model is that the population means differ. Viewed as linear regression, the slope is not zero. The goodness of fit of the two models is compared to see whether there is substantial evidence to reject the simpler (null hypothesis) model and accept the more complicated alternative model.

COMMON MISTAKES: COMPARING MODELS

Mistake: Comparing the fits of models that don't make scientific sense

Only use a statistical approach to compare models that are scientifically sensible. It rarely makes sense to blindly test a huge number of models. If a model isn't scientifically sensible, it probably won't be useful—no matter how high its R^2 for a particular data set.

Mistake: Using the F test method to compare unrelated models

The approach described in this chapter can only compare two related models. One model must be a simpler case of the other. The linear regression example does compare two related models, because the null hypothesis model is the same as the other model with the slope fixed to equal zero. Another way to say this is that the two models are nested. Nonnested models can be compared, but require methods that are beyond the scope of this book. To learn about alternative methods, start by reading Burnham and Anderson (2003).

Mistake: Comparing the fits of models whose predictions are indistinguishable in the range of the data

Figure 33.7 shows the predictions of three alternative models (straight line, hyperbola, and sine wave). In the range of the data ($X < 15$), the three models are indistinguishable. If you had scientific reason to compare the fits of these models, you'd be stuck. Spending your time struggling with statistical software wouldn't help a bit. The data simply cannot distinguish those three models.

At larger X values ($X > 15$), the predictions of the models diverge considerably. If you had reason to compare those models, it would be essential to collect data at X values (times) where the models predict substantially different outcomes (Y values).

Perspective

The alphabet soup of this chapter—SS, MS, df, F—can be overwhelming. Don't lose sight of the big picture. Every P value can be viewed as the result of comparing the fit of two models. One model is the null hypothesis. The other model is a more general alternative hypothesis. The P value answers the question: If the null hypothesis were really true, what is the chance that the data would be fit by the alternative model so much better? Interpreting P values is easy if you can identify the two models being compared.

CHAPTER 36

Nonlinear Regression

Models should be as simple as possible, but not more so.

A. EINSTEIN

Nonlinear regression is more general than linear regression. It can fit any equation that defines Y as a function of X and one or more parameters. The goal of nonlinear regression is to find the parameter values that generate the curve that comes closest to the data. Nonlinear regression is a topic excluded from most introductory statistics books, but it is a commonly used statistical method in many fields of science (such as pharmacology). Don't skip this chapter because it seems advanced and complicated. In fact, analyzing data with nonlinear regression is not much harder than using linear regression. Be sure to read Chapters 33 (linear regression) and 35 (comparing models) before reading this one.

FITTING A MODEL

Chapters 11 and 30 have already discussed data from Frazier et al. (2006), who measured the degree to which the neurotransmitter norepinephrine relaxes bladder muscle in old and young rats. Strips of bladder muscle were exposed to various concentrations of norepinephrine, and muscle relaxation was measured. The data from each rat were analyzed to determine the maximum relaxation and the concentration of norepinephrine that relaxes the muscle half that much (EC_{50}).

Table 36.1 and Figure 36.1 show the data from one young rat. Note that the X-axis of Figure 36.1 is logarithmic. Going from left to right, each tick on the axis represents a concentration of norepinephrine 10-fold higher than the previous tick.

The first step in fitting a model is choosing a model. In many cases, like this one, a standard model will work fine. Pharmacologists commonly model dose-response (or concentration-effect) relationships using the equation below.

$$Y = \text{Bottom} + \frac{\text{Top} - \text{Bottom}}{1 + 10^{(\text{LogEC50} - X) \cdot \text{HillSlope}}}$$

To enter this equation in a computer program, use the syntax below. Note that 2*3 means multiply 2 times 3, and 2^3 means take 2 to the third power.

Y = Bottom + (Top − Bottom)/(1 + 10^((LogEC50 − X)*HillSlope))

LOG[NOREPINEPHRINE, M]	% RELAXATION
−8.0	2.6
−7.5	10.5
−7.0	15.8
−6.5	21.1
−6.0	36.8
−5.5	57.9
−5.0	73.7
−4.5	89.5
−4.0	94.7
−3.5	100.0
−3.0	100.0

Table 36.1. Bladder muscle relaxation data for one young rat.

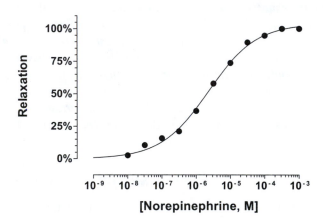

Figure 36.1. Bladder muscle relaxation data for one young rat.
The circles show the data from Table 36.1. The curve was fit by nonlinear regression.

In this equation, X represents the logarithm of the concentration of norepinephrine and Y is the response the investigators measured, the amount of muscle relaxation. Y is defined as a function of X and four parameters:

- Bottom. The value of Y when X is very low. This is the baseline value of Y when there is no drug added.
- Top. The value of Y when X is very high. As the concentration gets higher and higher, the response plateaus at a value called Top.
- $logEC_{50}$. The value of X (the logarithm of concentration) that provokes a response halfway between Bottom and Top.
- HillSlope. A measure of how steep the curve is. The two words ("Hill" and "slope") are smashed together to form a single parameter in the equation.

BEST-FIT VALUES

Bottom	=0.0
Top	104
$LogEC_{50}$	−5.64
HillSlope	0.622
EC_{50}	2.30e−006

STANDARD ERRORS

Top	2.06
$LogEC_{50}$	0.0515
HillSlope	0.0358

95% CI

Top	99.3 to 109
$LogEC_{50}$	−5.76 to −5.52
HillSlope	0.540 to 0.705
EC_{50}	1.75e−006 to 3.02e−006

GOODNESS OF FIT

df	8
R squared	0.997
Absolute sum of squares	43.0

Table 36.2. Results of nonlinear regression as reported by GraphPad Prism.

After choosing a model, the next step is to decide which of the parameters in the model should be fit to the data and which should be fixed to constant values. In this case, muscle relaxation must be zero with no added norepinephrine. So we'll tell the program not to find a best-fit value of Bottom, but rather to set it to a constant value of 0.0. We don't want to fix the top to 100, because the one goal of the study is to see whether that top plateau differs in old and young rats.

Once you pick the model (and choose which parameters to fit), the program is ready to go. The results calculated by GraphPad Prism are shown as the curve in Figure 36.1 and Table 36.2.

WEIGHTING

Regression usually assumes that scatter is the same, on average, in all parts of the curve. When this assumption is true, the best curve is found by minimizing the sum of squares of the vertical distances of the data from the line or curve.

In many experimental situations, you expect the average distance (or rather, the average absolute value of the distance) of the points from the curve to be higher when Y is higher. The points with the larger scatter would have much larger sum of squares and thus would dominate the calculations. To restore equal *weight* to all the data points, weighted nonlinear regression accounts for the expected inequality of scatter.

The most common form of weighted nonlinear regression assumes that the average scatter of points from the curve is proportional to Y. Although the average distance of the points from the curve is not consistent (it is larger where the curve goes higher), the average *relative* distance of points from the curve is consistent on average. Thus, weighted nonlinear regression doesn't minimize the sum of squares the actual distances of the points from the curve, but rather sums the squares of the relative distances.

HOW NONLINEAR REGRESSION WORKS

Both linear and nonlinear regression find the values of the parameters that make a model come as close as possible to the data. Linear regression fits one simple model. Nonlinear regression can fit any model you choose. Linear regression can be thought of as a special case of nonlinear regression.

Although linear and nonlinear regression have the same goal, they work differently. The linear regression method can be completely explained with simple algebra. In contrast, nonlinear regression uses a computationally intensive approach that can only be explained using calculus and matrix algebra.

Nonlinear regression works via an iterative or stepwise approach. The method is initially provided with an estimated value for each parameter. Nonlinear regression programs may provide these values automatically, or you may need to enter them yourself. The idea is to generate a an initial curve that goes somewhere in the vicinity of the data points. The nonlinear regression method then changes the values of the parameters to move the curve closer to the points. Then it changes the values again. It repeats, or iterates, these steps many times. That is why the method is called *iterative*. When any possible changes to the parameters would make the curve fit more poorly (or fit the same), the method finishes and reports the results.

Because the foundations of nonlinear regression cannot be understood without using matrix algebra and calculus, nonlinear regression has a reputation of being complicated and advanced. But this only applies to the mathematical foundation of the method. Using a nonlinear regression program and interpreting the results is just a tiny bit harder than using linear regression.

NONLINEAR REGRESSION RESULTS

Interpreting nonlinear regression results is quite straightforward. The whole point of nonlinear regression is to fit a curve to the data, so first look at the curve (Figure 36.1) and then look at the numerical results (Table 36.2).

Best-fit values of parameters
The best-fit values of the parameters should be interpreted in a scientific context.

For the bladder-relaxation example, let's focus only on the $logEC_{50}$. The program fits the $logEC_{50}$, and also transforms it back to the EC_{50}, which is reported as 2.3e–006. This notation is commonly used by many programs and means 2.3×10 to the power of -6. Because X values were the logarithms of concentration in molar, the $logEC_{50}$ is also expressed as the log of molar, and therefore the EC_{50} is in molar units (M). The best-fit EC_{50} is 0.0000023 M, which can also be written as 2.3 μM. This concentration of norepinephrine relaxes the bladder muscle half as much as the maximum possible relaxation.

CI of the parameters

The program also reports the standard error and the 95% CI of each parameter. The CIs are much easier to interpret and are an essential part of the nonlinear regression results. Given all the assumptions of the analysis (listed on the next page), you can be 95% confident that the interval contains the true parameter value.

The 95% CI for the $logEC_{50}$ ranges from –5.76 to –5.52. Pharmacologists are accustomed to thinking in log units of concentration. Most people prefer to see the values in concentration units. The 95% CI of the EC_{50} ranges from 1.75 to 3.02 μM. The CI is fairly narrow, and shows us that the EC_{50} has been determined to within a factor of two. That is more than satisfactory for this kind of experiment.

If the CI had been very wide, then you would not have determined the parameter very precisely, and would not be able to interpret its value. How wide is too wide? It depends on the context and goals of the experiment.

R^2

R^2 is the fraction of the total variance of Y that is explained by the model. In this example, the curve comes very close to all the data points so the R^2 is very high, 0.997.

When $R^2 = 0.0$, the best-fit curve fits the data no better than a horizontal line at the mean of all Y values. When $R^2 = 1.0$, the best-fit curve fits the data perfectly, going through every point. If you happened to fit a really bad model (maybe you made a mistake when choosing a model in a nonlinear regression program), R^2 can be negative. That tells you that the selected model fits the data more poorly than a horizontal line at the mean of all Y values.

Upper or lower case? With linear regression, you'll see both r^2 and R^2. This is just a matter of style, with no distinction. With nonlinear and multiple regression, it is always written R^2.

How high should R^2 be? There are no general guidelines. If you are performing a routine set of experiments, you will learn what range of R^2 values to expect, and then can troubleshoot if the value is too low. R^2 can be low for many reasons—the presence of outliers, fitting the wrong model, or the presence lots of experimental or biological variation.

ASSUMPTIONS: NONLINEAR REGRESSION

Assumption: The model is correct

When fitting one model, nonlinear regression assumes the model is correct. The next section explains how to compare the fits of two (or more) models.

Assumption: The independent variable has no variability, or at least much less variability than the dependent variable

This is quite reasonable for most experimental work. For example, there will be (or should be) very little error in pipetting different amounts of drugs into wells of a 96-well plate, or recording the time at which a blood sample is taken.

Assumption: The scatter of data around the curve is Gaussian

Nonlinear regression analysis assumes that the scatter of data around the curve is Gaussian. The CIs and P values cannot be interpreted if the distribution of scatter is far from Gaussian, or if some of the values are outliers from another distribution.

Assumption: The variability is the same everywhere

Nonlinear regression assumes that scatter of points around the best-fit line has the same standard deviation all along the curve. This assumption is referred to as *homoscedasticity*. This assumption is violated if the points with high or low X values tend to be further from the best-fit line that points with low X values. See the discussion of weighting earlier in this chapter.

Assumption: Data points are independent

Regression assumes that each point is randomly situated above or below the true curve and that no factor influences a batch of points collectively.

Assumption: The value of X is not used to compute Y

If the value of X is used to calculate Y (or the value of Y is used to calculate X), then linear regression calculations will be misleading. One example is a Scatchard plot, used by pharmacologists to summarize binding data. The Y value (drug bound to receptors divided by drug free in solution) is calculated from the X value (free drug), so linear regression is not appropriate. If a Scatchard plot is curved, it is a mistake to fit it with nonlinear regression. Instead, fit the raw data.

COMPARING TWO MODELS

Chapter 35 explained the general idea of comparing the fit of two models. Applying this idea to nonlinear regression is straightforward.

Figure 36.2 compares the fit of two dose-response models. The solid curve shows the fit explained above, where the program determined the best-fit value

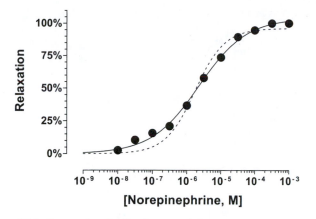

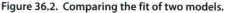

Figure 36.2. Comparing the fit of two models.
The solid curve is the same as Figure 36.1. The Hill slope was fit by non-linear regression and equals 0.622. The data were then fit again, but with the constraint that the Hill slope must equal 1.0. The dotted curve shows this fit, which does not do a good job of fitting the data.

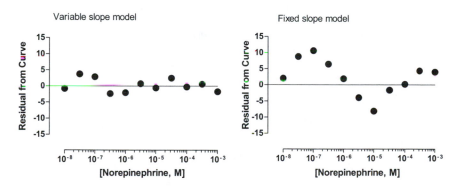

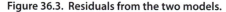

Figure 36.3. Residuals from the two models.
Each circle represents the residual (distance from the curve) of one data point. (Left) The residuals from the fit shown in Figure 37.1, with the Hill slope fit by nonlinear regression (variable slope). (Right) The residuals from the dotted curve of Figure 37.2, where the Hill slope was fixed to a standard value of 1.0.

of the Hill slope (0.622). The dotted curve represents a fit to a simpler model, where the Hill slope was fixed to a standard value of 1.0. It is obvious that this curve does not fit the data very well.

Figure 36.3 shows the residuals of the data points from each curve. You can see that the residuals from the fixed-slope model are, on average, much larger. You can also see that the residuals from that fit (on the right) are not random. In contrast, the residuals from the variable slope model are smaller (the curve comes closer to the points) and random (no obvious pattern).

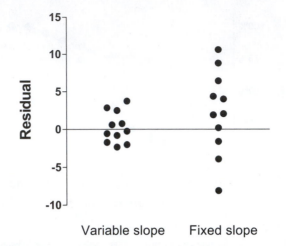

Figure 36.4. Residuals from the two models.

Each circle represents the residual (distance from the curve) of one data point. (Left) The residuals from the solid curve of Figure 36.2, with the Hill slope fit by nonlinear regression. (Right) The residuals from the dotted curve of Figure 36.2, where the Hill slope was fixed to a standard value of 1.0. This curve does not come as close to the points, so the residuals are larger. Note that the points are displaced horizontally to avoid overlap. Because the residuals from the full model are closer to each other, there is more potential for overlap, so those points have more horizontal displacement.

	HYPOTHESIS	SCATTER FROM	SUM OF SQUARES	DF
	Null	Fixed slope	358.1	9
–	Alternative	Variable slope	43.0	8
=	Difference	Improvement	315.1	1

Table 36.3. The variable slope model fits the data much better so the sum of squares is much smaller.

Figure 36.4 makes the comparison of the size of the residuals easier to see. Tables 36.3 and 36.4 compare the two fits, using a format similar to examples in Chapter 35. The null hypothesis is that the simpler model (fixed slope, one fewer parameter to fit) is correct. In fact, the alternative model fits much better (lower sum of squares) but has one fewer df. The calculations balance the difference in df with the difference in sum of squares.

If the fixed-slope model were correct, it is possible that random scatter of points made the curve fit so badly, but this would happen less than 0.01% of the time. This is strong evidence that the simple model is inadequate, so the more complicated model (in which the program fits the Hill slope) is preferred.

SOURCE OF VARIATION	SUM OF SQUARES	DF	MS	F RATIO	P VALUE
Difference	315.1	1	315.1	58.6	< 0.0001
Fixed slope model	43.0	8	5.4		
Variable slope model	358.1	9			

Table 36.4. Computing a F ratio and P value from the fits of the two models.
The F ratio is high, so the P value is tiny.

COMMON MISTAKES: NONLINEAR REGRESSION

Mistake: Choosing a polynomial model because it seems simpler

Some computer programs offer only one kind of curve fit, polynomial regression, which fits this model to data:

$$Y = \alpha + \beta_1 \cdot X + \beta_2 \cdot X^2 + \beta_3 \cdot X^3 + \beta_4 \cdot X^4 \ldots$$

If the equation ends with the β_2 term, it is called a second-order or quadratic equation. If you stop after the β_3 term, it is called a third-order or cubic equation.

Mathematicians and programmers prefer polynomial regression, because the method used to fit polynomial models is much more straightforward than the method used to fit nonlinear models. In fact, although a graph of the polynomial equation is curved, mathematicians consider it a linear model (because Y is linear with respect to each of the parameters). Any program that performs multiple linear regression can be used to fit polynomial regression.

Few biological or chemical processes follow models described by polynomial equations, so the parameters can rarely be interpreted in terms of chemistry or biology. Avoid using polynomial regression, because it seems simpler. Instead, to use nonlinear regression to fit the scientifically appropriate model.

Mistake: Transforming curved data to a linear form and then using linear regression

Before nonlinear regression became readily available in the early 1980s, scientists often transformed their data to make the graph linear, plotted the transformed linearized data by hand on a sheet of graph paper, drew a straight line by hand with a ruler, calculated the slope and Y intercept by hand, and then back-calculated the parameter estimates of the original nonlinear model. Later, scientists substituted computerized linear regression for the manual calculations.

Examples of linearizing transforms include Scatchard plots used by pharmacologists, double reciprocal Lineweaver–Burk plots used in enzymology, and the log transform used in kinetic studies. These methods are outdated and should not be used to analyze data. Nonlinear regression gives more precise results and is not much harder to perform.

Mistake: Letting a computer program choose the model

Choosing a model should be a scientific decision based on chemistry or physiology (or genetics, etc.). The choice should not be based solely on the shape of the graph.

Some people don't like thinking about equations, so they want a computer program to automatically fit thousands of equations and choose the model that fits the data best. Because a computer program cannot understand the scientific context of your experiment, a model chosen in this way is unlikely to be scientifically meaningful. The best-fit values of the parameters will probably have no scientific interpretation, so the fit is unlikely to be useful. Don't use a computer program as a way to avoid making scientific decisions.

Mistake: Fitting rolling averages, or smoothed data

As discussed in Chapter 33, smoothing the data (or computing rolling averages) violates the assumption that the residuals are independent and misleads the regression program about the amount of scatter. If you fit smoothed data, R^2 will be falsely high and the CIs will be falsely narrow. The results will be misleading.

Mistake: Using unweighted nonlinear regression when scatter increases as Y increases

It is common for biological data to violate the assumption that variability is the same for all values of Y. Instead, variability is often proportional to Y. Nonlinear regression programs offer weighting, and it is important to choose an appropriate weighting scheme.

Mistake: Using a standard model without thinking about which parameters should be fit

A crucial step in using nonlinear regression is to decide which parameters should be fit by nonlinear regression and which should be fixed to constant values based on control data. For example, in experiment discussed earlier in this chapter it made sense to constrain the Bottom parameter to a constant value of zero.

Mistake: Using R^2 to assess whether the fit is useful

A high value of R^2 tells you that the curve comes close to the data points. If your goal is to create a standard curve for interpolations, then this fit is useful. But if your goal is to determine best-fit values of parameters, a fit can have a high value of R^2, but still be quite useless. You need to look at whether the best-fit values have scientifically meaningful values and reasonably narrow CIs.

Mistake: Comparing two R^2 values to compare two fits

Comparing fits is tricky, and just choosing the fit with the larger R^2 is rarely appropriate. A model with more parameters will almost always fit with a larger R^2. You should not use R^2 to compare the fit of two models. Instead, use the method outlined in Chapter 35, which takes into account the number of parameters fit.

TIPS FOR UNDERSTANDING MODELS

The first step in nonlinear regression is to choose a model (equation). These tips will help you understand what an equation means. As an example, let's use the Michaelis–Menten equation that describes enzyme activity (Y) as a function of substrate concentration (X).

$$Y = \frac{V_{max} \cdot X}{K_m + X}$$

Tip: Make sure you know the meaning and units of X and Y
Here Y is enzyme activity, which can be expressed in various units, depending on the enzyme. X is the substrate concentration expressed in units of concentration.

Tip: Figure out the units of the parameters
In the example equation, the parameter K_m is added to X. It only makes sense to add things that are expressed in the same units, so K_m must be expressed in the same concentration units as X. This means that the units cancel in the term $X/(K_m + X)$, so V_{max} is expressed in the same units of enzyme activity as Y.

Tip: Figure out the value of Y at extreme values of X
Because X is concentration, it cannot be negative. But it can be zero. Substitute $X = 0$ into the equation and you will see that Y is also zero.

What happens when X is very large? As X gets large compared with K_m, the denominator $(X + K_m)$ has a value very similar to X. So the ratio $X/(X + K_m)$ approaches 1.0, and Y approaches V_{max}. So the graph of the model must level off at $Y = V_{max}$ as X gets very large. V_{max} is the maximum enzyme velocity.

Tip: Figure out the value of Y at special values of X
Because K_m is expressed in the same units as X, what is Y when X equals K_m? The ratio $X/(K_m + X)$ equals 0.5, so Y equals half of V_{max}. This means the K_m is the concentration of substrate that leads to a velocity equal to half the maximum velocity, V_{max}.

LEARN MORE ABOUT NONLINEAR REGRESSION

Few statistics texts even mention nonlinear regression, and the advanced texts on nonlinear regression tend to be very mathematical. Start with Glantz and Slinker (2000), who include a great chapter on nonlinear regression. If you like the style of this book, you'll also want to read my book on curve fitting (Motulsky & Christopoulos, 2004).

CHAPTER 37

━◢

Multiple, Logistic, and Proportional Hazards Regression

An approximate answer to the right problem is worth a good deal more than an exact answer to an approximate problem.

JOHN TUKEY

In laboratory experiments, you can generally control all the variables. You change one variable, measure another, and then analyze the data with one of the standard statistical tests. But in some kinds of experiments, and in many observational studies, you must analyze how one variable is influenced by several variables. Before reading this chapter, which introduces the idea of multiple regression, first read Chapters 33 and 34.

GOALS OF MULTIVARIABLE REGRESSION

In laboratory experiments, the experimenter usually changes one variable and measures something else. Prior chapters have explained how to analyze such data.

Often the situation is more complicated. In some kinds of experiments, and in most observational studies, the outcome you measure may be affected by multiple other variables. Fancier statistical methods are needed to untangle the data to figure out how multiple variables impact the outcome.

Multiple variable methods are powerful, versatile, and widely used. They really are beyond the scope of basic biostatistics, and this book only introduces you to the basic concepts behind these methods (Chapter 37) and the ways the results can be misleading (Chapter 38).

Multiple regression methods are used for several purposes:

- To assess the impact of one variable, while adjusting for others. Does a drug work, after adjusting for differences between the patients who received drug versus those who received placebo? Does a risk factor increase the risk of a disease, after adjusting for other differences between people who were and were not exposed to that risk factor?
- To create an equation for making useful predictions. Given the data we know now, what is the chance that this particular man with chest pain

TYPE OF REGRESSION	TYPE OF DEPENDENT (Y) VARIABLE	EXAMPLE Y VARIABLES
Linear	Continuous (interval or ratio)	Enzyme activity Renal function (creatinine clearance) Weight
Logistic	Binary or dichotomous	Death during surgery Graduation Recurrence of cancer
Polytomous	Discrete variable with more than two outcomes	
Proportional hazards	Elapsed time to a one-time event	Months until death Days until patient is weaned from ventilator Quarters in school before graduation
Anderson-Gill	Elapsed time to an event that can recur	Months until next seizure Days until next occurrence of atrial fibrillation
Poisson	Number of events in a time period	Number of hospitalizations Number of falls

Table 37.1. Different kinds of regression for different kinds of outcomes.

is having a myocardial infarction (heart attack)? Given several variables that can be measured easily, what is the predicted cardiac output of this patient?

- To understand scientifically how various variables impact an outcome. How do the concentrations of high-density lipoproteins (HDL, good cholesterol), low-density lipoproteins (LDL, bad cholesterol), triglycerides, C-reactive protein, and homocysteine predict the risk of heart disease? Part of the scientific (or clinical) goal might be to generate an equation that can predict the risk for individual patients. But part of that goal might be a basic understanding of the contributions of each risk factor, so as to aid public-health efforts and help prioritize future research.

These goals aren't always completely distinct, and the statistical methods used are the same regardless of goal.

LINGO

Different kinds of multiple regression

Methods that fit regression models with two or more independent variables are called *multiple regression* methods. Multiple regression is really a family of methods, with the specific type of regression used depending on what kind of outcome was measured (Table 37.1):

- *Multiple linear regression* is used when the outcome is continuous. Often this is shortened to *multiple regression.*
- *Multiple logistic regression* is used when the outcome is dichotomous. Often this is shortened to *logistic regression.*
- *Multiple polytomous logistic regression.*
- *Multiple proportional hazards regression* is used when the outcome is elapsed time until some event occurs. The event often is death, so proportional hazards regression is used to fit survival data. Often this method is shortened to *proportional hazards regression.* It is also called *Cox regression,* after the person who invented it.
- *Multiple Poisson regression* is used when the outcome is the number of events that occur in a certain time period. This book will not discuss Poisson regression further.
- *Anderson–Gill regression* is a modification of proportional hazards regression used when the event (unlike death) can happen more than once. So once an event occurs, the clock restarts for that subject and the time to the second event is recorded. This book will not discuss this method further.

Logistic and proportional hazards regression are almost always used with two or more independent variables, so the word "multiple" is often omitted.

All of the regression methods listed above (plus some more) are special cases of the *generalized linear model* (GLM). Beware of confusing lingo. The *general linear model* is a subset of the *generalized linear model.* The latter (generalized) has a broader meaning.

It can be further generalized to also fit nonlinear models, even with non-Gaussian random components (i.e., binomial or Poisson). Greco (1989) proposed the term *generalized nonlinear regression,* but this name is not widely used.

Variables

The models all predict an outcome, called the *dependent variable* (Y), from one or more predictors, called the *independent variables* (X).

When the independent variable has only two possible values, it is entered into the program as a *dummy variable.* For example, a dummy variable can code for gender by defining 0 to mean male and 1 to mean female. These codes, of course, are arbitrary.

It is also possible to use dummy variables when there are more than two categories (for example, four medical school classes). Consult more advanced books if you need to do this, because it is not straightforward. Several dummy variables are needed.

The term "multivariate"

Beware of the term *multivariate statistics,* because it is used inconsistently.

Sometimes the term *multivariate* refers to methods that simultaneously compare several outcomes at once. Factor analysis, cluster analysis, principal components analysis, and multiple ANOVA (MANOVA) are multivariate methods and are far beyond the scope of this book.

Sometimes the term *multivariate* is used to refer to the methods used when there is one outcome and several independent variables (i.e., multiple and logistic regression), but these methods are properly called *multivariable analyses*, rather than multivariate analyses.

MULTIPLE LINEAR REGRESSION

As you learned in Chapter 31, simple linear regression determines the best linear equation to predict Y from a single variable, X. Multiple linear regression finds the linear equation that best predicts Y from multiple independent variables.

An example: Does lead account for decreased kidney function with age?

Staessen and colleagues (1992) investigated the relationship between lead exposure and kidney function. Heavy exposure to lead can damage kidneys. Kidney function decreases with age and most people accumulate small amounts of lead as they get older. These investigators wanted to know whether accumulation of lead could explain some of the decrease in kidney function in with aging.

Staessen et al. studied 965 men and measured the concentration of lead in blood, as well as creatinine clearance to quantify kidney function. They also studied 1,016 women, but here we'll just discuss the analysis of the data from men. The people with more lead tended to have lower creatinine clearance, but this is not a useful finding. Lead concentration increases with age and creatinine clearance decreases with age. So differences in age confound any investigation between creatinine clearance and lead concentration. To adjust for this problem, the investigators used multiple regression to adjust for age and other factors.

The X variable they cared most about was the logarithm of lead concentration. They used the logarithm of concentration, rather than the lead concentration itself, because they expected the effect of lead to be multiplicative rather than additive—i.e., that a doubling of lead concentration (from any starting value) will have an equal effect on creatinine clearance. So why logarithms? The regression model is intrinsically additive. Note that the sum of the two logarithms is the same as the logarithm of the product: $\log(A) + \log(B) = \mathrm{Log}(A \cdot B)$. Therefore, transforming a variable to its logarithm converts a multiplicative effect to an additive one (Appendix E reviews logarithms).

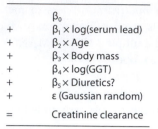

		β_0
+		$\beta_1 \times \log(\text{serum lead})$
+		$\beta_2 \times \text{Age}$
+		$\beta_3 \times \text{Body mass}$
+		$\beta_4 \times \log(\text{GGT})$
+		$\beta_5 \times \text{Diuretics?}$
+		ε (Gaussian random)
=		Creatinine clearance

Table 37.2. The multiple regression model for the example.

β_0 through β_5 are the six parameters fit by the multiple regression program. Each of these parameters has different units (listed in Table 37.3). The product of each parameter times the corresponding variable is expressed in the units of the Y variable (creatinine clearance), which are milliliters per minute (ml/min). The goal of multiple regression is to find the values for the six parameters of the model that make the predicted creatinine-clearance values come as close as possible to the actual values.

VARIABLE	MEANING	UNITS
X_1	log(serum lead)	Logarithms are unitless. Untransformed serum-lead concentration was in micrograms per liter.
X_2	Age	Years
X_3	Body mass	Kilograms per square meter
X_4	log(GGT)	Logarithms are unitless. Untransformed serum-GGT level was in units per liter.
X_5	Diuretics?	Unitless. 0 = Never took diuretics. 1 = Took diuretics.
Y	Creatinine clearance	Milliliters per minute

Table 37.3. Units of the variables used in the multiple regression examples.

Mathematical model

The multiple regression model is shown in Table 37.2. The dependent (Y) variable is creatinine clearance. The model predicts its value from a baseline value plus the effects of five independent (X) variables, each multiplied by a parameter.

The X variables were the logarithm of serum lead, age, body mass, logarithm of γ-glutamyl transpeptidase (a measure of liver function), and previous exposure to diuretics (coded as 0 or 1). This last variable is called a *dummy variable* (or indicator variable) because those two particular values were chosen arbitrarily to designate two groups (people who have not taken diuretics and those who have).

The final variable, ε, represents random variability (error). Like ordinary linear regression, multiple regression assumes that the random scatter follows a Gaussian distribution.

The model of Table 37.2 can be written as an equation that tries to predict the outcome by a weighted combination of inputs:

$$Y_i = \beta_0 + \beta_1 \cdot X_{i,1} + \beta_2 \cdot X_{i,2} + \beta_3 \cdot X_{i,3} + \beta_4 \cdot X_{i,4} + \beta_5 \cdot X_{i,5} + \epsilon_i$$

The subscript i refers to the particular patient. So Y_3 is the creatinine clearance of the third patient. The X values have two subscripts, because each patient has five different X values (Table 37.3). The parameters have only a single subscript. There are six population parameters, one for each independent variable (β_1 to β_5) and one baseline (β_0).

Goals of regression

Multiple regression fits the model to the data to find the values for the coefficients that make the model come as close as possible to predicting the actual data. These best-fit parameter values are called b_0, b_1, etc. (to distinguish the best-fit values in the sample from the ideal population values of the parameters, β_0, β_1, etc.)

Multiple regression reports the best-fit value of each parameter, along with a CI. Some programs report the standard error of each parameter instead of (or, in addition to) its CI.

One P value is reported for each independent variable. The null hypothesis is that the parameter provides no information to the model, so the β value for that parameter equals 0.0.

Interpret the coefficients

Multiple linear regression models do not distinguish between the X variable(s) you really care about and the other X variable(s) that you are adjusting for (called *covariates*). You make that distinction when interpreting the results. Here, the investigator's goal was to answer this question: After adjusting for effects of the other variables, is there a substantial linear relationship between the logarithm of lead concentration and creatinine clearance?

The best-fit value of β_1 (the coefficient for the logarithm of lead concentration) was –9.5 ml/min. After adjusting for all other variables, an increase in log(lead) of 1 unit (so that the lead concentration increases 10-fold) is associated with a decrease in creatinine clearance of 9.5 ml/min. The 95% CI ranged from –18.1 to –0.9 ml/min.

Understanding these values requires some context. The study participants' average creatinine clearance was 99 ml/min. So a 10-fold increase in lead concentrations would reduce renal function about 10%, with a 95% CI ranging from about 1 to 20%. Figure 37.1 illustrates this model.

Statistical significance

The CI of β_1 runs from a negative number to another negative number and does not include zero. Therefore, you can be 95% confident that increasing lead concentration is associated with a drop in creatinine clearance (poorer kidney function). Accordingly, the P value for this parameter must be less than 0.05. The authors don't quantify it more accurately than that, but most regression programs would report the exact P value.

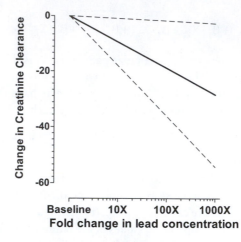

Figure 37.1. The prediction of multiple regression.
One of the variables entered into the multiple regression model was the logarithm of lead concentration. The best-fit value for its coefficient was –9.5. For every 1-unit increase in the logarithm of lead concentration, the predicted creatinine clearance is predicted to go down by 9.5 ml/min. For the logarithm to increase 1 unit, the lead concentration increases 10-fold. The solid line shows the best-fit value of that slope. The two dashed lines show the range of the 95% CI.

Note that this P value results from comparing the fit of two models (Chapter 35). It compares the full model (Table 37.2) with the same model where β_1 is fixed to 0.0 so the value of log(lead) does not enter into the calculations. The low P value leads to the conclusion to reject the latter model ($\beta1$ fixed to 0.0) and thus accept the full model.

The authors also report the values for all the other coefficients in the model. For example, the β_5 coefficient for the X variable "previous diuretic therapy" was -8.8 ml/min. That variable is coded as zero if the patient had never taken diuretics and 1 if the patient had taken diuretics. So that best-fit value means that after adjusting for all the other variables, subjects who had taken diuretics previously had a mean creatinine clearance that was 8.8 ml/min lower than subjects who had not taken diuretics. The authors state that the P value is less than 0.05, but they don't give the actual P value or CI. But if $P < 0.05$, we know the CI cannot include zero, so it must run from one negative number to another, centered on the best-fit value of –8.8 ml/min.

How well does the model fit the data?

Multiple regression reports that R^2 equals 0.27. This means that only 27% of the variability in creatinine clearance was explained by the model. The remaining 73% of the variability is random, associated with factors not included in this study, or is associated with variables included in this study but not in the forms entered in the model.

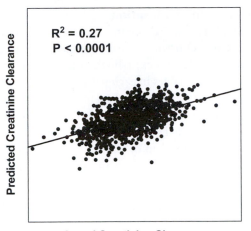

Figure 37.2. The meaning of R^2 in multiple regression.

The authors did not post the raw data, so this graph does not accurately represent the data in the example. Instead, I simulated some data that look very much like what the actual data would have looked like. Each of the 965 points represents one man in the study. The horizontal axis shows the actual creatinine clearance for each subject. The vertical axis shows the creatinine clearance computed by the multiple regression model from that subject's lead level, age, body mass, log γ-glutamyl transpeptidase, and previous exposure to diuretics. The prediction is somewhat useful, because generally people who actually have higher creatinine-clearance levels are predicted to have higher levels. But there is a huge amount of scatter. If the model were perfect, each predicted value would be the same as the actual value, all the points would line up on a 45-degree line, and R^2 would equal 1.00. Here the predictions are less accurate, and R^2 is only 0.27.

With linear regression, you can see the best-fit line superimposed on the data and visualize goodness of fit. This is not possible with multiple regression. With two independent variables, you could visualize the fit on a three-dimensional graph, but most multiple regression models have more than two independent variables.

Figure 37.2 shows a way to visualize how well a multiple regression model fits the data and to understand the meaning of R^2. Each point represents one subject. The horizontal axis plots each subject's measured creatinine clearance. The vertical axis plots the creatinine clearance value predicted by the model. This prediction is computed from the other variables in the model, but this calculation does not use the measured value of creatinine clearance. The actual values are not predicted perfectly. The two are correlated, with R^2 equal to 0.27. This is identical to the overall R^2 computed by multiple regression.

Correlation does not imply causation

In the example, the investigators chose to make creatinine clearance the dependent variable, so the model predicts creatinine clearance from the other variables. But this study included no experimental intervention. The investigators just measured a bunch of variables in each patient and looked for relationships.

The paper concludes that exposure to lead may impair renal function, but concedes that the data don't prove cause and effect. The data are also consistent with the hypothesis that reduced renal function (for other reasons) increases lead levels.

This is a fundamental problem of observational studies like this. The best way to overcome any doubts about cause and effect is to do an experiment. Of course, it wouldn't be ethical to expose people to lead to see what will happen to their renal function. But it would certainly be possible to do such an experiment with animals.

Is the model too simple?

Note how simple the model is. It predicts that log(lead) is linear with creatinine clearance, is linear with body mass, is linear with age, and is linear with log(GGT). It is easy to imagine other models. Maybe lead only affects creatinine clearance once it reaches a threshold value. Maybe low levels of lead affect renal function, but its effect plateaus at larger values. Maybe lead matters more in older people. There are many conceivable models, and the multiple linear regression model is only one possibility.

Compare alternative models

The authors collected more variables for each subject. They stated that the fit of the model was not improved when the model also accounted for smoking habits, mean blood pressure, serum ferritin level (a measure of iron storage), residence in urban versus rural areas, or urinary cadmium levels. So they omitted these variables from the model whose fit they reported.

Chapter 35 explained the idea behind comparing models, and this can be used to compare two models (with and without a questionable X variable). Including the extra variable in the model will almost certainly improve the fit. The extra sum of squares F test asks whether the improvement in fit is more than you'd expect by giving up 1 df (resulting from the additional variable in the model). The null hypothesis is that the simpler model, with fewer parameters, is correct.

Alternatively, the P value can also be computed by dividing the parameter value by its standard error to obtain a t ratio, and then determining the P value from that t ratio. The results will be the same.

It is easy to use that P value as a way to choose a model:

- If the P value is small (usually less than 0.05), reject the null hypothesis and accept the model with the extra parameter.
- If the P value is high, don't reject the null hypothesis. Keep the simpler model with fewer parameters.

VARIABLE	MEANING	UNITS
X_1	Place of residence	0 = Rural; 1 = Urban
X_2	Age	Years
X_3	Education	Years
X_4	Smoking	0 = No; 1 = Yes
X_5	Married	0 = No; 1 = Yes
X_6	Lower middle economic index	0 = No; 1 = Yes (lower middle)
X_7	Upper middle economic index	0 = No; 1 = Yes (upper middle)
X_8	Higher economic index	0 = No; 1 = Yes (higher)

Table 37.4. Variables used in the logistic regression example.

Chapter 38 explains a problem with variable selection methods: It is possible to overfit the data.

LOGISTIC REGRESSION

Logistic regression is used when there are two possible outcomes.

An example

Bakhshi and colleagues (2008) created a model to predict the prevalence of obesity in Iranian women. The outcome was obesity, considered a binary (dichotomous) variable (an alternative would be to use weight as an outcome in multiple regression). They created a model to predict the prevalence of obesity as a function of the various demographic variables listed in Table 37.4. The model contains three kinds of independent variables:

- Age and number of years of education are continuous.
- Smoking status, marital status, and place of residence are coded as binary variables. This required that they make some clear definitions to force all subjects into one of the two categories. For example: Is someone who used to be a heavy smoker considered a smoker or not? Is someone who is recently divorced after many years of marriage considered married or not?
- Economic index is divided into four categories: lower, lower middle, upper middle, and high. It is not an interval variable (see Chapter 8), so it would be a mistake to encode it as one variable with values ranging from 1 to 4. That approach would incorrectly imply that the distance between lower middle class and lower class is the same as the distance between lower middle class and upper middle class. Because class cannot be encoded as an interval variable, the investigators encoded the four economic classes as three separate binary variables. Note there is one fewer variable than categories.

They collected data from 14,176 women and fit the data with logistic regression.

Logistic regression model

Logistic regression fits a model that best predicts a binary (dichotomous) outcome variable from various independent variables. In many cases, the outcome has a natural definition. Here the definition is somewhat arbitrary. The investigators first computed the body mass index (BMI) from each subject's height and weight, and then classified the subjects with a BMI exceeding a selected threshold as "obese."

The model can be expressed in multiple ways. The equation below defines the model in the form that is easiest to understand. It calculates the logarithm of the odds ratio for any individual from the independent variables of that individual and from the odds ratios for each X variable:

$$\ln(OR_i) = X_{i,1} \cdot \ln(OR_1) + X_{i,2} \cdot \ln(OR_2) \ldots + X_{i,8} \cdot \ln(OR_8)$$

This same model can be rearranged so the left side is the probability that a subject with a certain set of X variables will have the outcome, instead of the equation above where the left side is the odds ratio for that subject.

For this example, the model has eight terms, corresponding to the eight independent variables listed in Table 37.4.

Why logarithms?

Odds ratios are lopsided. A decrease in risk is expressed as an odds ratio between 0 and 1, and an increase in risk is expressed as any odds ratio greater than 1. The logarithm of the odds ratio is symmetrical. Negative values indicate a decreased risk, and positives values indicate an increased risk. For example, if the odds ratio equals 2.0, the ln(OR) of is 0.69. And if the odds ratio is 0.5, the ln(OR) is of −0.69.

The logarithms are customarily computed as natural logarithms, with a base e, which is abbreviated above as *ln* (Appendix E reviews logarithms).

Odds ratios for each independent variable

The right side of the equation has one odds ratio for each independent variable. The example has eight independent variables, so the model has eight odds ratios. These are the main results of logistic regression.

Each odds ratio answers this question: If one particular X value were increased by 1.0 (keeping the others the same), how much would the logarithm of the odds ratio be expected to increase? That will make more sense in the next section when the results are interpreted in the context of this example.

If the odds ratio is near 1.0, then that independent variable has little impact on the outcome. If the odds ratio is much higher than 1.0, then an increase in that independent variable is associated with an increased likelihood of the outcome occurring. If the odds ratio is much less than 1.0, then an increase in that independent variable is associated with a decreased likelihood of the event occurring.

VARIABLE	MEANING	ODDS RATIO	95% CI
OR_1	Urban?	2.13	1.915 to 2.369
OR_2	Age	1.02	1.017 to 1.026
OR_3	Education	0.98	0.968 to 0.993
OR_4	Smoking?	0.65	0.468 to 0.916
OR_5	Married?	1.48	1.312 to 1.668
OR_6	Lower middle class?	1.37	1.206 to 1.554
OR_7	Upper middle class?	1.29	1.136 to 1.468
OR_8	Higher class?	1.25	1.994 to 1.425

Table 37.5. Results of logistic regression.

If the model is correct, there is an ideal population value for each of these odds ratios. From data from a sample of subjects, logistic regression estimates a value for each of these odds ratios, along with a 95% CI.

Predicted odds ratios for each individual subject

The odds ratios on the left side of the equation at the top of this page is for someone with a particular set of X values. Each predicts the odds the outcome occurring of a subject with that particular set of independent variables having the outcome (compared with a subject for whom all X variables equal zero). You can pretty much ignore these odds ratios. You don't need to enter these values when running a logistic regression analysis, and don't need to look at them when reviewing the results. The odds ratios you care about are the ones on the right side of the equation, one for each independent variable.

Interpreting the results

The results of logistic regression are shown in Table 37.5. Logistic regression computes an odds ratio for each independent variable along with a 95% CI (listed in Table 37.3).

The first independent variable is a binary, or dummy, variable that equals 1 when the subject lives in a city and otherwise equals zero. The corresponding odds ratio is 2.13. This means that a subject who lives in a city has a bit more than twice the odds of being obese as someone who doesn't, but whose other independent variables are identical. The model assumes that this odds ratio is the same regardless of age (within the range used in the study), regardless of education, regardless of smoking, etc. After correcting for effects of these variables, the results tell us that the odds ratio for living in a city is 2.13. The 95% CI ranges from 1.9 to 2.4.

If women who live in cities have the same risk of obesity as those who live in rural areas, then this odds ratio would equal 1.0. The 95% CI does not include 1.0, so the P value must be less than 0.05. And, because the CI doesn't even come close to 1.0, the P value must be much less than 0.05. These investigators did not report the P values, but most investigators do. The P value answers this question:

Assuming the model is correct and the population odds ratio (for this particular X variable) equals 1.0, what is the chance that random sampling would lead to an odds ratio as far from 1.0 (or father) as observed in this study?

The next independent variable is for age. The investigators don't say what age range they used, but they do say that the mean age was 37 with a standard deviation of 14, so they collected information from women with a wide range of ages. The odds ratio for this variable is 1.02. For every year increase in age, the risk of obesity goes up about 2%. The CI is very narrow and does not include 1.00. Therefore, the P value for age must be less than 0.05. Because an odds ratio of 1.0 indicates no effect, your first thought might be that an odds ratio of only 1.02 is trivial. But, in fact, this isn't trivial effect. Because the odds ratios multiply, the odds ratio for a 10-year increase in age is 1.02^{10}, or 1.22. That means that for every ten years increase in age, the risk of obesity increases about 22%.

Summary

It all seems complicated at first. Just the terms "logistic" and "multivariable" and "regression" are enough to scare away many people, and "logarithm" scares off many more. But you can look past all that and understand the results fairly easily. Logistic regression computes an odds ratio for each independent variable along with a CI. These are easy to interpret.

PROPORTIONAL HAZARDS REGRESSION

Proportional hazards regression is used when the outcome is elapsed time to an event, often used for analyses of survival times.

An example

Rosman and colleagues (1993) investigated whether diazepam (also known as Valium) would prevent febrile seizures in children. They recruited about 400 children who had had at least one febrile seizure. Their parents were instructed to give medication to the children whenever they had a fever. Half were given diazepam and half were given placebo (because there was no standard therapy).

They compared the two groups to see whether there was a difference in time until the first seizure. Note some confusing lingo. The method used to analyze these data is given the misleading name *survival analyses*, although the event they are tracking is *analysis*, even though the outcome in this example is not death.

The investigators asked whether treatment with diazepam would delay the time of first seizure, adjusting for differences in age, number of previous febrile seizures, and several other variables.

The proportional hazards model

A survival curve plots cumulative survival as a function of time. The slope of the survival curve is the rate of dying in a short time interval. This is termed the *hazard*. For example, if 20% of patients with a certain kind of cancer are expected to die this year, then the hazard is 20% per year. When comparing two groups, investigators often assume that the *ratio* of hazard functions is constant over time. For example, the hazard among treated patients might be one half the hazard in control patients. The death rates change over the course of the study, but at any particular time the treated patients' risk of dying is one half the risk of the control patients. Another way to say this is that the two hazard functions are proportional to one another. This is a reasonable assumption for many clinical situations.

The ratio of hazards is essentially a relative risk. If the ratio is 0.5, then the relative risk of dying in one group is half the risk of dying in the other group. *Proportional hazards regression*, also called *Cox regression* after the person who developed the method, uses regression methods to predict the relative risk based on one or more X variables.

The assumption of proportional hazards is not always reasonable. You would not expect the hazard functions of medical and surgical therapy for cancer to be proportional. You might expect surgical therapy to have the higher hazard at early times (because of deaths during the operation or soon thereafter) and medical therapy to have the higher hazard at later times. In such situations, proportional hazards regression should be avoided, or used only over restricted time intervals for which the assumption is reasonable.

Having accepted the proportional hazards assumption, we want to know how the hazard ratio is influenced by treatment or other variables. The model looks similar to the one used for logistic regression, except that it fits relative risks (RR) rather than odds ratios:

$$\ln(\text{hazard ratio}) = X_1 \cdot \ln(RR_1) + X_2 \cdot \ln(RR_2)\ldots$$

Interpreting the fit of the model

Rosman et al. fit the data using proportional hazards regression. The relative risk was 0.61, with a 95% CI ranging from 0.39 to 0.94. Compared with subjects treated with placebo, subjects treated with diazepam had only 61% of the risk of having a febrile seizure. This reduction was statistically significant with a P value of 0.027. If diazepam were truly ineffective, there would have been only a 2.7% chance of seeing such a low relative risk in a study of this size. This example shows that the results of proportional hazards regression are easy to interpret, although the details of the analysis are complicated.

ASSUMPTIONS

Assumption: Sampling from a population

This is a familiar assumption of all statistical analyses. The goal in all forms of multiple regression is to analyze a sample of data in order to make more general conclusions about the population from which the data were sampled.

Assumption: Linear effects with no interaction beyond what is specified in the model

The multiple regression model assumes that increasing a X variable by 1 unit increases (or decreases) the value of Y (multiple regression), or the log of the odds ratio (logistic regression), or the log of the relative risk (proportional hazards regression) by the same amount at all values of X.

In the multiple regression (lead-exposure) example, the model is that (on average) creatinine clearance would decrease by a certain amount when the logarithm of lead concentration increases by 1.0 (a for any 10-fold increase in lead concentration). For the example, the model assumes that the effect of lead and on kidney function is the same for the old and young, for the obese and slender, and for those who take diuretics and those who don't.

It is possible to extend the multiple regression model so as to bypass the assumption of no interaction, and this is very briefly explained in the next section.

Assumption: Independent observations

This is a familiar assumption, that data for each subject provide independent information about the links among the variables. In both examples, this assumption would be violated if some of the subjects were identical twins (or even siblings).

Assumption: Random component of model is correct

For any set of X values, multiple linear regression assumes that the random component of the model follows a Gaussian distribution, at least approximately. Furthermore, it assumes that the standard deviation of that scatter is always the same, unrelated to any of the variables. Logistic regression assumes that for any set of independent variables, the distribution of the two outcomes follows a binomial distribution.

Additional assumptions of proportional hazards regression

Proportional hazards regression also is based on all the assumptions of survival analysis listed in Chapters 5 and 29.

INTERACTING INDEPENDENT VARIABLES

Two of the independent variables in the multiple linear regression model are the logarithm of lead concentration and age. But what if those two variables are related? What if the effects of lead concentration matter more with older people? This kind of relationship is called an *interaction*.

To include interaction between age and the logarithm of serum lead concentration, add a new term to the model equation with a new parameter multiplied by the product of age (X_2) times the logarithm of lead (X_1):

$$Y = \beta_0 + \beta_1 \cdot X_1 + \beta_2 \cdot X_2 + \beta_3 \cdot X_3 + \beta_4 \cdot X_4 + \beta_5 \cdot X_5 + \beta_{12} \cdot X_1 \cdot X_2 + \epsilon$$

If the CI for the new parameter (β_{12}) does not include zero, then you would conclude that there is a significant interaction between age and log(lead). This means that the effects of lead change with age. Equivalently, the effect of age depends on the lead concentrations.

It is easy to include interaction terms in any of the multiple regression analyses (including logistic and proportional hazards regression). Interactions of three variables can be included by multiplying all three together.

Note that these interactions are simplistic. The interaction term above assumes that as people get older, there is a linear change in the effect of lead. But what if lead mattered a lot in the young and old, but not in people in between? This kind of nonlinear interaction would not be detected by the usual methods.

CORRELATED OBSERVATIONS

Nonindependent (correlated) observations are common

One of the assumptions of multiple regression is that each observation is independent. In other words, the deviation from the prediction of the model is entirely random. This assumption is violated in many experimental designs, where observations are correlated as part of the experimental design. Here is a partial list of such designs, adapted from Katz (2006):

- Longitudinal studies. These involve multiple observations of the same subject at different times. This is also called a repeated-measures design.
- Crossover studies. These involve multiple observations of the same subject, after receiving different treatments.
- Multiple observations on each individual. For example, a study of arthritis might include measurements from both knees of each subject. This provides more information than a measurement from only a single knee, although the two measurements in each subject are highly correlated.
- Clusters. Some subjects are recruited from one group (family, hospital, country) and other subjects are recruited from another group. Many groups can be used. One example is a multicenter clinical trial. The observations within each center are likely to be closer to each other than to observations from a different center.
- Case-control. Subjects are recruited into the study as a matched set. See Chapter 28.

- Meta-analyses. The best medical evidence is often obtained by combining the results of many studies. The difficult part of a meta-analysis is deciding which studies to include or exclude from the analysis and how to express all of the treatment effects on the same scale. The results can then be combined using a multiple regression method that takes into account how the data were pooled, and the fact that some studies used more patients than others.

These are all very useful experimental designs, but they complicate data analysis. With all of these designs, observations are correlated or clustered. Observations within a cluster will be more similar to each other than to observations in a different cluster.

In some cases, the correlation can be hierarchical. A clinical study of a surgical procedure can use patients from three different medical centers. Because the centers may serve very different populations, the results within each center will be closer to each other than to results from other centers. Within each center, several different surgeons may do the procedure. Patients will tend to have results more similar to other patients of that surgeon than to patients operated on by a different surgeon. For each patient, results might be collected at several time points. The multiple measurements of one patient will be closer to each other than to measurements from other patients.

It is essential to account for clustering when analyzing data

What happens if data from any of the experimental designs discussed in this chapter are analyzed using the usual regression (or ANOVA) techniques, without accounting for the clustering or correlation? The usual regression methods assume that each value is independent of the others, so the variation among all the values is viewed as a measure of overall variability. When the values are in fact correlated, the overall variability will probably be underestimated. The best-fit values of the regression coefficients won't be affected much, but the CIs will likely to be too narrow and the P values will probably be too small. It is easy to be fooled by an invalid regression analysis.

Simple alternatives are often adequate

With some experimental designs, straightforward approaches let you analyze the data simply. Examples include the following:

- If each subject has drug concentrations measured at multiple times, compute the area under the concentration-versus-time curve for each subject. Enter those areas (and not the individual drug concentrations) as the dependent variable into a regression model.
- If a clinical study is done in three different medical centers, analyze the data for each center separately. If all three analyses reach similar conclusions, a fancier analysis may not be needed.

Q & A

Do you always have to decide which variable is the outcome (dependent variable) and which variables are the predictors (independent variables) at the time of data collection?	No. In some cases, the independent and dependent variables may not be distinct at the time of data collection. The decision is sometimes made only at the time of data analysis. But beware of these analyses. The more ways you analyze the data, the more likely you are to be fooled by overfitting (see Chapter 38).
Does it make sense to compare the value of one best-fit parameter with another?	No. The units of each parameter are different, so they can't be directly compared. If you want to compare, read about standardized parameters in a more advanced book. Standardizing rescales the parameters so they are unitless. Standardized parameters can then be compared. A variable with a larger standardized parameter has a more important impact on the dependent variable.
Do all the independent variables have to be expressed in the same units?	No. Usually they are in different units.
What units are the parameters expressed in?	The product of each parameter times the corresponding independent variable is expressed in the same units as Y. So the parameters are expressed in the Y units divided by the X units.
How is regression related to other statistical methods?	Chapter 35 pointed out that an unpaired t test can be recast as linear regression. Similarly, one-way ANOVA can be recast as multiple regression. It is also possible to use logistic or proportional hazards regression to compare two groups, replacing the methods explained in Chapters 27–29 (the results won't be exactly the same, but should be close). Essentially all of statistics can be recast as a form of fitting some kind of model using an appropriate kind of regression.
How does ANCOVA fit in?	This book does not discuss ANCOVA. It is a model that is equivalent to multiple linear regression when at least one independent variable is categorical and at least one is continuous.
How are the CIs calculated?	Some programs report the standard error of each parameter, instead of its CI. Computing the CI of the best-fit value of a model parameter works just like computing the CI of the mean (Chapter 12).

Continued

Compute the margin of error by multiplying the reported standard error times a value obtained from the t distribution (see Appendix D). This value depends only on the level of confidence desired (95% is standard) and the number of df (equal to the number of subjects in the study minus the number of parameters fit by the model). For 95% confidence and with plenty of df (common in multiple regression), the multiplier approximates 2.0. Add and subtract this margin of error from the best-fit value to obtain the CI.

Fancier methods are sometimes needed

The methods used to properly analyze correlated data are far beyond the scope of this book. Here is a list of some of the methods:

- General estimating equations (GEE)
- Mixed effects models, also called random effects models
- Conditional logistic, or proportional hazards regression
- Repeated-measures ANOVA, or analysis of covariance (ANCOVA)
- Hierarchical or multilevel regression models (Gelman and Hill, 2007)

HOW IT WORKS

Multiple linear regression is an extension of linear regression. The goals are the same: to adjust the values of the parameters in the model to minimize the sum of the squares of the discrepancies between the actual and predicted Y values.

The computations of logistic regression and proportional hazards regression are more difficult than linear regression and will not be explained here. The method of least squares does not apply. Instead, these approaches use an iterative maximum likelihood method. The details are far beyond the scope of this book, but the general idea of maximum likelihood was explained in Chapter 34.

LEARNING MORE ABOUT MULTIPLE REGRESSION

The texts by Katz (2006) and Campbell (2006) are concise, clear, practical, and nonmathematical. The books by Glantz and Slinker (2000) and Vittinghoff and colleagues (2007) have more depth and more math, while remaining clear and practical.

CHAPTER 38

$\rightharpoondown$

Multiple Regression Traps

If your experiment needs statistics, you ought to have done a better experiment.

LORD ERNEST RUTHERFORD

*T*he results of multiple, logistic, and proportional hazards regression *can be misleading. The goal, as in all of statistics, is to analyze data from a sample and make valid inferences about the population. With multiple regression, it is too easy to reach invalid conclusions. This chapter explains what you need to beware of when evaluating the results of multiple regression.*

BEWARE OF OVERFITTING

The goal of regression, like all of statistics, is to analyze data from a sample and make valid inferences about the overall population. With multiple regression techniques, that goal is not always met. It is too easy to reach conclusions that apply to the fit of the sample data, but do not really exist in the population. When the study is repeated, the conclusions will not be reproducible.

This problem is called *overfitting* (Babyak, 2004). It happens when you ask more questions than the data can answer.

Cause of overfitting: Too many independent variables

One cause of overfitting is including too many independent variables in the model, compared to the number of subjects.

How many independent variables is too many? For multiple regression, a rule of thumb is that there should be at least 10–15 subjects per independent variable (see Chapter 43). Fitting a model with 5 independent variables thus requires 50–75 subjects. For logistic and proportional hazards regression, the dependent variable is the occurence of an event, and the rule of thumb refers to the number of subjects to whom the event occurs, rather than to the total number of subjects. For example, say that logistic regression is used to model the occurrence of stroke, you expect that about 10% of the subjects will have a stroke during the study period, and the model has 5 independent variables. In this situation, the sample size would need to be 500–750. With that many subjects, you expect that

50–75 will have a stroke (10% of 500-750). Divide by the number of independent variables (5) to see that the rule of thumb is met, with equals 10–15 events per independent variable.

One way to reduce the impact of overfitting is to account for any relationship between the independent variables when you create the model. Read about *multilevel* and *hierarchical regression* in Gelman and Hill (2007).

Cause of overfitting: Too many model variations

Multiple regression analyses offer the investigator lots of choices, making it easy to overfit data by fitting many variations of the same model:

- With and without interaction terms
- With and without transforming some independent variables
- With and without transforming the dependent variable
- Including and excluding outliers or influential points
- Pooling all the data or analyzing some subsets separately
- Rerunning the model, defining a different variable to be the dependent, outcome, variable

When you fit the data many different ways and then report only the model that fits the data best, you are likely to make conclusions that are not valid.

Cause of overfitting: Variable selection

When thinking about overfitting, what counts is not only the number of variables included in the final model, but also the other variables that the investigators collected but decided not to include.

Before entering data into a multiple regression program, some investigators first look at the degree of correlation or association of each possible independent variable with the outcome. They then enter into the multiple regression program only those variables that are strongly correlated or associated with the outcome. This kind of manual screening can lead to overfitting (Babyak, 2004).

Multiple regression programs can choose variables automatically. One approach (*all subsets regression*) is to fit the data to every possible model (each model includes some X variables and may exclude others). With many variables and large data sets, the computer time required is prohibitive. To conserve computer time with huge data sets, other algorithms use a stepwise approach. One approach (*forward stepwise selection*, also called a *step-up* procedure) is to start with a very simple model and add new X variables one at a time, always adding the X variable that most improves the model's ability to predict Y. Another approach (*backward stepwise selection*, also called a *step-down* procedure) is to start with the full model (include all X variables) and then sequentially eliminate the X variable that contributes the least to the model.

The appeal is clear. You just put all the data into the program, and it makes all the decisions for you. How many models does a multiple regression program compare when given data with k independent variables and instructed to use the all subsets method to compare the fit of every possible model? Each variable can be included or excluded from the final model, so the program will compare 2^k models. For example, if the investigator starts with 20 variables, then automatic variable selection compares 2^{20} models (more than a million), even before considering interactions.

Simulated example of overfitting

Chapter 23 already referred to a simulated study by Freedman (1983) that demonstrated the problem with this approach. His paper was reprinted within a text by Good and Hardin (2006). He simulated a study with 100 subjects, with data from 50 independent variables recorded for each. All values were simulated, so it is clear that the outcome is not associated with any of the simulated independent variables. As expected, the overall P value from multiple regression was high, as were most of the individual P values (one for each independent variable).

He then chose the 15 independent variables that had the lowest P values (less than 0.25) and reran the multiple regression program using only those variables. Now the overall P value from multiple regression was tiny (0.0005). The contributions of 6 of the 15 independent variables were statistically significant (P < 0.05).

If you didn't know these were all simulated data with no associations, the results might seem impressive. The tiny P values beg you to reject the null hypotheses and conclude that the independent variables can predict the dependent variable.

The problem is essentially one of multiple comparisons, already discussed in Chapter 23. With lots of variables, it is too easy—way too easy—to be fooled. You can be impressed with high R^2 values and low P values, even though there are no real underlying relationships in the population.

Should you mistrust all analyses with variable selection?

No. It certainly makes sense to use statistical methods to decide whether to include or exclude a few carefully selected independent variables. But it does not make sense to let a statistics program test dozens or hundreds (or thousands) of possible models in hopes that the computer can work magic.

In some cases, the goal of the study is exploration. The investigators are not testing a hypothesis, but rather are looking for a hypothesis to test. Variable selection can be part of the exploration. But any model that emerges from an exploratory study must be considered a hypothesis to be tested with new data.

BEWARE OF MULTICOLLINEARITY

What is multicollinearity?

The term *multicollinearity* is as hard to understand as it is to say. But it is important to understand, because multicollinearity can interfere with proper interpretation of multiple regression results. Multicollinearity is a common problem with multiple (and logistic and proportional hazards) regression, and it can frustrate your ability to make sense of the data.

When two X variables are highly correlated, they both convey essentially the same information. For example, one of the variables included in the multiple regression example of the Chapter 37 is BMI, which is computed from an individual's weight and height. If the investigators had entered weight and height separately into the model, they probably would have encountered multicollinearity, because people who are taller also tend to be heavier.

The problem is that neither variable adds much to the fit of the model after the other one is included. If you removed either height or weight from the model, the fit would not change much. But if you removed both height and weight from the model, the fit would be much worse.

Lingo: Two (or more) related X variables are *collinear*. When they are included in a multiple regression model, the results show *collinearity*. When three or more X variables are tangled, the results demonstrate *multicollinearity*.

The effects of multicollinearity

The multiple regression model assesses the *additional* contribution of each variable, after accounting for all the other independent variables. When variables are collinear, each variable makes little individual contribution. This creates three problems:

- The CIs for the parameters become wider and the P values for each parameter become larger.
- P values can seem paradoxical. The fit of a multiple regression model with two independent variables could result in a low overall P value. This leads to the conclusion that the model is useful, and that the independent variables can predict the dependent variable. The paradox is that the P value for each independent variable could be high. After accounting for the other independent variables, neither variable can predict the outcome.
- Automatic variable selection can be arbitrary, depending on the order in which the variables are entered (or removed) from the model. If weight is entered into the model first, height may not make a significant contribution. Conversely, if height is entered first, weight may not make a significant contribution. The results of automated variable selection methods depend in part on the order in which it sees the collinear variables.

Quantifying multicollinearity

Multicollinearity is quantified with either *variance inflation factor* (VIF) or *tolerance* (they are reciprocals of each other). One value for VIF (and tolerance) is computed for each independent variable in the model. A high VIF (say >0.90) is a sign of multicollinearity, as is a low (<0.10) tolerance.

Avoiding multicollinearity

The best way to reduce multicollinearity is to reduce the number of independent variables. One approach is simply to leave out one of the related variables.

Another approach was mentioned in the example in Chapter 37. The investigators combined height and weight into a single variable (BMI, body mass index). They avoided multicollinearity and reduced the number of independent variables in the model. This wasn't a mathematical trick, but a sensible way to analyze the data.

BEWARE OF OVERINTERPRETING R^2

R^2 is commonly used as a measure of goodness of fit in multiple linear regression, but it can be misleading. Even if the independent variables are completely unable to predict the dependent variable, R^2 will be greater than zero. The expected value of R^2 increases as more independent variables are added to the model. This limits the usefulness of R^2 as a way to quantify goodness of fit, especially with small sample sizes.

In addition to reporting R^2, which quantifies how well the model fits the sample data, some programs also report an *adjusted R^2*, which estimates how well the model is expected to fit new data. It accounts for the number of independent variables and is always smaller than R^2. How much smaller depends on the relative numbers of subjects and variables. The multiple regression example in Chapter 37 (regarding kidney function) had far more subjects (965) than independent variables (5), so the adjusted R^2 is only a tiny bit smaller than the unadjusted R^2. The two are equal to two decimal places (0.27).

BEWARE OF CORRELATION VERSUS CAUSATION

Correlation cannot prove causation.

Chapter 37 already pointed out this problem. The investigators chose to place creatinine clearance (a measure of kidney function) on the left side of the model (Y), and the concentration of lead on the right (X). But that doesn't prove that lead poisons the kidney. It is conceivable that the relationship goes the opposite direction, with changes in kidney function somehow affecting lead accumulation.

Also beware of confounding variables. An absurd example mentioned by Katz (2006) makes the concept clear. People who carry matches in their pocket are more likely to get lung cancer than people who don't. A multiple regression model to find risk factors associated with lung cancer might identify carrying matches as a significant risk factor. Of course, carrying matches doesn't cause cancer. Rather, people who smoke are also likely to carry matches.

REGRESSION MODELS SHOULD BE VALIDATED

All scientific results are tentative, and important work is always worth repeating. For all the reasons explained above, one should be especially skeptical about results obtained via multiple regression.

The best way to validate a finding is to repeat the entire study. Define the model with one set of data, and test the model with an entirely different set of data. Confirmation by a different group of investigators makes the finding even more believable.

It is also possible to validate a finding by splitting a sample. Three methods are used:

- Holdout validation. Divide the sample into two groups, which don't need to be equal in size. Fit a model on the larger sample, and test that model on the other sample.
- Leave-one-out cross validation. The idea is pretty simple, although the details are daunting. Remove the first subject and fit all the rest. Use that fit to predict the result of the first subject (using its independent variables) and record the discrepancy between the prediction and actual outcome. Now take out only the second subject, and analyze all the rest (including the first). Again record the discrepancy between the predicted and actual result for that second subject. Repeat for all subjects, and then analyze the set of discrepancies. If the discrepancies are small, the model works well. This method can also be used to quantify how much the parameter estimates change when a data point is eliminated (rather than looking at how well the model predicts the missing value). In this context, the method is called a *jackknife procedure.*
- Bootstrapping. The idea is to randomly sample subjects from your sample to create a new sample. This sampling is done in such a way that some subjects may get selected more than once, and other subjects may be excluded. When a subject is selected twice, his data simply enter the computer program twice as if he were two different subjects (no new data are collected). Bootstrapping produces many pseudosamples, each the same size as the original sample. Similar results from the analysis of many bootstrapped samples gives you confidence that the findings are real.

The Rest of Statistics

CHAPTER 39

Analysis of Variance

In science, consensus is irrelevant. What is relevant is
reproducible results. The greatest scientists in history are
great precisely because they broke with the consensus.

MICHAEL CRICHTON (2005)

*O*ne-way *ANOVA compares the means of three or more groups,*
assuming that all values are sampled from Gaussian populations.
This chapter explains the idea of ANOVA and the specifics of one-way
ANOVA. Chapter 40 will explain the follow-up multiple comparisons
tests.

COMPARING THE MEAN OF THREE OR MORE GROUPS

Example data

Hetland and coworkers (1993) were interested in hormonal changes in women
runners. Among their investigations, they measured the level of luteinizing
hormone (LH) in nonrunners, recreational runners, and elite runners. Because
the distribution of hormone levels appeared to be lognormal (see Chapter 11),
the investigators transformed all the values to the logarithm of concentration
and performed all analyses on the transformed data. This was a smart decision,
because it made the values actually analyzed (the logarithms) come closer to
approximating a Gaussian distribution.

They didn't publish the raw data, but the summarized data are shown in
Table 39.1 and Figure 39.1. The left side of Figure 39.1 shows the mean and SD.
Assuming the data (as shown, already converted to logarithms) are sampled from
a Gaussian distribution, the SD error bars should include approximately two
thirds of the data points. You can see that there is a lot of variation within each
group and a huge amount of overlap between groups. Certainly, you could not
use the LH level to predict whether someone was a runner.

The right side of Figure 39.1 shows the mean with SEM error bars. Because
the sample sizes are fairly large, you can view these SEM error bars as approximately 68% CIs (see Chapter 14). Looked at this way, it seems as though the
mean of the nonrunners might be distinct from the mean of the two groups of
runners.

GROUP	LOG(LH)	SD	SEM	N
Nonrunners	0.52	0.25	0.027	88
Recreational runners	0.38	0.32	0.034	89
Elite runners	0.40	0.26	0.049	28

Table 39.1. LH levels in three groups of women.

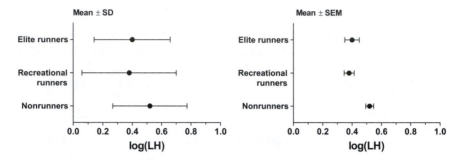

Figure 39.1. Data from Table 39.1 shown as a graph of the mean with SD (left) or SEM (right).

What's wrong with computing several t tests?

Your first thought when analyzing these data might be to use unpaired t tests (Chapter 30). You'd need one t test to compare nonrunners with recreational runners, another to compare nonrunners with elite runners, and yet another to compare recreational runners with elite runners. The main problem with this approach is multiple comparisons (Chapters 22 and 23). As you include more groups in the study, you increase the chance of observing one or more significant P values by chance. If the null hypothesis was true (all three populations have the same mean), there would be a 5% chance that each particular t test would yield a significant P value. But with three comparisons, the chance that any one (or more) of them will be significant would be far higher than 5%.

Interpreting a P value from one-way ANOVA

The data were not analyzed with t tests, but rather with one-way ANOVA, which compares all the groups at once.

The one-way ANOVA reports that the P value is 0.0039.

To interpret any P value, the first step is to articulate the null hypothesis. Here, the null hypothesis is that the mean concentration of LH is the same in all three populations. The P value answers the following question:

> Assuming the null hypothesis is true, what is the chance of randomly picking samples with mean values as different (or more different) than observed in this study?

If the three sets of data were really sampled from identical populations, there is only a 0.4% chance that the three means would be as far apart as actually observed.

ASSUMPTIONS: ONE-WAY ANOVA

One-way ANOVA is based on the same assumptions as the unpaired t test:

- The samples are randomly selected from, or at least representative of, the larger populations.
- The observations within each sample were obtained independently. The relationships between all the observations in a group should be the same. You don't have independent measurements if some of the LH measurements were from the same person measured on several occasions or if some of the subjects are twins (or even sisters).
- The data are sampled from populations that approximate a Gaussian distribution. In this case, the assumption applies to the logarithms actually analyzed.
- The SD of all populations are identical. This assumption is less important with large samples and when the sample sizes are equal. In this example, the data were all transformed to logarithms before the analysis was done, so the assumption refers to the log-transformed values.

HOW IT WORKS: ONE-WAY ANOVA

You can interpret ANOVA without knowing how it works, but you are less likely to use ANOVA inappropriately if you have some idea how it works. The descriptions below give you a general idea for how it works.

The first two sections below explain alternative ways to look at the method. The two are equivalent and produce exactly the same results. I find the first approach easier to understand, but the second is more traditional.

Determine sum of squares by fitting alternative models

Comparing three or more means with one-way ANOVA can be viewed as comparing the fit of the data to two models using the ideas presented in Chapter 35. The two models are as follows:

- Null hypothesis: All populations share the same mean, and any differences between sample means are caused by random sampling.
- Alternative hypothesis: All populations do not share the same means. At least one population has a mean different than the rest.

The top row of Table 39.2 quantifies how well the null hypothesis fits the data. Goodness of fit is quantified by the sum of squares of the difference between each value and the grand mean (totally ignoring any distinction among the three groups).

The second row of Table 39.2 shows how well the alternative hypothesis fits the data. Table 39.2 reports the sum of squares of the difference between each value and the mean of the sample that value came from.

The third row of Table 39.2 shows the difference. Of all the variation (sum of squares from the null hypothesis grand mean), 94.7% is the result of scatter

	HYPOTHESIS	SCATTER FROM	SUM OF SQUARES	PERCENTAGE OF VARIATION	
	Null	Grand mean	17.38	100.0	
−	Alternative	Group means	16.45	94.7	
=	Difference	Improvement	0.93	5.3	$R^2 = 0.053$

Table 39.2 One-way ANOVA as a comparison of models.

SOURCE OF VARIATION	SUM OF SQUARES	df	MS	F RATIO	P VALUE
Between groups	0.93	2	0.46	5.69	0.0039
Within groups (error, residual)	16.45	202	0.081		
Total	17.38	204			

Table 39.3 ANOVA table showing the F ratio.

within the groups, leaving 5.3% of the total variation as resulting from a difference between the group means.

To determine the P value requires more than dividing the variance into its components. It also requires accounting for the number of values and the number of parameters fit by each model. This is done in Table 39.3, which will be discussed after first explaining an alternative approach to thinking about the sum of square values.

Alternative approach: Partitioning the sum of squares

A more common way to think about ANOVA is portioning the variability into different components.

The example data come from three groups. The first step in ANOVA is to compute the total variability among all the values (ignoring which value came from which group). This is done by summing the squares of the differences of each value from the *grand* mean. This is shown in the bottom row of Table 39.3. The total sum of squares is 17.38.

Some of the variation comes from differences *among* the group means because the group means are not all the same. Sum the squares of each group mean from the grand mean and weight by sample size to get the sum of squares resulting from treatment. This is shown in the top row of Table 39.3. The sum of squares between group means is 0.93.

The rest of the variation comes from variably *within* each group, quantified by summing the squares of the differences of each value from its group mean. This is shown in the second row of Table 39.3. The sum of squares within groups is 16.45. This is also called the residual sum of squares or the error sum of squares.

It isn't obvious (but can be proven with simple algebra), but the sum of squares resulting from treatment and the sum of squares within the groups always add up to the total sum of squares.

Determining P from F

The third column of Table 39.3 shows the number of df. The bottom row labeled total is for the null hypothesis model. There are 205 values and only 1 parameter was fit (the grand mean), which leaves 204 df. The next row up shows the sum of squares from the group means. Three parameters were fit (the mean of each group), so there are 202 df (205 data points minus 3 parameters). The top row shows the difference. The alternative model (three distinct means) has 2 more parameters than the null hypothesis model (one grand mean), so there are 2 df in this row. The df, like the sums of squares, can be partitioned so the bottom row is the sum of values in the rows above.

The fourth column divides the sum of squares by the number of df to compute the MS, which could also be called variances. Note that it is not possible to add the MS in the top two rows to obtain a meaningful MS for the bottom row. Because the MS for the null hypothesis is not used in further calculations, it is left blank.

To compute a P value, you must take into account the number of values and the number of groups. This is done in the last column of Table 39.3.

If the null hypothesis were correct, each MS value would estimate the variance among values, so the two MS values would be similar. The ratio of those two MS values is called the F ratio, after Fisher (a pioneering statistician who invented ANOVA and much of statistics).

If the null hypothesis were true, F would be likely to have a value close to 1. If the null hypothesis were not true, F would probably have a value greater than 1. The probability distribution of F under the null hypothesis is known for various df and can be used to calculate a P value that answers the question: If the null hypothesis was true, what is the chance that randomly selected data (given the total sample size and number of groups) would lead to an F ratio this large or larger? For this example, $F = 5.690$ with 2 df in the numerator and 202 df in the denominator, and $P = 0.0039$.

R^2

Look at the first column of Table 39.2, which partitions the total sum of squares into its two component parts. Divide the sum of squares resulting from differences between groups (0.93) by the total sum of squares (17.38) to determine the fraction of sum of squares resulting from differences between groups, 0.053. This is eta squared, $\tilde{\eta}^2$, which is interpreted the same as R^2. Only 5.3% of the total variability in this example is the result of differences between group means. The remaining 94.7% of the variability is within the groups.

The low P value means that the differences among group means are very unlikely to be caused by chance. The low R^2 means that those differences among group means are only a tiny fraction of the overall variability. You also saw this on the left side of Figure 39.1, where the SD error bars overlap so much.

REPEATED-MEASURES ANOVA

The difference between ordinary and repeated-measures ANOVA is the same as the difference between the unpaired and paired t tests. Use repeated-measures ANOVA to analyze data collected in three kinds of experiments:

- Measurements are made repeatedly in each subject, perhaps before, during, and after an intervention.
- Subjects are recruited as matched sets (often called *blocks*), matched for variables such as age, zip code, or diagnosis. Each subject in the set receives a different intervention (or placebo).
- A laboratory experiment is run several times, each time with several treatments (or a control and several treatments) handled in parallel. More generally, you should use a repeated-measures test whenever the value of one subject in the first group is expected to be closer to a particular value in the other group than to a random subject in the other group.

When the experimental design incorporates matching, use the repeated-measures test, because it is usually more powerful than ordinary ANOVA. Of course the matching must be done as part of the protocol, before the results are collected. The decision about pairing is a question of experimental design and should be made long before the data are analyzed.

Although the calculations for the repeated-measures ANOVA are different from those for ordinary ANOVA, the interpretation of the P value is the same. The same kind of multiple comparisons tests are performed.

Q & A: One-Way ANOVA

Can one-way ANOVA be done with two groups?	One-way ANOVA is usually only done for three or more groups, but it could be done for only two groups. Many programs won't allow this, but it certainly is mathematically possible. Although the approach seems very different, one-way ANOVA for two groups is mathematically equivalent to an unpaired t test and will compute an identical P value.
Are the results valid if sample size differs between groups?	Yes. ANOVA does not require that all samples have the same number of values. Two of the assumptions of ANOVA—that the data come from Gaussian populations and that these populations have equal standard deviations—matter much more when sample size varies a lot between groups. If you have very different sample sizes, a small P value from ANOVA may be caused by non-Gaussian data (or unequal variances) rather than differences among means.

Continued

Q&A Continued

Is the F ratio always positive?	Yes. Because the ANOVA calculations deal with sums of squares, the F ratio is always positive.
Does ANOVA really compare variances?	Don't get misled by the term *variance*. The word variance refers to the statistical method being used, not the hypothesis being tested. ANOVA tests whether group means differ significantly from each other. ANOVA does not test whether the variances of the groups are different.
If the P value is small, can we be sure that all the means are distinct?	No. A small P value means it is extremely unlikely that the data were sampled from populations where all the means were identical. A P value can be small when all groups are distinct, or if one is distinct whereas the rest are indistinguishable. Chapter 40 will show how to compare individual pairs of means.
Does ANOVA account for the order of groups?	No. The order of the groups is entirely irrelevant when computing the ANOVA table and P value. In the example, the three groups have a natural order. The ANOVA calculations do ***not*** take into account this order. ANOVA treats the groups as categories, and the calculations don't take into account how the groups are related to each other. Chapter 40 briefly explains a posttest for trend that does consider the group order.
Is the P value from one-way ANOVA one- or two-tailed?	Neither. With ANOVA, the concept of one- and two-tail P values does not really apply. Because the means of the groups can be in many different orders, the P value has many tails.
If I need to use a program to compute a P value from F, does it matter in which order the two df values are entered?	Yes. The calculation of a P value from F requires knowing the number of df for the numerator of the F ratio and also the number of df for the denominator. If you mistakenly swap the two df values, the P value will be incorrect.
Do the one-way ANOVA calculations require raw data?	No. One-way ANOVA (but not repeated-measures ANOVA) can be computed without raw data, so long as you know the mean, sample size, and SD (or SEM) of each group.
Can all kinds of ANOVA also be done using regression techniques?	Yes. ANOVA compares the fit of several models to the data, and this can be done with regression techniques as well. The answers will be fundamentally identical, but will look very different.
Can all kinds of regression be done using ANOVA techniques?	No.

TWO-WAY ANOVA AND BEYOND

Although Chapter 39 only explained one-way ANOVA, many other forms of ANOVA are used. This section will briefly describe two-way ANOVA, without a full example.

The term *one-way* means that the subjects are categorized in one way. In the example above, they were categorized by how much exercise they did. If they were also divided into age groups, the data would be analyzed by two-way ANOVA, also called two-factor ANOVA. If they were simultaneously divided into a group that is pregnant and a group that is not pregnant, you'd need three-way ANOVA.

Two-way ANOVA simultaneously tests three null hypotheses and so computes three P values:

1. *Interaction.* The null hypothesis is that there is no interaction between the two factors. In our example, the null hypothesis is that the difference in log(LH) caused by exercise is the same for all age groups. Equivalently, the null hypothesis is that the difference in log(LH) among age groups is consistent for all levels of exercise. If the interaction P value is small, then there usually is no point trying to interpret the other two P values. If you know the effect of exercise differs for different age groups, then trying to quantify one P value for the effects of age and one for the effect of exercise is usually pointless.

2. *First factor.* The null hypothesis is that the population means are identical for each category of the first factor. In our example, the null hypothesis is that the mean log(LH) is the same for each level of exercise in the overall population and that all observed differences are caused by chance.

3. *Second factor.* The null hypothesis is that the population means are identical for each category of the second factor. In our example, the null hypothesis is that the mean log(LH) is the same for all age groups in the overall population and that all observed differences are caused by chance.

As with one-way ANOVA, special methods have been developed to deal with repeated measures in one or both factors.

CHAPTER 40

Multiple Comparison Tests After ANOVA

When did "skeptic" become a dirty word in science?
MICHAEL CRICHTON (2003)

*O*ne-way ANOVA computes a single P value testing the null hypothesis that all groups were sampled from populations with identical means. This chapter explains how multiple comparison tests let you dig deeper to see which pairs of groups are statistically distinguishable. Before reading this chapter, read Chapters 22 and 23 (multiple comparisons) and 39 (one-way ANOVA).

MULTIPLE COMPARISON TESTS FOR THE EXAMPLE DATA

Goal

Chapter 39 analyzed a sample data set comparing LH levels (actually their logarithms) in three groups of women. One-way ANOVA reported a very small P value. If the null hypothesis that all groups were sampled from populations with equal means were true, it would be quite rare for random sampling to result in so much variability among the sample means.

Multiple comparison tests dig deeper to find out which groups differ from which other groups, taking into account multiple comparisons (Chapter 22). To prevent getting fooled by bogus statistically significant conclusions, the significance level is redefined to apply to an entire family of comparisons, rather than to each individual comparison (Table 40.1). This is one of the most confusing parts of statistics. Using this new definition of statistical significance will reduce the chance of obtaining false reports of statistical significance (fewer Type I errors) but at the cost of reducing the power to detect real differences (more Type II errors).

For this example, the goal is to compare every mean with every other mean, and the appropriate test is called *Tukey's* test (more generally, the Tukey–Kramer test, which allows for unequal sample size). The results include both CIs and conclusions about statistical significance.

SITUATION	MEANING OF A 5% SIGNIFICANCE LEVEL	ERROR RATE
One comparison	If the null hypotheses were true, there is a 5% chance that random sampling would lead to the incorrect conclusion that there is a real difference.	Per comparison
A family of comparisons	If all null hypotheses were true, there is a 5% chance that random sampling would lead to one or more incorrect conclusions that there is a real difference.	Per experiment or Familywise

Table 40.1. Statistical significance is redefined for multiple comparisons.

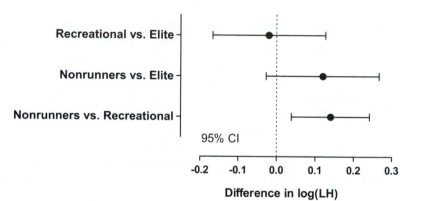

Figure 40.1. Tukey's multiple comparisons 95% CIs from Table 41.1.

The 95% confidence level applies to the entire family of comparisons, rather than to an individual comparison.

TUKEY'S MULTIPLE COMPARISON TEST	DIFFERENCE BETWEEN MEANS	95% CI OF DIFFERENCE
Nonrunners versus recreational runners	0.1400	0.038 to 0.24
Nonrunners versus elite runners	0.1200	−0.027 to 0.27
Recreational runners versus elite runners	−0.0200	−0.17 to 0.13

Table 40.2. Multiple comparison posttests CIs.

The 95% confidence level applies to the entire family of intervals, rather than to each interval individually. The original data were expressed as the logarithm of LH concentration, so the mean differences and both confidence limits shown here are in those same units (logarithm of concentration).

Multiple comparison confidence intervals

Figure 40.1 plots the 95% CI for the difference between each mean and every other mean. These are tabulated in Table 40.2.

These are multiple comparisons CIs, so the 95% confidence level applies to the entire family of comparisons, rather than to each individual interval. Given

TUKEY'S MULTIPLE COMPARISON TEST	RATIO	95% CI OF RATIO
Nonrunners versus recreational runners	1.38	1.09 to 1.74
Nonrunners versus elite runners	1.32	0.94 to 1.86
Recreational runners versus elite runners	0.96	0.68 to 1.35

Table 40.3. Multiple comparisons CIs, expressed as ratios rather than differences.
The values in Table 40.2 are the differences between two logarithms, which is mathematically identical to the logarithm of the ratio. Transforming to antilogarithms creates the table of ratios and CIs of ratios, shown here.

the assumptions of the analysis (listed in Chapter 39), there is a 95% chance that all three of these CIs include the true population value, leaving only a 5% chance that any one or more of the intervals does not include the population value.

Because these are multiple comparison CIs, it makes no sense to show just one. The 95% confidence level applies to the entire set of intervals, and it is impossible to correctly interpret any individual interval without seeing the entire set.

CIs as ratios

The data entered into the ANOVA program (shown in Chapter 39) are expressed as the logarithm of the concentration of LH, so Figure 40.1 and Table 40.2 show differences between two logarithms. Many find it easier to think about these results without logarithms, and it is easy to convert the data to a more intuitive format.

The trick is to note that the difference between the logarithms of two values is mathematically identical to the logarithm of the ratio of those two values (logarithms and antilogarithms are reviewed in Appendix E). Transform each of the differences (and each confidence limit) to its antilogarithm, and the resulting values can be interpreted as the ratio of two LH levels. Written as equations,

$$\log(A) - \log(B) = \log\left(\frac{A}{B}\right)$$

$$10^{(\log(A)-\log(B))} = \frac{A}{B}.$$

To convert a logarithm base 10 back to the original value requires taking that value to the power of 10, which many calculators do with the button labeled 10^Y. Table 40.3 and Figure 40.2 shows the results. Each row shows the ratio of the mean LH level in one group divided by the mean in another group, along with the 95% CI of that ratio. A dotted line marks a ratio of 1.0.

Statistical significance

If a 95% CI for the difference between two means includes zero (the value specified in the null hypothesis), then the difference is not statistically significant ($P > 0.05$).

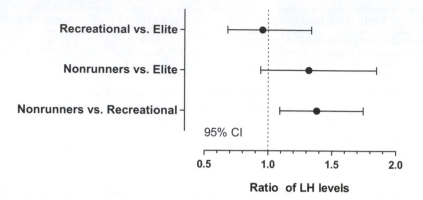

Figure 40.2 Tukey's multiple comparisons 95% CIs, expressed as ratios of LH levels rather than difference between mean log(LH) concentrations.
The values correspond to Table 40.2.

Two of the three 95% CIs shown in Table 40.2 and Figure 40.1 include zero, and so those comparisons are not statistically significant at the 5% significance level. The CI for the remaining comparison (nonrunners versus recreational runners) does not include zero, so that difference is significantly significant.

The same conclusion can be reached using the ratios in Table 40.3 and Figure 40.2. The null hypothesis of identical populations corresponds to a ratio of 1.0. Only one comparison (nonrunners versus recreational runners) does not include 1.0, so that comparison is statistically significant.

The 5% significance level applies to the entire set or family of comparisons. It is a familywise significance level (defined in Chapter 22). If the overall null hypothesis were true (values from all groups are sampled from populations with identical means), there is a 5% chance that one or more of the comparisons would be declared statistically significant and thus a 95% chance that none of the comparisons would be statistically significant.

It is hard to think about significance levels that apply to a family of comparisons. Don't think about whether one particular comparison is statistically significant. Instead, think about dividing the family of comparisons into two piles—statistically significant and not statistically significant.

Table 40.4 shows the conclusions about statistical significance at three different significance levels.

THE LOGIC OF MULTIPLE COMPARISON TESTS

Multiple comparisons tests account for multiple comparisons

If all null hypotheses are true and you make several comparisons without any special corrections, then 5% of all those comparisons will generate a statistically significant result. The chance of making one or more Type I error

		STATISTICALLY SIGNIFICANT?		
	DIFFERENCE	α=0.05	α=0.01	α=0.001
Nonrunners-recreational	0.1400	Yes	Yes	No
Nonrunners-elite	0.1200	No	No	No
Recreational-elite	−0.02000	No	No	No

Table 40.4. Statistical significance of multiple comparisons.

The significance levels (alpha) apply to the entire family of comparisons, not to each individual comparison.

(declaring statistical significance when really the null hypotheses are all true) would be greater than 5%. This problem of multiple comparisons was discussed in Chapter 22.

As their name suggests, multiple comparisons tests account for multiple comparisons by making the confidence level apply to the entire family of CIs. Given certain assumptions, there is a 95% chance that all of the CIs include the true population value, leaving only a 5% chance that one or more of the intervals do not include the population value.

Similarly, the 5% significance level applies to the entire family of comparisons. If the null hypothesis is true (all data sampled from populations with identical means), there is a 95% chance that none of the comparisons would be declared statistically significant, leaving a 5% chance that one or more comparisons would (erroneously) be declared statistically significant.

With more groups, CIs between means become wider

The example had three groups, and there were three possible pairwise comparisons of means. If there were five groups, then there would be 10 possible comparisons between sample means (AB, AC, AD, AE, BC, BD, BE, CD, CE, DE). Table 40.5 and Figure 40.3 show how the number of possible comparisons increases with the number of groups.

The multiple comparisons define the significance level (for declaring differences to be statistically significant) and confidence level (for CIs for the difference between two means) to apply to the entire family of comparisons. This requires making the CIs wider than they would be if only a single comparison were made. Accordingly, if you have more groups, a difference must be larger before it will be deemed statistically significant. This cost of controlling the significance level (risk of making a Type I error and finding a significant result by chance) is decreasing the power to detect real differences.

Multiple comparisons tests use data from all groups, even when comparing two

One-way ANOVA is based on the assumption that all the data are sampled from populations with the same SD, even if their means differ. If this assumption is

NO. OF GROUPS	NO. OF PAIRWISE COMPARISONS
3	3
4	6
5	10
6	15
7	21
8	28
9	36
10	45
11	55
12	66
13	78
14	91
15	105
16	120
17	136
18	153
19	171
20	190
k	$k(k-1)/2$

Table 40.5. Number of possible pairwise comparisons between group means as a function of the number of groups.

The number of possible pairwise comparisons is very large when you have many groups.

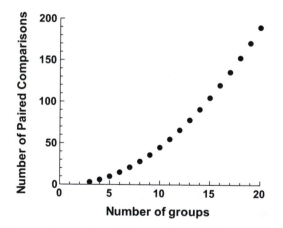

Figure 40.3 Number of possible pairwise comparisons between group means as a function of the number of groups.

valid, it is used to give the multiple comparisons test more power than they would otherwise have.

One-way ANOVA reports the mean square within groups, which the best estimate of the population variance considering all the values in all groups. The square root of this value (not usually reported by ANOVA) is the best estimate of the population SD.

The multiple comparisons tests work by comparing the difference between two means to that estimate of the population SD, while also taking into account the number of values in the two groups being compared. Quantifying the variation among all values within all groups, and not just the two being compared, gives the test more statistical power than it would have if each comparison considered only the values in the two groups being compared.

Multiple comparisons tests account for intertwined comparisons

Once you have compared the mean of group A with the mean of group B and the mean of group A with the mean of group C, you already know something about the comparison of group B with group C. Consider three groups (with equal n) where the mean of A is greater than the mean of B and the mean of B is greater than the mean of C, and both comparisons are statistically significant. Without any calculations, you know that the mean of A must be significantly greater than the mean of C. The multiple comparisons methods account for this interlinking of comparisons.

Multiple comparisons tests can declare the difference between pairs of means to be statistically significant, but they do not compute exact P values

When a t test compares two means, it reports an exact P value. You can then decide, optionally, to compare that P value to a preset significance level to decide whether the test concludes that the difference is statistically significant.

Multiple comparisons tests following ANOVA are different. Statistical significance is determined accounting for multiple comparisons. The significance level doesn't apply to any one particular comparison, but rather to the entire family of comparisons. Accordingly, exact P values are not computed for each comparison. It is common, however, for statistics programs to report statistical significance at several different familywise significance levels (as is done in Table 40.4).

OTHER MULTIPLE COMPARISON TESTS

Statisticians have developed numerous methods to follow one-way ANOVA. The example above used Tukey's test, which compares the mean of each group with the mean of every other group. This section explains some (but certainly not all) alternative tests.

Dunnett's test: Compare each mean with the mean of a control group

Dunnett's test compares the mean of each group to the mean of a control group, without comparing the other groups among themselves. For example, it would be used in an experiment that tests the effects of six different drugs and with a goal to define which drugs have any effect and not to compare the drugs with each other.

Because Dunnett's test makes fewer comparisons than Tukey's method, it generates narrower CIs and has more power to detect differences. It is very useful.

The decision to use Dunnett's test (along with a definition of which group is the control group) should be part of the experimental design. It isn't fair to first do Tukey's test to make all comparisons and then switch to Dunnett's test to get more power.

Bonferroni's test: Compare preselected pairs of means

Bonferroni's approach was explained in Chapter 22. Although it can be used to compare all pairs of means, it should not be used in this way because Tukey's test has more power. Similarly, it should not be used to compare each group against a control, because Dunnett's test has more power for that purpose. Bonferroni's multiple comparison tests should be used when the experiment design requires comparing only selected pairs of means. By making a limited set of comparisons, you get narrower CIs and more statistical power to detect differences.

It is essential that you select those pairs based on experimental design, before collecting the data. It is not fair to first look at the data and then decide which pairs you want to compare. By looking at the data first, you have implicitly compared all groups.

Holm's test: Powerful, but no confidence intervals

The Holm multiple comparison is a powerful and versatile multiple comparison test. It can be used to compare all pairs of means, compare each group mean to a control mean, or compare preselected pairs of means. It is not restricted to being used as a follow up to ANOVA, but can be used in any multiple comparison context. The test is quite logical and easy to understand.

The test is powerful, understandable and versatile. What's not to like? The Holm test can only be used to decide which comparisons are statistically significant and which are not. Unlike the tests developed by Tukey, Bonferroni, and Dunnett, it cannot also compute a set of confidence intervals (Westfall et al. 1999; page 40).

The Holm-Sidak test is a modified version of Holm's test that is slightly more powerful.

Scheffe's test: More general comparisons

Scheffe's multiple comparison test can make more elaborate comparisons than the other tests. For example, you might want to compare the mean of all treated groups with the mean of a control group. Or you might want to compare the mean of groups A and B with the mean of groups C, D, and E. These comparisons are sometimes called *contrasts*.

Scheffe's method can test any number of this kind of comparison. This increased versatility comes with a price. To allow for the huge number of possible comparisons, the CIs generated by Scheffe's method are wider than those generated by other methods. Accordingly, the test has less statistical power to detect differences than do the other multiple comparison tests. The precise comparisons do not need to be defined as part of the experimental design. It is OK to test comparisons that you didn't think of until you saw the data.

Posttest for a trend: Is group mean correlated with group order?

The different groups compared by ANOVA often have a natural order—for example, ages, time intervals, or doses. However, one-way ANOVA calculations completely ignore this order. ANOVA analyzes data from different doses or different ages exactly the same as it analyzes data from different species or different drugs. If you randomly shuffled the doses or ages, the ANOVA results wouldn't change.

The *posttest for trend* computes the correlation coefficient between the outcome and group order, along with a P value testing the null hypothesis that there is no trend. If this P value is small, there is a statistically significant trend (correlation) between group order and the outcome.

To learn more, see Altman (1990). Fancier tests for trend can look for nonlinear trends. Look up "polynomial contrasts" in advanced ANOVA texts for more details.

HOW IT WORKS: MULTIPLE COMPARISONS TESTS

Chapter 12 briefly explained how a CI of a mean is computed. The margin of error of the CI of a mean is the product of two values. The first is the SEM, which is computed from the SD and sample size. The second is a critical value from the t distribution, which depends on the desired confidence level (95%) and the number of df $(n-1)$.

Chapter 30 extended that idea to the CI for the difference between two means. The standard error of the difference between means is computed from both SDs and both sample sizes.

When computing a multiple comparisons test, the standard error for the difference between two means is not computed from the SDs of those two groups, but rather from the SDs of all the groups. ANOVA software rarely reports this pooled SD, but instead reports the pooled variance (the square of the pooled SD), which is labeled "mean square within groups" or "mean square residual." The standard error of the difference between two means is computed from that value (the same for all comparisons) and the sample size of the two groups being compared (which might not be the same for all comparisons).

The margin of error of the CI is computed by multiplying the standard error of the difference times a critical value that depends on the choice of test, the number of df, the degree of confidence desired, and the number of comparisons.

Q & A: Multiple Comparison Tests Following One-Way ANOVA

What is the difference between a multiple comparison test and a post hoc test?	The term *multiple comparison test* applies whenever several comparisons are performed at once, with a correction for multiple comparisons. The term *post hoc test* refers to situations where you can decide which comparisons you want to make after looking at the data. Often, however, it is used informally as a synonym for multiple comparisons test. Posttest is an informal, but ambiguous, term. It can refer to either all multiple comparisons tests or only to post hoc tests.
If one-way ANOVA reports a P value less than 0.05, are multiple comparison tests sure to find a significant difference between group means?	Not necessarily. The low P value from the ANOVA tells you that the null hypothesis that all data were sampled from one population with one mean is unlikely to have produced these data. But the difference might be a subtle one. It might be that the mean of A and B is significantly different than the mean of groups C, D, and E. Scheffe's post test can find such differences (called "contrasts"), and if the overall ANOVA is statistically significant, Scheffe's posttest is sure to find a significant contrast.
	The other posttests compare group means. Finding that the overall ANOVA reports a statistically significant result does not guarantee that any of these multiple comparisons will find a statistically significant difference. It seems surprising, but it is possible for the overall ANOVA to reject the null hypothesis that all data are sampled from populations with the same mean, while none of the posttests find a statistically significant difference between pairs of means.
If one-way ANOVA reports a P value greater than 0.05, is it possible for a multiple comparison test to find an statistically significant difference between some group means?	Yes, it is possible.
Are the results of multiple comparisons tests valid if the overall P value for the ANOVA is greater than 0.05?	It depends on which multiple comparisons test you use. Tukey's, Dunnett's, and Bonferroni's tests mentioned above are valid even if the overall ANOVA yields a nonsignificant P value.
Does it make sense to focus only on multiple comparison results and ignore the overall ANOVA results?	It depends on the scientific goals. ANOVA tests the overall null hypothesis that all the data come from groups that have identical means. If that is your experimental question—do the data provide convincing evidence that the means are not all identical—then ANOVA is exactly what you want.

Continued

Q&A Continued

	If the experimental questions are more focused and answered by multiple comparison tests, you can safely ignore the overall ANOVA results and jump right to the results of multiple comparisons. Note that the multiple comparison calculations all use the mean-square result from the ANOVA table. So even if you don't care about the value of F or the P value, the multiple comparisons tests still require that the ANOVA table be computed.
Can I assess statistical significance by observing whether two error bars overlap?	If two SE error bars overlap, you can be sure that a posttest comparing those two groups will find no statistical significance. However, if two SE error bars do not overlap, you can't tell whether a posttest will or will not find a statistically significant difference. If you plot SD error bars, rather than SEM, the fact that they do (or don't) overlap does not let you reach any conclusion about statistical significance.
Do multiple comparison tests take into account the order of the groups?	No. With the exception of the posttest for trend, mentioned above, multiple comparisons tests do not consider the order that the groups were entered into the program.
Do all CIs between means have the same length?	If all groups have the same number of values, then all the CIs for the difference between means will have identical lengths. If the sample sizes are unequal, then the standard error of the difference between means depends on sample size. The CI for the difference between two means will be wider when sample size is small and narrower when sample size is larger.
Why wasn't the Newman-Keuls test used for the example?	Like Tukey's test, the Newman–Keuls test (also called the Student–Newman–Keuls test) compares each group mean with every other group mean. Some prefer it because it has more power. I prefer Tukey's test, because the Newman-Keuls test does not really control the error rate as it should (Seaman, Levin, & Serlin 1991) and cannot compute CIs.

MULTIPLE INDIVIDUAL COMPARISONS

Is is not always wise to correct for multiple comparisons so that the significance level applies to the entire family of comparisons rather than to each individual comparison.

Risk of Type I error (Labeling a chance difference as statistically significant)	Lower
Risk of Type II error (Missing a real difference)	Higher
Width of CIs	Wider

Table 40.6. Consequences of correcting for multiple comparisons compared to individual comparisons.

Never correct for multiple comparisons?

Correcting for multiple comparisons reduces the risk of a Type I error, but at the cost of increasing the risk of a Type II error (Table 40.6). Rothman (1990) argues that this tradeoff is not worth it and recommends that correcting for multiple comparisons should not be used. This recommendation is sensible, but not mainstream.

Don't correct when only a few comparisons were planned

Correcting for multiple comparisons can lead to ambiguous situations. Imagine that you are running a research program to investigate the mechanism of action of a drug. You want to know whether it blocks a certain receptor. You set up the proper assay and ran some test experiments to make sure everything works. Now imagine two alternative scenarios.

Scenario 1: You run an experiment testing only your one drug against a control. The difference is statistically significant. The drug worked as you predicted, and the results are statistically significant. Your research moves forward.

Scenario 2: You run an experiment testing not only your drug, but also two additional drugs. There is no reason to expect these drugs to block the receptor you are studying, but it would be very interesting if they did. Setting up the assay and running various controls was a lot of work, but testing three drugs is not a whole lot harder than testing one drug, so you give it a try. Every once in a while, this kind of exploratory experiment can move research forward. Not this time. The two extra drugs don't work. Not a big disappointment and not too much time wasted.

The data for the main drug are exactly the same in both scenarios. In the second scenario, two other drugs were tested at the same time. To account for multiple comparisons, the comparisons used Dunnett's method, so the 5% significance level applied to the family of three comparisons, rather than to each individual comparison. With this analysis, the result for the main drug was not statistically significant. Because more comparisons were made, the method became more cautious about concluding statistical significance.

In this example, the correction for multiple corrections didn't really make sense. The experiment was done to test one main hypothesis, and the other two hypotheses were add-ons. When one or a few comparisons are clearly defined in advance as being critical, some statisticians advocate not using any correction for multiple comparisons for these few comparisons. This approach is called *planned comparisons*, but that term is ambiguous because many multiple comparisons are planned in advance.

The statistical principles are fairly straightforward, without much controversy. But that doesn't make it easy to decide what to do in this situation. Reasonable statisticians disagree.

CHAPTER 41

Nonparametric Methods

Statistics are like a bikini. What they reveal is suggestive, but what they conceal is vital.

AARON LEVENSTEIN

*M*any *of the methods discussed in this book are based on the assumption that the values are sampled from a Gaussian distribution. Another family of methods makes no such assumption about the population distribution. These are called* nonparametric methods. *The nonparametric methods used most commonly work by ignoring the actual data values and instead analyze only their ranks. Computer-intensive resampling and bootstrapping methods also do not assume a specified distribution, so they are also nonparametric.*

NONPARAMETRIC TESTS BASED ON RANKS

The idea of nonparametric tests

The unpaired t test and ANOVA are based on the assumption that the data are sampled from populations that follow a Gaussian distribution. Similarly, the paired t test assumes that the differences between pairs are selected from a Gaussian population. Because these tests are based on an assumption about the distribution of values in the population that can be defined by parameters, they are called *parametric tests.*

Nonparametric tests make no assumptions about the distribution of the populations. The most popular forms of nonparametric tests are based on a really simple idea. Rank the values from low to high and analyze only those ranks, ignoring the actual values. This ensures that the test isn't affected much by outliers (see Chapter 25) and doesn't assume any particular distribution.

Comparing two unpaired groups: Mann–Whitney test

The Mann–Whitney test is a nonparametric test to compare two unpaired groups to compute a P value. It works by following these steps:

1. Rank all the values without paying attention to which of the two groups the value comes from. In the example from Chapter 30 (bladders of old

OLD	YOUNG
3.0	10.0
1.0	13.0
11.0	14.0
6.0	16.0
4.5	15.0
8.0	17.0
4.5	9.0
12.0	7.0
2.0	

Table 41.1. Ranks of the data shown in Table 30.1.

The smallest value has a rank of 1, and the largest value has a rank of 17. Note that two values tie for ranks of 4 and 5, so both are assigned a rank of 4.5. These ranks are plotted in Figure 41.1.

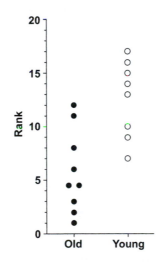

Figure 41.1. The data (ranks) of Table 41.1 are plotted here.

vs. young rats), two values tie for ranks of 4 and 5, so both are assigned a rank of 4.5. Table 41.1 and Figure 41.1 show the ranks.

2. Sum the ranks in each group. In the example data, the sum of the ranks from the old rats is 52; the sum of the ranks of the young rats is 101. The values from younger rats tend to be larger, so tend to have higher ranks.

3. Calculate the mean rank of each group.

4. Compute a P value for the null hypothesis that the distribution of ranks is totally random.

Under the null hypothesis, it would be equally likely for either of the two groups to have the larger mean ranks, and more likely to find the two mean ranks close together than far apart. Based on this null hypothesis, the P value is computed by answering this question: If the distribution of ranks between two groups were distributed randomly, what is the probability that the difference between the mean ranks would be this large or even larger? The answer is 0.0061. It certainly is not impossible that random shuffling of values from two identical populations would lead to sums of ranks this far apart, but it would be very unlikely. Accordingly, we conclude the difference between the young and old rats is statistically significant.

Although the Mann–Whitney test makes no assumptions about the distribution of values, it is still based on some assumptions. Like the unpaired t test, the Mann–Whitney test assumes that the samples are randomly sampled from (or representative of) a larger population and that each value was obtained independently. But unlike the t test, the Mann–Whitney test does not assume anything about the distribution of values in the populations from which the data were sampled.

Lingo: This test developed by Mann and Whitney is equivalent to one developed by Wilcoxon. So the same test is sometimes called the *Wilcoxon rank-sum test*. Don't mix that up with the nonparametric test for paired data discussed in the next section.

Comparing two paired groups: Wilcoxon matched-pairs signed-rank test

The Wilcoxon matched-pairs signed-rank test (often referred to simply as Wilcoxon's test) compares two paired groups. It tests the null hypothesis that there is no difference in the populations, so the differences between matched pairs will be randomly positive or negative.

Like the paired t test (Chapter 31), it can be used in several situations:

- A variable is measured in each subject before and after an intervention.
- Subjects are recruited as pairs matched for variables such as age, postal code, or diagnosis. One of each pair receives one intervention, whereas the other receives an alternative treatment.
- Twins or siblings are recruited as pairs. Each receives a different treatment.
- Each run of a laboratory experiment has a control and treated preparation handled in parallel.
- A part of the body on one side is treated with a control treatment, and the corresponding part of the body on the other side is treated with the experimental treatment (e.g., right and left eyes).

It works via the following steps:

1. Calculate the difference between each matched pair, keeping track of the sign. A decrease is negative and an increase is positive.
2. Rank the absolute value of the differences, temporarily ignoring the sign.
3. Add up the ranks of all the positive differences and the ranks of all negative differences. For the example data (Chapter 31, Darwin's plants), the sums of ranks are 96 and 24.

4. Compute the difference between those two sums, 72.
5. Computing a P value answers the question: If the null hypothesis was true, what would be the chance of randomly choosing samples such that the sums of positive and negative ranks would differ by 72 or more? The answer is 0.0413.

Like the paired t test, Wilcoxon's test assumes that the pairs are randomly selected from (or at least representative of) a larger population and that each pair is selected independently from the others. Unlike the paired t test, Wilcoxon's test does not assume a Gaussian distribution of differences.

Nonparametric correlation

One nonparametric method for quantifying correlation is called *Spearman's rank correlation*. Spearman's rank correlation is based on the same assumptions as ordinary (Pearson) correlations listed in Chapter 32, with two exceptions. Rank correlation does not assume Gaussian distributions and does not assume a linear relationship between the variables. However, Spearman's nonparametric correlation does assume that any underlying relationship between X and Y is monotonic (either always increasing or always decreasing).

Spearman's correlation separately ranks the X and Y values and then computes the correlation between the two sets of ranks.

For the insulin sensitivity example of Chapter 32, the nonparametric correlation coefficient, called r_S, is 0.74. The P value, which tests the null hypothesis that there is no rank correlation in the overall population, is 0.0036.

Nonparametric ANOVA

The nonparametric test analogous to one-way ANOVA is called the *Kruskal–Wallis test*. The nonparametric test analogous to repeated-measures one-way ANOVA is called *Friedman's test*. These tests first rank the data from low to high and then analyze the distribution of the ranks among groups.

THE ADVANTAGES AND DISADVANTAGES OF NONPARAMETRIC TESTS

The advantage of nonparametric tests is clear. They don't require the assumption of sampling from a Gaussian population and so can be used when the validity of that assumption is dubious. And when that assumption is false, nonparametric tests have more power than parametric tests to detect differences.

So why not always use nonparametric tests? There are three reasons.

Nonparametric tests are less powerful when the data are Gaussian

Because nonparametric tests only consider the ranks and not the actual data, they essentially throw away some information, so they are less powerful. If there truly is a difference between Gaussian populations, the P value is likely to be higher with a nonparametric test. How much higher? It depends on sample size.

With large samples, the nonparametric tests are nearly as powerful as the parametric tests when the data are really sampled from Gaussian populations. This is assessed by a value called the *asymptotic relative efficiency*. For example, with large samples drawn from Gaussian populations, the asymptotic relative efficiency of the Mann–Whitney test is 95%. This means that the power of a Mann–Whitney test is equal to the power of a t test with 95% as many data points. The other nonparametric tests have similarly high asymptotic relative efficiencies.

With small samples from Gaussian populations, nonparametric tests have much less power than parametric tests. And with tiny samples, nonparametric tests have zero power:

- With seven or fewer values, the Mann–Whitney test always reports a two-tail P value greater than 0.05.
- With five or fewer data pairs, Wilcoxon's matched pairs test always reports a two-tail P value greater than 0.05.
- With four or fewer XY pairs, Spearman's correlation always reports a two-tail P value greater than 0.05.

When the populations are not Gaussian, nonparametric tests can be much more powerful than parametric tests (Sawilowsky, 2005).

Nonparametric results are usually not reported with CIs
This book has emphasized the importance of CIs. As implemented by most programs, however, nonparametric tests usually report only P values and not CIs.

Some nonparametric tests can be extended to compute CIs. But this requires additional assumptions. For example, the Mann–Whitney test can be extended to provide a CI for the difference between medians. But this requires assuming that the distributions of the two populations have the same shape, with the distributions shifted (and thus having different medians). This assumption is not needed to interpret the P value.

Nonparametric tests are not readily extended to regression models
Chapter 34 showed that t tests can be recast as regression. A t test compares two means. So can simple linear regression. Multiple regression can compare two means after adjusting for differences in other variables. Nonparametric tests cannot be readily extended in this way.

DON'T AUTOMATE THE DECISION OF WHEN TO USE A NONPARAMETRIC TEST

The decision of when to use a nonparametric test is not straightforward, and reasonable people can disagree about when to use nonparametric tests.

Many think that the choice of using a nonparametric test can be automatic. First, perform a normality test (Chapter 24). If the data pass, use a parametric test. If the data fail the normality test, then use a nonparametric test.

This approach is not recommended for the following reasons:

- When analyzing data from a series of experiments, they should all be analyzed the same way (unless there is some reason to think they aren't comparable). In this case, results from a single normality test should not be used to decide whether to use a nonparametric test.
- Data sometimes fail a normality test because the values were sampled from a lognormal distribution (Chapter 11). In this case, transforming the data to logarithms will create a Gaussian distribution. In other cases, transforming to reciprocals or other transformations can often convert a non-Gaussian distribution to a Gaussian distribution.
- Data can fail a normality test because of the presence of an outlier (Chapter 25). In some cases, it can sometimes make sense to analyze the data without the outlier using a conventional parametric test, rather than using a nonparametric test.
- The decision of whether to use a parametric or nonparametric test is most important with small data sets (because the power of nonparametric tests is so low). But with small data sets, normality tests have little power. So an automatic approach would give you false confidence.

The decision of when to use a parametric test and when to use a nonparametric test is a difficult one. It really is difficult, requiring thinking and perspective. This decision should not be automated.

CHOOSING BETWEEN PARAMETRIC AND NONPARAMETRIC TESTS: DOES IT MATTER?

Does it matter whether you choose a parametric or nonparametric test? The answer depends on sample size. There are four cases to think about (Table 41.2):

Using a parametric test with data from a large non-Gaussian population

The central limit theorem (discussed in Chapter 10) ensures that parametric tests work well with large samples even if data are sampled from non-Gaussian populations. In other words, parametric tests are robust to mild deviations from Gaussian distributions, so long as the samples are large. But there are two snags:

- It is impossible to say how large is large enough, because it depends on the nature of the particular non-Gaussian distribution. Unless the population distribution is really weird, you are probably safe choosing a parametric test when there are at least two dozen data points in each group.

DISTRIBUTION	TEST	SMALL SAMPLES	LARGE SAMPLES
Gaussian population	Nonparametric	Misleading. Nonparametric tests have little power with small samples.	Little problem. With large samples, nonparametric tests are nearly as powerful as parametric tests.
Non-Gaussian population	Parametric	Misleading. With small samples, parametric tests are not very robust to violations of the Gaussian assumption.	Little problem. With large samples, parametric tests are robust to violations of the Gaussian assumption.
Not sure	Normality tests	Not very helpful with small samples.	Helpful.

Table 41.2. The problem with small samples.

- If the population is far from Gaussian, you may not care about the mean or differences between means. Even if the P value provides an accurate answer to a question about the difference between means, that question may be scientifically irrelevant.

Using a nonparametric test with data from a large Gaussian population

Nonparametric tests work well with large samples from Gaussian populations. The P values tend to be a bit too large, but the discrepancy is small. In other words, nonparametric tests are only slightly less powerful than parametric tests with large samples.

Using a parametric test with data from a small non-Gaussian population

The central limit theorem doesn't apply with small samples, so the P value may be inaccurate.

Using a nonparametric test with data from a small Gaussian population

The nonparametric tests lack statistical power with small samples. The P values will tend to be high.

Summary

Large data sets present no problems. It is usually easy to tell whether the data come from a Gaussian population (and normality tests can help), but it doesn't matter much because the nonparametric tests are so powerful and the parametric tests are so robust.

Small data sets present a dilemma. It is difficult to tell whether the data come from a Gaussian population, but it matters a lot. The nonparametric tests are not powerful and the parametric tests are not robust.

Q & A: Nonparametric Tests Based on Rank

Can data be nonparametric?	No. Nonparametric is an adjective that can only be applied to statistical tests, not to data.
If I am sure my data are not Gaussian, should I use a nonparametric test?	Not necessarily. It may be possible to transform the data in a way that makes the population Gaussian. Most commonly, a log transform of data from a lognormal distribution (Chapter 11) will create a Gaussian population.
Are the chi-square test and Fisher's exact test nonparametric?	The distinction between parametric and nonparametric tests doesn't apply to tests that deal with dichotomous outcomes. The term nonparametric is sometimes used for these tests, but there is no distinction between parametric and nonparametric tests when analyzing dichotomous data.
Is it OK to run both a parametric and a nonparametric test and pick the P value I like?	No. P values can only be interpreted when the test is chosen as part of the experimental design.
Does the Mann–Whitney test compare medians?	Only if you assume that the two populations have identically shaped distributions. The distributions don't have to be Gaussian or even specified, but you do have to assume that the shapes are identical. Given that assumption, the only possible way for two populations to differ is by having different medians (the distributions are the same shape, but shifted). If you don't make that assumption, then it is not correct to say that a Mann–Whitney test compares medians.
Can nonparametric tests be used when some values are "off scale"?	If some values are too high or too low to quantify, parametric tests cannot be used because those value are not known. If they simply are ignored, the test results will be biased because the largest (or smallest) values were thrown out. In contrast, a nonparametric test can work well when a few values are too high (or too low) to measure. Assign values too low to measure an arbitrary very low value and assign values too high to measure an arbitrary very high value. Because the nonparametric test only knows about the relative ranks of the values, it won't matter that you didn't enter those extreme values precisely.

Continued

My data violate the assumption of an unpaired t test that the two populations have the same standard deviation. Should I use the Mann–Whitney test instead?	No. If the groups are sampled from populations with distinct SDs, then the nonparametric tests simply test whether the distributions are different. You already know that the distributions are different. What you want to know is whether the means or medians are distinct. But when the data are sampled from populations with different shaped distributions (which you already know), the Mann–Whitney test does not test whether the medians differ.
When the decision isn't clear, should I choose a parametric test or nonparametric test?	When in doubt, some people choose a parametric test because they aren't sure the Gaussian assumption is violated. Others choose a nonparametric test because they aren't sure the Gaussian assumption is met. Reasonable people disagree.

NONPARAMETRIC TESTS THAT ANALYZE VALUES (NOT RANKS)

There is another approach to analyzing data without making assumptions about the shape of the population distribution, and that also avoids the need to analyze ranks. These tests go by the names *permutation tests*, *randomization tests*, and *bootstrapping*.

The idea of all these tests is to analyze the actual data, not ranks, but not to assume any particular population distribution. All of these tests require intensive calculations that require computers and so are called *computer-intensive methods*. Because they don't make any assumptions about population distributions, these tests are nonparametric (but often that term is used to only refer to the tests that analyze ranks).

To compute a P value, the parametric methods start with an assumption (usually Gaussian distribution) about the population and then use math to figure out the distribution of all possible samples from that population.

The computer-intensive nonparametric methods have a completely different outlook. They make no mathematical assumption about the population, beyond the fact that the sample data were selected from it. They work by brute force rather than elegant math.

Randomization or permutation tests work by shuffling. Computers run many simulated "experiments." Each use the sample data. What changes are the labels for the groups. These labels are randomly shuffled among the values. If you are comparing a control and treated group, each shuffling changes the selection of which values are labeled "control" and which are labeled "treated." Analyzing this set of pseudosamples can lead to valid insights into your data.

With small data sets, these methods can systematically inspect every possible way to shuffle the labels among values. With large data sets, the number of possible rearrangements becomes astronomical, and so these software programs examine a large number (often 1,000 to 10,000) of randomly chosen permutations, which is enough to get valid results.

Another approach called *bootstrapping* or *resampling* has already been mentioned briefly in Chapters 13 and 38. The idea of bootstrapping is that all you know for sure about the population is that the sample was obtained from it. Statistical inference requires thinking about what would happen if you picked many samples from that population. Without making any parametric assumptions, this can be approximated by resampling from that single sample.

This resampling is done with replacement. Imagine you write each value on a card and place all of the cards in a hat. Mix well, pick a card, and record its value. Then put it back in the hat before mixing and picking the next card. Note that some values may get selected more than once, and other values may not be selected. Of course, it is actually done with computerized random-number generators. Bootstrapping produces many pseudosamples, each the same size as the original sample. The samples are different because some values are duplicate (or more) and others are omitted. Comparing the actual data with the distribution of bootstrap samples can lead to statistical conclusions via P values and CIs.

It seems like magic. It sure doesn't seem that useful statistical conclusions will emerge by analyzing sets of pseudosamples created by *bootstrapping*. That accounts for the strange name, *bootstrapping*. At first glance, analyzing data this way seems about as (un)helpful as trying to get out of a hole by pulling up on the straps of your boots.

The theorems have been proven, the simulations have been run, and plenty of real-world experience has validated these approaches. They work! Many think computer-intensive methods are the future of statistics because they are so versatile. They can be easily adapted to be used in new situations and don't require making or believing assumptions about the distribution of the population (except that the sample is representative). To learn more, start with a short text by Wilcox (2001) and then a longer book by Manly (2006).

CHAPTER 42

Sensitivity, Specificity, and Receiver-Operator Characteristic Curves

Reports that say that something hasn't happened are always interesting to me, because as we know, there are known knowns; there are things we know we know. We also know there are known unknowns; that is to say we know there are some things we do not know. But there are also unknown unknowns—the ones we don't know we don't know.

DONALD RUMSFELD

This chapter explains how to quantify false-positive and false-negative results from laboratory tests. Although this topic is rarely found in basic statistics texts, deciding whether a clinical laboratory result is normal or abnormal uses logic very similar to deciding whether a finding is statistically significant or not. Learning the concepts of sensitivity and specificity presented here is a great way to review the ideas of statistical hypothesis testing and Bayesian logic.

DEFINITIONS OF SENSITIVITY AND SPECIFICITY

The accuracy of a diagnostic test is quantified by its sensitivity and specificity.

- The *sensitivity* is the fraction of all those with the disease who get a positive test result. In Table 42.1, sensitivity equals $C/(C + D)$.
- The *specificity* is the fraction of those without the disease who get a negative test result. In Table 42.1, specificity equals $B/(B + A)$.

It is easy to mix up these two values.

Sensitivity measures how well the test identifies those with the disease, that is, how sensitive it is. If a test has a high sensitivity, it will pick up nearly everyone with the disease.

Specificity measures how well the test identifies those who don't have the disease, that is, how specific it is. If a test has a very high specificity, it won't mistakenly give a positive result to many people without the disease.

	DECISION: ABNORMAL TEST RESULT	DECISION: NORMAL TEST RESULT	TOTAL
Disease absent	A	B	A+B
Disease present	C	D	C+D
Total	A+C	B+D	A+B+C+D

Table 42.1. The results of many hypothetical lab tests, each analyzed to reach a decision to call the results normal or not.

The top row tabulates results for patients without the disease, and the second row tabulates results for patients with the disease. You can't actually create this kind of table from a group of patients unless you run a "gold standard" test that is 100% accurate.

THE PREDICTIVE VALUE OF A TEST

Definitions of positive and negative predictive values

Neither the specificity nor the sensitivity answers the most important questions: If the test is positive (abnormal test result, suggesting the presence of disease), what is the chance that the patient really has the disease? If the test is negative (normal test result), what is the chance that the patient really doesn't have the disease? The answers to those questions are quantified by the *positive predictive value* and the *negative predictive value*. Based on Table 42.1,

$$\text{Positive Predictive Value} = \frac{\text{True positives}}{\text{All positive results}} = \frac{C}{A+C}$$

$$\text{Negative Predictive Value} = \frac{\text{True negatives}}{\text{All negative results}} = \frac{B}{B+D}.$$

The sensitivity and specificity are properties of the test. In contrast, the positive predictive value and negative predictive value are determined by the characteristics of the test and the prevalence of the disease in the population being studied. The lower the prevalence of the disease, the lower the ratio of true positives to false positives. This is best understood by example.

Background to porphyria example

Acute intermittent porphyria is an autosomal dominant disease that is difficult to diagnose clinically. It can be diagnosed by reduced levels of porphobilinogen deaminase. But the levels of the enzyme vary in both the normal population and patients with porphyria, so the test does not lead to an exact diagnosis.

Using the definition that levels less than 98 units are abnormal, 82% of patients with porphyria have an abnormal test result. This means that the sensitivity of the test is 82%. Additionally, 3.7% of normal people have an abnormal test result. This means that the specificity of the test is $100 - 3.7\% = 96.3\%$.

What is the likelihood that a patient with <98 units of enzyme activity has porphyria? In other words what is the positive predictive value of the test? The answer depends on who the patient is. We'll work through two examples.

	DECISION: ABNORMAL TEST RESULT	DECISION: NORMAL TEST RESULT	TOTAL
Disease absent	36,996	962,904	999,900
Disease present	82	18	100
Total	37,078	962,922	1,000,000

Table 42.2. Expected results of screening one million people with the porphyria test from a population with a prevalence of 0.01.

Most of the abnormal test results are false positives.

Test used in random screening

In this example, the test was done to screen for the disease, so the people being tested have no particular risk for the disease. Porphyria is a rare disease with a prevalence of about 1 in 10,000. Because the people being tested were not selected because of family history or clinical suspicion, you expect about 0.01% to have the disease.

The test gave a positive result. Knowing the test result, what is the probability that this patient has the disease? To find out, we must enter numbers into Table 42.1 to create Table 42.2.

1. Assume a population of 1,000,000 (arbitrary). All we care about are ratios of values, so the total population size is arbitrary. $A + B + C + D = 1,000,000$.
2. Because the prevalence of the disease is 1/10,000, the total number in the disease-present column is $0.0001 \times 1,000,000$, or 100. $C + D = 100$.
3. Subtract the 100 diseased people from the total of 1,000,000, leaving 999,900 disease-absent people. $A + B = 999,900$.
4. Calculate the number of people with disease present who also test positive. This equals the total number of people with the disease (100) times the sensitivity (0.82). $C = 82$.
5. Calculate the number of people without disease who test negative. This equals the total number of people without the disease (999,900) times the specificity (0.963). $B = 962,904$.
6. Calculate the number of people with the disease who test negative: $D = 100 - 82 = 18$.
7. Calculate the number of people without the disease who test positive: $A = 36,996$.
8. Calculate the two column totals. $A + C = 37,078$. $B + D = 962,922$.

If you screen 1 million people, you expect to find an abnormal test result in 37,078 people. Only 82 of these cases will have the disease. When someone has a positive test, the chance is only $82/37,078 = 0.22\%$ that he or she has the disease. That is called the positive predictive value of the test. Because only about 1 in about 500 of the people with positive test results have the disease, the other 499 of 500 positive tests are false positives.

Of the 962,922 negative tests results, only 18 were false negative. The predictive value of a negative test is 99.998%.

	DECISION: ABNORMAL TEST RESULT	DECISION: NORMAL TEST RESULT	TOTAL
Disease absent	19	481	500
Disease present	410	90	500
Total	429	571	1,000

Table 42.3. Expected results of testing 1,000 siblings of someone with porphyria.
In this group, the prevalence will be 50%, and few of the abnormal test results will be false positives.

	DECISION: ABNORMAL TEST RESULT	DECISION: NORMAL TEST RESULT
Disease absent	False positive	
Disease present		False negative
	DECISION: REJECT NULL HYPOTHESIS	**DECISION: DO NOT REJECT NULL HYPOTHESIS**
Null hypothesis is true	Type I error	
Null hypothesis is false		Type II error

Table 42.4. False-positive and false-negative lab results are similar to Type I and Type II errors in statistical hypothesis testing.

	IF ...	WHAT IS THE CHANCE THAT ...
Sensitivity	The patient has disease...	...a lab result will be positive?
Power	There is a difference between populations...	...a result will be statistically significant?
	IF ...	**WHAT IS THE CHANCE THAT ...**
Specificity	The patient does not have the disease...	...a lab result will be negative?
1-alpha	There is no difference between populations...	...a result will not be statistically significant?

Table 42.5. Relationships between sensitivity and power and specificity and alpha.

Testing siblings

The disease is autosomal dominant, so there is a 50% chance that each sibling has the gene. If you test many siblings of people who have the disease, you expect about half will have the disease. Table 42.3 shows the predicted results when you test 1,000 siblings of patients. Positive results are expected in 429 of the people tested. Of these individuals, 410 will actually have the disease and 19 will be false positives. The predictive value of a positive test, therefore, is 410/429, which is about 96%. Only about 4% of the positive tests are false positives.

Analogy to statistical tests

The analogies between interpreting laboratory tests and statistical hypothesis testing are shown in Table 42.4 and Table 42.5.

Interpreting a positive or negative test requires knowing who is tested (what the prevalence is). Similarly, as explained in Chapters 18 and 19, the interpretation of statistical significance depends on the scientific context (the prior probability).

RECEIVER-OPERATOR CHARACTERISTIC (ROC) CURVES

When evaluating a diagnostic test, it is often difficult to decide where to set the threshold that separates a clinical diagnosis of "normal" from one of "abnormal."

If the threshold is set high (assuming that the test value increases with disease severity), some individuals with low test values or mild forms of the disease will be missed. The sensitivity will be low, but the specificity will be high. Few of the positive tests will be false positives, but many of the negative tests will be false negatives.

On the other hand, if the threshold is low, most individuals with the disease will be detected, but the test will also mistakenly diagnose many normal individuals as abnormal. The sensitivity will be high, but the specificity will be low. Few of the negative tests will be false negatives, but many of the positive tests will be false positives.

The threshold can be set to have a higher sensitivity or a higher specificity, but not both (until a better diagnostic test is developed).

An ROC curve visualizes the tradeoff between high sensitivity and high specificity (Figure 42.1). Why the odd name? ROC curves were developed during World War II, within the context of determining whether a blip on a radar screen represented a ship or an extraneous noise. The radar-receiver operators used this method to set the threshold for military action.

BAYES REVISITED

Interpreting clinical laboratory tests requires combining what you know about the clinical context and what you learn from the lab test. This is simply Bayesian logic at work. Bayesian logic has already been discussed in Chapter.

Probability versus odds
Likelihood can be expressed either as a probability or as odds.

- The *probability* that an event will occur is the fraction of times you expect to see that event in many trials.
- The *odds* are defined as the probability that the event will occur divided by the probability that the event will not occur.

A probability is a fraction and always ranges from 0 to 1. Odds range from 0 to infinity. Any probability can be expressed as odds. Any odds can be expressed

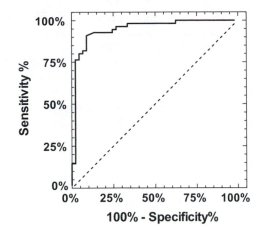

Figure 42.1. An ROC curve.

The solid line shows the tradeoff of sensitivity versus specificity. Each point along the curve represents a different possible threshold value defining an abnormal test result. The dotted line shows the expected ROC curve for a method (like flipping a coin) that has no predictive value.

as a probability. Convert between odds and probability (for situations where there are only two possible outcomes):

$$Odds = \frac{probability}{1 - probability}$$

$$Probability = \frac{odds}{1 + odds}.$$

If the probability is 0.50 or 50%, then the odds are 50:50 or 1. If you repeat the experiment often, you expect to observe the event (on average) in one of two trials (probability = 1/2). That means you'll observe the event once for every time it fails to happen (odds = 1:1).

If the probability is 1/3, the odds equal 1/3/(1 – 1/3) = 1:2 = 0.5. On average, you'll observe the event once in every three trials (probability = 1/3). That means you'll observe the event once for every two times it fails to happen (odds = 1:2).

The likelihood ratio

The *likelihood ratio* is the probability of obtaining a positive test result in a patient with the disease divided by the probability of obtaining a positive test result in a patient without the disease. The probability of obtaining a positive test result in a patient with the disease is the sensitivity. The probability of obtaining a positive test result in someone without the disease is (1-specificity). So the likelihood ratio equals sensitivity divided by (1-specificity).

Using this equation, we can rework the examples. The test used in the intermittent porphyria example has a sensitivity of 82% and a specificity of 96.3%.

| WHO WAS TESTED? | PRETEST | | POSTTEST | |
	PROBABILITY	ODDS	ODDS	PROBABILITY
Random screen	0.0001	0.0001	0.0022	0.0022
Sibling	0.50	1.0000	22.2	0.957

Table 42.6. The porphyria calculations computed using Bayes's equation.

The pretest probability is first converted to odds. Then the posttest odds are computed by multiplying the pretest odds by the likelihood ratio, which equals 22.1. Then the odds are converted to probabilities.

Thus, the likelihood ratio is $0.82/(1.0 - 0.963) = 22.2$. A person with the condition is 22.2 times more likely to get a positive test result than a person without.

Bayes as an equation

Bayes's equation for clinical diagnosis can be written as follows:

$$\text{Posttest Odds} = \text{Pretest odds} \cdot \frac{\text{sensitivity}}{1 - \text{specificity}} = \text{Pretest odds} \cdot \text{Likelihood ratio.}$$

The posttest odds are the odds that a patient has the disease, taking into account both the test results and your prior knowledge about the patient. The pretest odds are the odds that the patient has the disease determined from information you know before running the test.

Using this equation, we can rework the examples with intermittent porphyria, which has a likelihood ratio of 22.2. Table 42.6 redoes the calculations shown earlier using the compact equation.

BAYES, GENETIC LINKAGE, AND LOG OF ODDS (LOD) SCORES

When two loci (genes or DNA sequences) are located near each other on the same chromosome, they are said to be linked. If the two loci are very close, crossing over or recombination between the two loci occurs rarely. Thus, alleles of linked loci tend to be inherited together. If the loci are further apart, recombination (a normal process) occurs more frequently. If the loci are very far apart, the two loci segregate independently, just as if they were on different chromosomes.

Linkage is useful in genetic diagnosis and mapping. Because it is not possible to detect all abnormal genes directly, geneticists try to identify a marker gene (such as those for variable antigens or isozymes) or a variable DNA sequence that is linked to the disease gene. Once you know that the disease gene is linked to a marker, the presence of the marker (which you can identify) may often predict the presence of the disease gene (which you cannot identify directly). This allows detection of genetic diseases prenatally or before they cause clinical problems. It also allows the diagnosis of unaffected heterozygotes (carriers) who can pass the abnormal gene on to their children. This method works best for diseases caused by an abnormality of a single gene.

Before linkage can be useful in diagnosis, you must identify a marker linked to the gene. This is usually done by screening lots of potential markers. How can you tell whether a marker is linked to a disease gene? Geneticists study large families and observe how often the disease and marker are inherited together and how often there is recombination. If there are few recombination events between the marker and the disease, there are two possible explanations. One possibility is that the two are linked. The other possibility is that the two are not linked, but— just by coincidence—there were few recombination events.

Geneticists don't use the terms sensitivity or specificity. But linkage studies, like clinical lab tests, can have false-positive and false-negative results.

Bayesian logic combines the experimental data with the prior probability of linkage to determine the probability that the gene is truly linked to the disease. To calculate Bayes's equation, we must define the likelihood ratio in the context of linkage. When calculating the predictive values of lab tests, we defined the likelihood ratio as the probability that someone with the disease will have an abnormal test result divided by the probability that someone without the disease will have an abnormal test result. For studies of linkage, therefore, the likelihood ratio is the probability of obtaining the observed data if the genes really are linked divided by the probability of observing those data if the genes are really not linked. The details of the calculations are beyond the scope of this book. When you read papers with linkage studies, you'll rarely see reference to the likelihood ratio. Instead you'll see the *log of odds (LOD) score*, which is simply the logarithm (base 10) of the likelihood ratio.

A LOD score of 3 means that the likelihood ratio equals 1,000 (because $10^3 = 1,000$). This means that the data are 1,000 times more likely to be observed if the marker is linked to the disease than if the marker is not linked. A higher LOD score is stronger evidence for linkage.

To calculate the probability that the marker is linked to the gene requires accounting for the prior probability of linkage using Bayesian logic.

Posttest odds of linkage = pretest odds of linkage · likelihood ratio.

To calculate Bayes's equation, you must know the prior (or pretest) odds of linkage. Using common definitions of linkage, 2% of randomly selected markers are linked to any particular disease gene. Converting to odds, the pretest odds of linkage is about 0.02. If you pick a marker known to be on the same chromosome as the disease, then the pretest odds of linkage will be higher.

If a LOD score equals 3, what is the probability that the marker and disease are truly linked? The posttest odds equal the pretest odds (0.02) times the likelihood ratio ($10^3 = 1000$), which is 20. Converting to a probability, the posttest probability equals 20/21, which is about 95%. If you observe a LOD score of 3.0, you will conclude that the marker and gene are linked. When you make that conclusion, there is a 95% chance that you will be correct, leaving a 5% chance that you will be wrong.

If a LOD score equals or exceeds 3, geneticists usually conclude that the marker and disease are linked. If a LOD score is less than or equal to –2, geneticists conclude that the marker and disease are not linked. If the LOD score is between –2 and 3, geneticists conclude that the evidence is not conclusive.

CHAPTER 43

Sample Size

The aim of science is to seek the simplest explanation of complex facts.... Seek simplicity and distrust it.

A. N. Whitehead

Many experiments and clinical trials are run with too few subjects. An underpowered study is a wasted effort because even substantial treatment effects are likely to go undetected. Even if the treatment substantially changed the outcome, the study would have only a small chance of finding a statistically significant effect. When planning a study, therefore, you must choose an appropriate sample size.

THREE APPROACHES TO CHOOSING SAMPLE SIZE

Ad hoc (not recommended)
It seems so simple, so tempting. Collect and analyze some data. If the CIs are not as narrow as you like or the results are not statistically significant, collect some more data and reanalyze. Keep collecting more data until the CI is narrow enough or you obtain a statistically significant result (or until you run out of money, time, or curiosity).

If you use this *ad hoc* approach, the P values and CIs simply cannot be interpreted. The problem is that you'll keep going if you don't like the result, but stop if you do like the result. As explained on pages 169–170, if the null hypothesis is true, the chance of obtaining a statistically significant result (P<0.05) using an ad hoc approach is much greater than 5%. Therefore, the resulting P values and CIs are not valid. It is too easy to fool yourself if an *ad hoc* method is used to choose sample size.

Conventional
The usual approach is simple: Choose a sample size, collect data from that many subjects, and then analyze the data. The rest of this chapter explains this approach.

Adaptive trials
The idea behind adaptive trials is simple: Interim analyses, performed while the trial is proceeding, are used to decide the course of the study. This approach to designing large clinical trials is gaining acceptance (Kuehn, 2006).

The simplest adaptive designs may only analyze the data once at the middle of a trial and then decide to stop the trial if patients in one group are having substantially better outcomes than those in the other. This approach is also called *sequential analysis*. Newer adaptive techniques decide when to stop adding new patients to the study, when to stop the study, and what proportion of new subjects are assigned to each alternative treatment. These decisions are based on clearly designed protocols that ensure that the statistical results are meaningful.

In some cases, the adaptive design can lead investigators to end a study early when it is clear that one treatment is much better than the other, or it becomes clear that the difference between the treatments is, at best, trivial. In other cases, the adaptive design can prolong a study until it reaches a crisp conclusion.

The methods used to adapt a study to interim findings are not straightforward, have some drawbacks (Fleming, 2006), and are not yet standard, so they won't be explained here.

SAMPLE SIZE AND CIs

This section shows a simple way to think about choosing sample size. Later sections explain a more complicated approach that takes into account statistical power.

Previous chapters have shown you how to calculate CIs for many kinds of results. In all cases, the width of the CI depends on sample size. Everything else being equal, a larger sample size produces a narrower CI. Therefore, if you can state the desired width of the CI, you can calculate how many subjects you need.

One mean

Let's start with the simplest case. You plan to measure a variable in n subjects and calculate the mean and 95% CI of the mean. How large must you make n to reduce the width of the 95% CI to a certain precision?

A simplified equation is shown below. It starts with an equation from Chapter 12 that defines the margin of error of the CI, w, which is computed from n, s (the SD), and t^* (the critical value of the t distribution, which is close to 2.0 for large samples and 95% confidence). Rearrange to define n.

$$w = \frac{t^* \cdot s}{\sqrt{n}}$$
$$t^* \approx 2$$
$$n \approx 4\left(\frac{s}{w}\right)^2$$

The only trick is that n depends upon the value of t^*, which itself depends on n. The way out of this loop is to realize that t^* (for 95% confidence) is nearly equal to 2.0, unless the sample size is very small.

For example, if the SD of blood pressure is 10 mmHg and you wish to measure the blood pressure of a large enough sample to define the mean value with a margin of error of 5 mmHg, how large must our sample be? The answer is approximately 16.

Difference between two means

To compute the difference between two means, more data are needed. The uncertainty in each mean contributes toward uncertainty in their difference. Each group requires twice as many values.

$$n \approx 8 \left(\frac{s}{w} \right)^2 \quad \text{(per group)}$$

Continuing the example, how many values are needed so that that the 95% CI for the difference between the two means has a margin of error of 5 mmHg? Keeping the assumption that the SD of blood pressures is about 10 mmHg, 32 values are needed in each group, or 64 in total.

One proportion

How many subjects are needed to determine a proportion with a specified margin of error? Use equations from Chapter 4, simplified a bit assuming a large n.

$$w \approx 2 \sqrt{\frac{p(1-p)}{n}}$$

$$n \approx \frac{4p(1-p)}{w^2}$$

If you can estimate the proportion (p) and specify the desired precision, the sample size is readily calculated.

When reading or watching the news, you've undoubtedly heard the phrase "this poll has a margin of error of 3%." How many subjects were used in such a poll? It depends on the expected size of p. First, let's set $w = 0.03$ and $p = 0.5$, and n is then 1,111. Indeed, many polls use a sample of about that size. What if p is expected (from earlier polls) to equal about 0.10? Set $w = 0.03$ and $p = 0.10$, and n is then 400.

Note that the quantity $p(1-p)$ is maximum when $p = 0.5$. If you can't estimate the value of p, set it equal to 0.5, which is the worst-case assumption requiring the largest sample size.

Two proportions

The number of subjects needed in each group to determine the difference between two proportions with a specified precision is as follows, where p_{av} is the anticipated average of the two proportions:

$$n \approx \frac{8 \cdot p_{av}(1-p_{av})}{w^2} \quad \text{(in each group)}$$

For example, how many values are needed to determine the difference in incidence rates of hypertension in two populations, when you expect the incidences to be about 0.10 and you want the margin of error to be 0.02? Set $p_{av} = 0.11$ (the average of the two expected incidences) and $w = 0.02$. You need about 1,958 subjects in each group.

If estimating p_{av} is impossible, calculate a worst-case sample size by setting p_{av} equal to 0.5. Any other value would require a smaller sample size.

General comments on calculating sample size for estimation

Two notes on the equations presented above follow:

- If the assumptions are correct and you perform many experiments using the calculated sample size, the average margin of error will equal the value you specify. If you run one experiment with the calculated sample size, the chance is 50% that the margin will be wider, and 50% that it will be narrower, than the value you specified.
- The calculated sample sizes are the number of subjects you will need at the end of the experiment. It is usually wise to start with a larger number to allow for subjects who drop out and for experimental problems.

SAMPLE SIZE AND STATISTICAL
HYPOTHESIS TESTING

The four questions

The approach above is logical and simple, but sample-size calculations usually use a more complicated approach that answers the overall question: How many values are needed to obtain statistical significance? The calculations require the investigator to answer four questions:

- What significance level? Statistical significance is usually defined as a P value less than 0.05. If the threshold is stricter (say a P value less than 0.01), then a larger sample size is needed.
- How much power? Power (explained in Chapter 20) is the answer to this question: If there truly is an effect of a defined size, what is the chance that random sampling will result in statistically significant results? If the goal is to have lots of power, then the sample size must be large. If moderate power is adequate, then the sample size can be smaller.
- How large an effect are you looking for? It takes a huge sample size to reliably detect a tiny effect, but a smaller sample size can detect a huge effect.
- What is the context? When comparing means, you must estimate the expected value of the SD. If the data have lots of variability, a large sample size is needed. If the data are very consistent (tiny SD), a smaller sample size will suffice. When comparing proportions, you must estimate how far the proportions will be from 50:50. If you expect the two outcomes to each occur about half the time, the sample size must be larger than if you expect the two proportions to be very different.

Interpreting a statement regarding sample size and power

Papers often include a statement that goes something like this:

> We chose to study 313 subjects in each group in order to have 80% power of detecting a 33% reduction in the recurrence rate from a baseline rate of 30% with a significance level of 0.05 (two tailed).

To obtain this sample size, the following values would be entered into a sample-size program:

- $\alpha = 0.05$. This is the standard definition of statistical significance. If the null hypothesis is true, there will be a 5% chance of obtaining a significant result, leaving a 95% chance that the result will not be statistically significant.
- Baseline probability of the outcome (here, recurrence): 30%, or 0.30.
- Desired effect: $\Delta = 10\%$ (from 30% down to 20%, a risk reduction of 33%).
- Power = 80%. The investigators assume that the recurrence rate is normally 30% and hypothesize that the new treatment reduces the recurrence rate by one third. Assuming this hypothesis is true, the sample size was chosen so that the chance of obtaining a statistically significant result is 80%. Some programs ask you to enter β instead of power. It equals 1.0-power. For this example, $\beta = 0.20$, or 20%.

Although a statement regarding sample-size calculations sounds very precise ("we calculated that we need 313 subjects in each group"), consider these ambiguities:

- Different programs use different equations, giving slightly different sample sizes.
- The calculations tell you how many subjects you need at the end of the study. You will usually need to begin the study with additional subjects to allow for dropouts and experimental problems.
- The values of α and β are arbitrary. Ideally, the values should be based on the relative consequences of Type I and Type II errors, but more often α and β are simply set to conventional values.
- The value of Δ is arbitrary. Ideally, Δ is the smallest difference that would be clinically (or scientifically) important. In practice, this value is hard to define.
- Sample-size calculations assume that you will only measure and analyze one outcome. Common sense tells you that you should appraise all relevant clinical variables, and most clinical investigators do so. Although it seems like this should increase the power of a study, current statistical methods are not well designed to cope with multiple outcome variables.

A calculation or a negotiation?

Although it always sounds like the investigator calculated sample size from α, β, and Δ, often the process is more of a negotiation. The investigators first specifies ideal values for α, β, and Δ and then is horrified at the enormous number of subjects required. They then adjust those values until n seems "reasonable."

Parker and Berman (2003) point out that this approach is very useful. In many situations, the goal isn't to calculate the number of subjects needed, but rather to ask: If I use n subjects, what information can I learn?

In some cases, the calculations may convince you that it is impossible to find what you want to know with the number of subjects you are able to use. This can be very helpful. It is far better to cancel such an experiment in the planning stage than to waste time and money on a futile experiment that won't have sufficient power. If the experiment involves any clinical risk or expenditure of public money, performing such a study can even be considered unethical.

Standard effect sizes are not very helpful

Computing sample size requires that you decide how large an effect you are looking for—how large a difference (association, correlation...) would be scientifically interesting.

J. Cohen (1988) makes some recommendations for what to do when you don't know what effect size you are looking for. He limits these recommendations to the behavioral sciences (his area of expertise) and warns that all general recommendations are more useful in some circumstances than others. Here are his guidelines for an unpaired t test:

- A "small" difference between means is equal to one fifth the SD.
- A "medium" effect size is equal to one half the SD.
- A "large" effect is equal to 0.8 times the SD.

So if you are having trouble deciding what effect size you are looking for (and therefore are stuck and can't determine a sample size), J. Cohen would recommend you choose whether you are looking for a small, medium, or large effect and then use the standard definitions.

Lenth (2001) argues that you should avoid these "canned" effect sizes, and I agree. You must decide how large a difference you care to detect based on understanding the experimental system you are using and the scientific questions you are asking. J. Cohen's recommendations seem a way to avoid thinking about the goals of the experiment. It doesn't make sense to only think about the difference you are looking at in terms of the scatter you expect to see (anticipated SD), without even considering what the mean value might be.

If you choose standard definitions of alpha (0.05), power (80%), and effect size (see above), then there is no need for any calculations. If you accept those standard definitions for all your studies, then all studies need a sample size of 26 in each group to detect a large effect, 65 in each group to detect a medium effect, and 400 in each group to detect a small effect. Choosing standard effect sizes is really the same as picking standard sample sizes. Choosing sample size is more complicated than that, and you must take into account the scientific goals, the consequences of missing a real effect, the consequences of mistakenly reporting an effect that doesn't really exist, and the cost and risk of the experiments.

The winner's curse can lead to underestimating needed sample size

All sample size calculations require you to specify how large a difference (or effect) you are looking for. It takes a huge sample size to reliably detect a tiny effect, but a smaller sample size to detect a huge effect. But specifying the size of a difference you care about is not easy.

Many people prefer to use results from a prior study and then calculate a sample size large enough to detect an effect that large. This approach seems to make sense, but it leads to a big problem: The published difference or effect is likely to inflate the true effect (Ioannidis, 2008). This is similar to a phenomenon that economists call the *winner's curse*, where the person who wins an auction usually ends up paying too much (Zollner & Pritchard, 2007).

The origin of the winner's curse is easy to understand. If many studies are performed, the average of the effects detected in these studies should be close to the true effect. Some studies will happen to find larger effects, and some studies will happen to find smaller effects. But studies with small effects tend not to get published (or the analysis gets tweaked to make a larger effect). Studies with larger effects are more likely to get published. This means that the results in published studies tend to overestimate the actual effect size.

What happens if you use the published effect size to compute necessary sample size for a repeat experiment? You'll have a large enough sample size to have 80% power (or whatever power you specify) to detect that published effect size. But if the real effect size is smaller, the power of the study to detect that real effect will be less than the power you chose.

SAMPLE SIZE RULES OF THUMB

Comparing two means

The equation below computes the sample size (n) needed per group to compare two means with a standard significance level of 0.05 (two tailed) and a standard power of 80%:

$$n \approx 16 \left(\frac{s}{w} \right)^2 \text{ (per group)}$$

Continuing the example from the first part of this chapter, how many values are needed to compare two groups when the SD of blood pressures is about 10 mmHg (s) and we want to be able to detect a difference of 5 mmHg (w)? If we choose to define significance as a P value less than 0.05 and to obtain 80% power, 64 values are needed in each group, or 128 in total.

Let's review exactly what this means:

- Assume that the true difference between means is 5.00 mmHg.
- Now imagine that you perform many experiments, with n = 64 per group in each experiment.
- Because of random sampling, you won't find that the difference between means equals 5.00 mm in every experiment. Instead, you'll find that the

difference between means will be greater than 5.00 mmHg in about half the experiments and less than 5.00 mmHg in the other half.

- In 80% (the power) of those experiments, the P value will be less than 0.05 (two tailed), so the results will be deemed statistically significant. In the remaining 20% of the experiments, the difference between means will be deemed not statistically significant, so you will have made a Type II (beta) error.
- This can be summarized as follows: A sample size of 64 in each group has 80% power to detect a difference between means of 5.00 mmHg with a significance level (alpha) of 0.05 (two tailed).

Earlier in this chapter, this same example was used to compute the sample size needed so that the margin of error of the 95% CI for the difference between two means would be 5.0 mmHg. The sample size, computed in that way, was half of what was computed in the discussion immediately above. Why the difference? The CI calculations implicitly assumed a power of 50%. With the computed sample size, there is a 50% chance that the margin of error would be the value you specified or smaller. If you want a 80% chance that the margin of error would be the value you specified or smaller, the sample size would be 64 per group, just as computed above.

The calculation above is for 80% power. A sample size about half as large will suffice if you only need 50% power and a sample size twice as large is needed for 99% power.

Comparing two proportions

The number of subjects needed in each group to determine the difference between two proportions with a specified significance level is as follows, where p_{av} is the anticipated average of the two proportions:

$$n \approx \frac{16 \cdot p_{av}(1-p_{av})}{w^2} \text{ (in each group)}$$

For example, how many values are needed to determine the difference in incidence rates of hypertension in two populations when you expect the incidence to be about 0.10 and you want to be able to detect a difference in incidence rates as small as 0.02? Set $p_{av} = 0.09$ (the average of the two expected incidences), and $w = 0.02$. You need about 3,276 subjects in each group.

If estimating p_{av} is impossible, calculate a worst-case sample size by setting p_{av} equal to 0.5. Any other value would require a smaller sample size.

Nonparametric tests

Nonparametric tests, reviewed in Chapter 41, are used when you are not willing to assume that your data come from a Gaussian distribution. Commonly used nonparametric tests are based on ranking values from low to high and then comparing the distribution of the ranks between groups. This is the basis of tests named after Wilcoxon, Mann–Whitney, and Friedman.

When calculating a nonparametric test, you don't have to make any assumption about the distribution of the values. That is why it is called nonparametric. But if you want to calculate necessary sample size for a study to be analyzed by a nonparametric test, you must make an assumption about the distribution of the values. It is not enough to say the distribution is not Gaussian; you must say what kind of distribution it is. If you are willing to make such an assumption (say, assume an exponential distribution of values, or a uniform distribution), you should consult an advanced text or use a more advanced program to compute sample size.

But most people choose a nonparametric test when they don't know the shape of the underlying distribution. Without making an explicit assumption about the distribution, detailed sample-size calculations are impossible. But all is not lost! Depending on the nature of the distribution, the nonparametric tests might require either more or fewer subjects. But they never require more than 15% additional subjects if the following two assumptions are true:

- You are looking at reasonably high numbers of subjects (how high depends on the nature of the distribution and test, but figure at least a few dozen).
- The distribution of values is not unusual (e.g., it doesn't have infinite tails, in which case its SD would be infinitely large).

So a general rule of thumb is this: If you plan to use a nonparametric test, compute the sample size required for a parametric test and add 15% (Lehman, 2007).

Multiple or logistic regression

How many subjects are needed to perform a useful multiple regression analysis? It depends on the goals of the study and your assumptions about the distributions of the variables. The calculations are tricky and require you to enter values you will probably find very difficult to estimate.

The only firm rule is that you need more cases than variables, a lot more. Here are some published rules of thumb, where m is the number of independent variables, and n is the number of subjects required:

- $n > 10 \cdot m$
- $n > 20 \cdot m$ (without any variable selection)
- $n > 40 \cdot m$ (with variable selection)
- $n > 50 + 8 \cdot m$ (Green, 1991)

Note that m is the number of independent variables you start with, even if only a smaller number of variables are included in the final model.

If the outcome is binary (logistic or proportional hazards regression), n is the number of events, not the number of subjects. If the specified outcome happens to 5% of the subjects, then the number of subjects needed equals $20 \cdot n$, where n is computed via one of the equations above. If the event happens to 20% of the subjects, then the number of subjects needed is $5 \cdot n$. If the event modeled by logistic regression happens to 75% of the subjects, then the required number of subjects is 4n (the calculations are based on the less frequent of the two outcomes).

Q & A: Sample Size

Does 80% power mean that 80% of the subjects would be improved by the treatment and 20% would not?	No. Power refers to the fraction of hypothetical studies that would report statistical significance. This is the same as asking what the chances are that one planned study will reach statistical significance. Power has nothing to do with the fraction of patients who benefit from a treatment.
How much power do I need?	Sample-size calculations require you to choose how much power the study will have. If you want more power, you'll need a larger sample size. Often power is set to a standard value of 80%. Ideally, the value should be chosen to match the experimental setting, the goals of the experiment, and the consequences of making a Type II error (Chapter 16).
What are Type I and Type II errors?	See Table 16.2. A Type I error occurs when the null hypothesis is true, but your experiment gives a statistically significant result. A Type II error occurs when the alternative hypothesis is true, but your experiment yields a result that is not statistically significant.
What's wrong with always using the standard definitions of statistical significance and power?	Almost all researchers set alpha to 0.05. This means that if the null hypothesis were true and you did lots of experiments, then in 5% of the experiments where there really is no difference at all, you'd incorrectly conclude that the difference is statistically significant. The chance of a Type I error is 5%. There isn't such a strong tradition for a particular value of power, but many researchers choose a sample size to achieve a power of 80%. That means that if the effect you want to see really exists, there is an 80% chance that your experiment will result in a statistically significant result, leaving a 20% chance of missing the real difference. The chance of a Type II error is 20%. Using these standard definitions, you are four times more likely to make a Type II error

Continued

	(miss a real effect) than a Type I error (falsely conclude that an effect is significant). This makes sense if the consequences of making a Type I error are four times as bad (as costly) as making a Type II error. But the relative consequences of Type I and II errors depend on the context of the experiment. In some situations, making a Type I error has more serious consequences than making a Type II error. In other situations, the consequences of a Type II error might be worse.
	Although it is tempting to simply choose standard values for alpha and power, it is better to choose values based on the relative consequences of Type I and Type II errors.
When comparing two groups, should the sample size of each group be the same?	Consider using unequal sample sizes when one treatment is much more expensive, difficult, or risky—or when it is hard to find appropriate subjects for one group (for example, when comparing patients with a rare disease to controls).
	If you choose unequal sample sizes, the total number of subjects must increase. You can reduce the number of subjects in one group (but never to less than half of what the size would have been if the sample sizes were equal), but you must increase the number of subjects in the other group even more. This makes sense if one treatment is more expensive, difficult, or risky than the other.
What is beta?	Beta is defined as 100% minus power. A power of 80% means that if the effect size is what you predicted your experiment has an 80% chance of obtaining a statistically significant result, and thus a 20% chance of obtaining a not significant result.
	In other words, there is a 20% chance that you'll make a Type II error (missing a true effect of a specified size). Beta, therefore, equals 20%, or 0.20.
Why don't the equations that compute sample size to achieve a specified margin of error require you to enter a value for power?	This chapter began with simple rules for calculating sample size to obtain a specified margin of error (width of CI). If the assumptions are all true and you use the computed sample size, there is a 50% chance that the computed margin of error will be less than the desired value, and a 50% chance that it will be larger. Essentially, these methods are preset for 50% power.
	If you double the sample sizes the power increases to 80%. If the assumptions are all true

Continued

Q&A Continued

	and you use this larger computed sample size, there will be an 80% chance that the computed margin of error will be less than the desired value and a 20% chance that it will be larger.
Can a study ever have 100% power?	No.
Why does power decrease if you set a smaller value for α?	When you decide to make α smaller, you set a stricter criterion for finding a significant difference. The advantage of this decision is that it decreases the chance making a Type I error. The disadvantage is that it will now be harder to declare a difference significant, even if the difference is real. By making α smaller, the chance is increased that a real difference will be declared not significant. Statistical power is decreased.
Why does power increase if you choose a larger n?	If you collect more evidence, conclusions will be more certain. Collecting data from a larger sample size decreases sampling error and thus increases statistical power.

PART I

Putting It All Together

CHAPTER 44

Statistical Advice

> When the data don't make sense, it's usually because you have
> an erroneous preconception about how the system works.
> ERNEST BEUTLER

*T*his chapter summarizes some of the statistical advice presented earlier in the book. For more practical advice, read the excellent book on
statistical rules of thumb by van Belle (2008).

DON'T FORGET THE BIG PICTURE

Statistics lets you make general conclusions from limited data

The whole point of statistics is to extrapolate from limited data to make a general
conclusion. "Descriptive statistics" simply describes data without reaching any
general conclusions. But the challenging and difficult aspects of statistics are all
about making inferences, reaching general conclusions from limited data. These
inferences are always presented in terms of probability. If a statistical conclusion
ever seems 100% certain, you probably are misunderstanding something.

Garbage In, Garbage Out

Statistical analyses are only useful if the data have been collected properly.
Thinking about experimental design is the challenging part of science. Perfect
studies are rare, so we must draw conclusions from imperfect studies. This
requires judgment and intuition, and the statistical considerations are often
minor.

Correlation or association does not imply causation

A significant correlation or association between two variables may indicate that
one variable causes the other. But it may just mean that both are related to a third
variable that influences both. Or it may be a coincidence.

Distinguish between studies that measure an important outcome and studies that measure a proxy or surrogate outcome

Measuring important outcomes (i.e., survival) can be time consuming and
expensive. It is often far more practical to measure proxy or surrogate variables

		RESULTS FROM...	
INTERVENTION	INCIDENCE OF	OBSERVATIONAL STUDIES	EXPERIMENT
Hormone replacement therapy after menopause	Cardiovascular events	Decrease	Increase
Megadose vitamin E	Cardiovascular events	Decrease	No change
Low-fat diet	Cardiovascular events and cancer	Decrease	No change
Calcium supplementation	Fractures and cancer	Decrease	No change
Vitamins to reduce homocysteine	Cardiovascular events	Decrease	No change

Table 44.1. Hypotheses suggested by observational studies proven not to be true by experiment

Adapted from Spector and Vesell (2006a). "Cardiovascular events" include myocardial infarction, sudden death, and stroke.

(i.e., white cell count). But, although the relationship between the proxy variable and the real variable may be "obvious," it may not be true. Treatments that improve results of lab tests may not improve health or survival.

Beware of very large and very small samples

The problem with very large sample sizes is that tiny differences will be statistically significant, even if they are scientifically or clinically trivial. Make sure you look at the size of the differences and not just their statistical significance.

The problem with small studies is that they have very little power. With small sample sizes, large and important differences can be insignificant. Before accepting the conclusion from a study that yielded a P value greater than 0.05 (and thus not significant), you should look at the CI and calculate the power of the study to detect the smallest difference that you think would be clinically or scientifically important.

Distinguish experiments from observational studies

Experiments give much stronger evidence than observational studies. With observational studies, it is difficult to untangle cause and effect and to deal with confounding covariates. Observational studies require more complicated analyses and yield less certain results.

To emphasize this point, Spector and Vesell (2006a) review five hypotheses suggested by observational studies that turned out not to be valid when tested with clinical experiments (Table 44.1).

INTERPRET P VALUES WISELY

$P < 0.05$ is not sacred

There really is not much difference between $P = 0.045$ and $P = 0.055$! By convention, the first is statistically significant and the second is not, but this is completely arbitrary.

A rigid cutoff for significance is useful in some situations, but is not always needed. Don't be satisfied when someone tells you whether the P value is greater or less than some arbitrary cutoff, ask for its exact value. More important, ask for the size of the difference or association and for a CI.

Statistically significant does not mean scientifically important

If the P value is less than 0.05 (an arbitrary, but well accepted threshold), the results are deemed to be statistically significant. That phrase sounds so definitive. But all it means is that, by chance alone, the difference (or association or correlation...) you observed (or one even larger) would happen less than 5% of the time. That's it. A tiny effect that is scientifically or clinically trivial can be statistically significant (especially with large samples).

Spector and Vesell (2006b) give an example. Use of montelukast for treatment of allergic rhinitis reduces symptoms, and the results are statistically significant. However, the drug reduces allergy symptoms by only 7%, so is clinically not useful.

P values (and statistical significance) are purely the result of arithmetic. Conclusions about importance require judgment and context. "In the end, patients and physicians want to know the magnitude of the benefit or lack thereof, not the statistical significance of individual studies" (Spector and Vesell, 2006b).

Not statistically significant does not mean no difference

If a difference is not statistically significant, the observed results are not inconsistent with the null hypothesis. That does *not* mean that the null hypothesis is true.

Papers often conclude that there is no evidence that A causes B. This is not the same as concluding that A doesn't cause B. The study may have used few subjects and had little power to find a difference.

Don't forget: Absence of evidence is not evidence of absence.

Published P values tend to be optimistic

By the time you read a paper, a great deal of selection has occurred. When experiments are successful, scientists continue the project. Lots of other projects get abandoned. And when the project is done, scientists are more likely to write up projects that lead to significant results. And journals are more likely to publish "positive" studies. If the null hypothesis were true, you would get a significant result 5% of the time. But those 5% of studies are more likely to get published than the other 95%.

BEWARE OF MULTIPLE COMPARISONS

If you compute enough P values, some are likely to be small

When analyzing random data, on average 1 of 20 comparisons will be statistically significant by chance. Beware of large studies that make dozens or hundreds of comparisons, because you are likely to encounter spurious significant results. When reading papers, ask yourself how many hypotheses the investigators tested.

Distinguish between studies designed to generate a hypothesis and studies designed to test one

If you look at enough variables, or subdivide subjects enough ways, some significant relationships are bound to turn up by chance alone. Such an approach can be a useful way to generate hypotheses. But such a hypothesis then must be tested with new data.

Decisions about how to analyze data should be made in advance

Analyzing data requires many decisions. Which test? What to do with outliers? Transform the data first? Should the data be normalized to external control values? All of these decisions (and more) should be made at the time you design an experiment. If you make analysis decisions after you see the data, there is a danger that you will pick and choose among analyses to get the results you want. It is easy to be fooled by this approach.

Beware of variable selection in multiple regression

Selecting which independent variables to include in multiple regression models is a form of multiple comparisons and can easily lead to overfitting (results that won't reproduce).

Don't pick and choose from the results of multiple tests

It's tempting. Look at both the results of a t test and a nonparametric test. A resampling test too! Then report the P value you like the best, usually the smallest one. This approach leads to results that cannot be interpreted.

THINK ABOUT THE DATA

Look at the data

Statistical tests are useful because they objectively quantify uncertainty and help reduce data to a few values. Although such calculations are helpful, inspection of statistical calculations should never replace looking at the data. The data are primary; statistics merely summarize.

Look behind the data

In some cases, the data shown in graphs and entered into statistics programs have already been processed. In some cases, the adjustments, exclusions, and smoothing done before the data are actually analyzed have a huge impact on the conclusions.

Outliers may be important

Statistical tests (t tests, ANOVA) compare averages. Variability in biological or clinical studies is not always primarily caused by measurement uncertainties. Instead, the variability in the data may reflect real biological diversity.

Appreciate this diversity! Don't get mesmerized by averages; the extreme values can be more interesting. Nobel prizes have been won from studies of individuals whose values were far from the mean.

Don't ask only whether the means are different; ask whether the SDs are different

"Math Scores Show No Gap for Girls, Study Finds," reported the New York Times (Lewin, 2008). Not quite (Briggs, 2008). In addition to showing essentially no difference in the average math scores between boys and girls, the study showed that there was a difference in variation (Hyde, Lindberg, Linn, Ellis, & Williams, 2008). The scores of boys were more variable, and twice as many boys as girls were in the top 1%. To fully understand the data, you must consider more than just the averages.

Here is another example. Steven Jay Gould wondered about changes in professional baseball from 1870 to 1970 (Gould, 1997). Why have there been no players with batting averages over 0.400 since 1941? Although the mean batting average has been consistent, he discovered a remarkable drop in the SD, especially in the first half of that period. This decrease in variability, he concludes, occurred because players, coaching, refereeing, and equipment have all become more consistent. With the same mean and a lower SD than in earlier times, a batting average greater than 0.400 would be expected to be much more rare.

Non-Gaussian distributions are normal

Many statistical tests depend on the assumption that the data points come from a Gaussian distribution, and scientists often seem to think that nature is kind enough to see to it that all interesting variables are so distributed. This isn't true. Many interesting variables are not scattered according to a Gaussian distribution.

Don't ignore pairing

Paired (or repeated-measures) experiments are very powerful. The use of matched pairs of subjects (or before and after measurements) controls for many sources of variability. Special methods are available for analyzing such data, and they should be used when appropriate.

	ACCEPTED	DENIED	% ACCEPTED
Men	3,738	4,704	44.3
Women	1,494	2,827	34.6

Table 44.2. Admissions to the graduate programs in Berkeley, 1973.
At first glance, this seems to be evidence of sexism.

BEWARE OF MISSING VARIABLES

Statistics is only a small part of doing science. Many puzzles in data analysis are solved by clever scientific thinking, not by fancier analyses. Here are two examples.

Pooled data can hide important findings

Admission was offered to 44.3% of the men and 34.6% of the women who applied to a graduate school (Table 44.2; Bickel, Hammel, & O'Connell, 1975). The ratio is 1.28, with a 95% CI ranging from 1.22 to 1.34. The P value is less than 0.0001. This seems to be proof of sexism, but it is not.

Because admissions decisions are made by individual program, the data for each program should be looked at individually. In 75 of the 85 programs, the difference between men and women was not statistically significant. In 4 programs, the difference was statistically significant, and women were less likely to be admitted. In 6 programs, the difference was statistically significant, and men were less likely to be admitted.

What's going on? Why do the pooled data suggest sexism?

Some graduate programs accept a high fraction of applicants and others accept a low fraction of applicants. The two departments most popular among women admitted only 34 and 24% of the applicants, whereas the two departments most popular among men admitted 62 and 63% of the applicants (Freedman, 2007). A smaller fraction of women were admitted overall for a simple reason: Women tended to apply to more selective programs than did men.

This is a classic example of *Simpson's paradox*. Analysis of pooled data can lead to misleading results.

The same problem probably happens in some medical studies. Imagine how little progress you'd make if you tested whether drugs cure cancer if the studies included patients with all kinds of cancers. Cancer is a group of many diseases that respond to different drugs. Combining all those diagnoses into one study would lead to frustration and inconclusive results. Most likely, many medical conditions (perhaps septic shock and autism) really are combinations of distinct disorders. Until we figure out how to identify the individual diseases, studies of therapies are likely to be ambiguous.

Beware of lurking variables

This example (extended from one presented by Freedman, 2007) is a bit silly but makes an important point. Everyone knows what determines the area of a

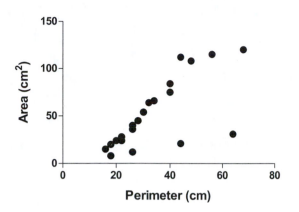

Figure 44.1. This graph plots area of rectangles as a function of their perimeter.

The raw data are in Table 47.1.

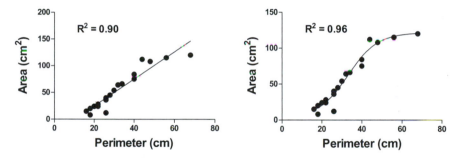

Figure 44.2. We removed two outliers from Figure 47.1 and fit the curve to a straight line (left) or a sigmoidal shaped curve (right).

rectangle, but pretend you don't. Your goal is to find a model that predicts the area of a rectangle from its perimeter.

Figure 44.1 shows that rectangles with larger perimeters also tend to have larger areas, with two outliers. Figure 44.2 fits the remaining points (after removing the "outliers") to possible models. The straight-line model (Figure 44.2, left) might be adequate, but the sigmoid shaped model (Figure 44.2, right) fits the data better.

Figure 44.3 adds data from more rectangles. Now it seems that those two outliers were really not so unusual. Instead, it seems that there are two distinct categories of rectangles. The right side of Figure 44.3 tentatively identifies the two types of rectangles with open and closed circles and fits each to a different model.

This process sort of seems like real science. In fact, of course, it is nonsense. Two rectangles with the same perimeter can have vastly different areas,

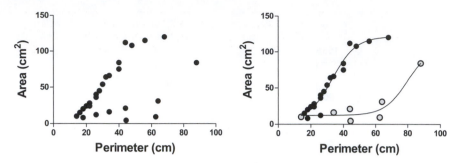

Figure 44.3. Now we collected data from more rectangles and realize those two outliers were not really so unusual (left).

Instead, it seems that there are two different kinds of rectangles requiring two different models (right).

depending on their shape. Predicting the area of a rectangle from its perimeter is simply impossible. The area must be computed from both height and weight. An important variable was missing (lurking). Understanding these data required simple thinking to identify the missing variable, rather than fancy statistical analyses.

CONCENTRATE ON CIs

CIs are easier to understand than P values
The whole idea of statistics is to make general conclusions from data, to extrapolate from the sample being analyzed to the overall population. CIs are the most straightforward way to do this. P values and conclusions about statistical significance can be helpful too, but should not replace the use of CIs.

CIs are optimistic (too narrow)
The "real" CI is nearly always wider than the CI calculated from a particular experiment. The strict interpretation of a CI assumes that your samples are randomly sampled from the population of interest. This is often not the case. Even if the sample were randomly selected, the population of interest (all patients) is larger and more heterogeneous than the population of patients studied (limited to certain ages, without other disease, living in a certain area and receiving medical care from a certain medical center). Thus, the true 95% CI (which you can't calculate) is often wider than the interval you calculate.

BE SKEPTICAL

Many (perhaps most) published research findings are false
Chapter 22 pointed out that statistically significant results can occur by chance, even when the null hypothesis is true. This is called making a Type I error. Chapter 18 showed you how to compute the fraction of all statistically significant

	STATISTICALLY SIGNIFICANT: REJECT NULL HYPOTHESIS	NOT STATISTICALLY SIGNIFICANT: DO NOT REJECT NULL HYPOTHESIS	TOTAL
No real effect (null hypothesis true)	47	893	940
Effect is real	48	12	60
Total	95	905	1,000

Table 44.3. Results of 1,000 comparisons with 80% power, a 5% significance level, and a prior probability = 6%.

Of the 60 comparisons where there really is an effect, 80% (the power), or 48, will be statistically significant. Of the remaining 940 experiments where there is really no effect, 5%, or 47, will be statistically significant. Thus, half (47/95) of the statistically significant results are false.

findings that are Type I errors based on three values:

- Definition of statistical significance, α. If this is set to a tiny value (say 0.001 rather than the usual 0.05), it is much more likely that statistically significant findings will be real.
- Power. When the experiment has low power, a smaller fraction of statistically significant results will be true.
- The scientific context. Consider the two extreme cases. If you do a series of positive control experiment, where you know for sure that the effect is real, then every single statistically significant result will definitely be real. There can be no false positives. On the other hand, if you run a series of negative controls, where you know for sure the null hypothesis is true, than every single statistically significant result must be a Type I error, a false positive. Actual experiments are between these two extremes. Statistically significant results from focused experiments based on solid science and prior data are more likely to be true. Statistically significant results from unfocused experiments are more likely to be false positives.

Table 44.3 shows one scenario, using the standard definition of statistical significance (P < 0.05) and a standard goal for power (80%). Table 44.3 assumes that given the scientific context of that series of experiments, in 6% of the experiments there is a real difference (or effect) and in 94% there is not. Of those 6%, 80% (the power) will yield a statistically significant result. Of the other 94%, random sampling will lead to a statistically significant conclusion in 5%. In this situation, only about half of the statistically significant effects are in experiments where there in fact is a true difference and half of the statistically significant results are false positives.

Many experiments are designed to have less than 80% power, and the prior probability of a true effect could possibly be less than 6%. Thus, it is quite possible to report statistical significance in a situation where the chance is greater than 50% that the finding is a false positive.

Chapters 22 (multiple comparisons) and 38 (overfitting in multiple regression) point out the many ways in which investigators can fool themselves and

FACTOR	EXPLANATION
Small sample size	Small studies have less power than large ones. Statistically significant results from studies with lower power are more likely to be false than studies with lots of power.
Reported effect is small	Studies have less power to detect small effects than large ones. Statistically significant results from studies with lower power are more likely to be false than studies with lots of power.
Many comparisons; only report the ones that are statistically significant	Chapter 23 has explained how easy it is to be fooled by multiple comparisons.
Flexible data analysis without a plan	Analyze data flexibly, without a rigid analysis protocol established before the data were collected. Chapter 23 already warned about this problem.
Biased investigators; financial	If the investigators have a financial motive for the results to be statistically significant, they will try harder to extract a statistically significant conclusion from the data.
Biased investigators; opinionated	Investigators with strong opinions about how the result is supposed to come out may tend to accept and publish results that go the "right way" and reanalyze or ignore data that go the "wrong way." These investigators are more likely to publish work that turns out to be wrong than are open-minded investigators.
Hot field	When a field is hot, investigators may rush to publish statistically significant findings and tend to spend less time running all the needed controls.

Table 44.4. Factors that increase the chance that a published statistically significant finding will turn out to not be true (inspired by Ioannidis, 2005).

boost the chance of bogus statistically significant results. Ioannidis (2005) argues that *most* published statistically significant research findings are false. Table 44.4 lists factors that increase the chance that a published result is false.

The winner's curse: True published findings tend to be inflated

What about the published findings that are true and not false positives? As pointed out in Chapter 43, these studies tend to inflate the size of the difference or effect.

The explanation is simple. If many studies are performed, the average of the effects detected in these studies will usually be close to the true effect. By chance, some studies will happen to find larger effects, and some studies will happen to find smaller effects. But studies with small effects tend not to get published (publication bias was mentioned in Chapter 23). On average, therefore, the studies that do get published tend to have effect sizes that overestimate the true effect (Ioannidis, 2008). This is called the winner's curse (Zollner, 2007). This term was coined by economists to describe the winner of an auction, who tends to overpay.

CHAPTER 45

Choosing a Statistical Test

The greatest challenge facing mankind is the challenge of
distinguishing reality from fantasy, truth from propaganda.
MICHAEL CRICHTON (2003)

I f you are not sure which statistical test to use, the tables in this chapter
may help you decide. Reviewing these tables is also a good way to
review your understanding of statistics.

OUTCOME: CONTINUOUS DATA FROM
GAUSSIAN DISTRIBUTION

Examples	Cholesterol plasma level (mg/dL)
	Change in systolic blood pressure (mmHg)
	Number of headaches in a week (not really continuous, but perhaps close enough so all the analyses below are still useful)
Test Gaussian assumption	Normality tests
	Outlier tests
Describe one sample	Frequency distribution
	Sample mean
	Minimum and maximum value and range
	25th and 75th percentiles
	Sample SD
Make inferences about one population	One-sample t test
Compare two unmatched (unpaired)groups	Unpaired t test
Compare two matched (paired) groups	Paired t test
Compare three or more unmatched (unpaired) groups	One-way ANOVA, followed by multiple comparison tests
Compare three or more matched (paired) groups	Repeated-measures ANOVA followed by multiple comparison tests

Quantify association between two variables	Pearson's correlation
Explain/predict one variable from another	Simple linear regression
	Simple nonlinear regression
	("Simple" means you are predicting the outcome from a single independent variable)
Explain/predict one variable from several others	Multiple linear regression
	Multiple nonlinear regression

OUTCOME: CONTINUOUS DATA FROM NON-GAUSSIAN DISTRIBUTION (OR RANKED DATA)

Examples	17β-estradiol levels (pg/mL)
	IIEF-5 scoring system (5–25)
	Gleason score for prostate cancer (2–10)
	Confidence (5 = *very high*, 4 = *high*, 3 = *moderate*, 2 = *low*, 1 = *very low*)
Describe one sample	Frequency distribution
	Sample median
	Minimum and maximum value and range
	25th and 75th percentiles
Make inferences about one population	Wilcoxon's rank-sum test
Compare two unmatched (unpaired) groups	Mann–Whitney test
Compare two matched (paired) groups	Wilcoxon's matched pairs test
Compare three or more unmatched (unpaired) groups	Kruskal–Wallis test
	Dunn's posttest
Compare three or more matched (paired) groups	Friedman's test
	Dunn's posttest
Quantify association between two variables	Spearman's correlation

OUTCOME: SURVIVAL TIMES (OR TIME TO AN EVENT)

Examples	Time to death for prostate cancer patient
	Time to end of cold symptoms
	Time to REM sleep
Describe one sample	Kaplan–Meier survival curve
	Median survival time
	Five year survival percentage

Make inferences about one population	Confidence bands around survival curve CI of median survival
Compare two unmatched (unpaired) groups	Log-rank test Gehan–Breslow test CI of ratio of median survival times CI of hazard ratio
Compare two matched (paired) groups	Conditional proportional hazards regression
Compare three or more unmatched (unpaired) groups	Log-rank test Gehan–Breslow test
Compare three or more matched (paired) groups	Conditional proportional hazards regression
Explain/predict one variable from one or several others.	Cox's proportional hazards regression

OUTCOME: BINOMIAL

Examples	Cure of acute myeloid leukemia within a specific time period, yes or no Success (yes/no) of preventing motion sickness Recurrence of infection, yes or no
Describe one sample	Proportion
Make inferences about one population	CI of proportion Binomial test to compare observed distribution with a theoretical (expected) distribution
Compare two unmatched (unpaired) groups	Fishers' exact test
Compare two matched (paired) groups	McNemar's test
Compare three or more unmatched (unpaired) groups	Chi-square test Chi-square test for trend
Compare three or more matched (paired) groups	Cochrane Q
Explain/predict one variable from one or several others.	Logistic regression

CHAPTER 46

Capstone Example

He uses statistics as a drunken man uses lamp-posts—for
support rather than illumination.

ANDREW LANG

This chapter was inspired by Bill Greco, who is its narrator and coauthor. One definition of capstone is "a final touch," and this chapter reviews many of the statistical principles presented throughout this book. It also demonstrates the usefulness and versatility of simulations. Although based on a true situation, many of the elements of the storyline, person names, and drug name have been changed to protect the innocent.

THE CASE OF THE EIGHT NAKED IC$_{50}$s

Then

It is Friday, May 2, 1975. It is a chilly spring day in Buffalo, New York. Gerald Ford is the president of the United States. There are no PCs on the desks of scientists. The Internet hadn't been invented yet. I was a new graduate student, who had just received an A in a beginning biostatistics course.

An interim chairman, Dr. Jeremy Bentham, asked me for help. Two months ago, he had submitted a manuscript that compared the potency of two drugs to block the proliferation of cultured cancer cells. The key results are shown in Table 46.1, which tabulates the amount of drug needed to inhibit cell growth 50% (the IC$_{50}$).

The average IC$_{50}$ for trimetrexate (TMQ) was 21 nM and that for methotrexate (MTX) was 2.4 nM. A smaller IC$_{50}$ corresponds to a more potent drug, because less drug is needed to inhibit growth. MTX was 8.8-fold (21 nM/2.4 nM) more potent than TMQ. MTX was the standard dihydrofolate reductase (DHFR) inhibitor used in the clinic; TMQ was a new lipophilic DHFR inhibitor with "better" cellular uptake properties.

The investigator was sure of the conclusion based on his experience with these types of agents and the specific cell growth inhibition assay. He was very confident that, in this KB cell line, TMQ is about 10-fold less potent than is MTX. Each of the eight experiments had taken 1 week to conduct. All eight experiments

TMQ (NM)	MTX (NM)
5.5	0.83
12	1.1
19	1.9
47	5.8

Table 46.1. Sample data for this example.

Human KB cells were grown in monolayer culture in glass T-25 flasks with RPMI 1640 medium and 10% fetal calf serum for 7 days. Each IC_{50} was calculated from the concentration-effect curve from a separate experiment, consisting of five control flasks (no added drug) and three flasks at each of 7 different logarithmically spaced concentrations of TMQ or MTX. Cell growth was assessed by measuring total protein content with the Lowry assay.

were conducted with the same passage of the KB cell line over the 6-month period preceding the submission of the manuscript. The IC_{50}'s for TMQ and MTX of 19 and 1.9 nM, respectively, were determined from a joint experiment, with the sharing of controls. The other 6 IC_{50} determinations were made at different times and preceded this last "paired experiment." The overall theme of the manuscript was a comparison of the two DHFR inhibitors against the single KB human cell line regarding antiproliferative potency, cellular uptake, metabolism, and inhibition of the target enzyme, DHFR.

As part of the usual process of peer review, the journal's editor sent the manuscript to several anonymous reviewers. The paper was rejected largely because of the following comment by one reviewer:

"This reviewer performed an unpaired Student's t test on the data (see Table 46.1), and found that there is no significant difference between the mean IC_{50} of TMQ and MTX (P = 0.092) against KB cells. The data do not support your conclusion."

Not believing the reviewer, he asked me to check the calculations.

Using the formulas and tables in my biostatistics text and a scientific calculator, I performed a standard unpaired two-tail Student's t test (with the usual assumption of equal error variance for the two populations). I found that $t = 2.01$ and $P = 0.092$, in total agreement with the reviewer. Because $P > 0.05$, I informed the investigator that the reviewer was correct, the difference in potency was not statistically significant.

Because the P value was 0.092, the investigator asked, doesn't that mean there is a (1.000−0.092), which equals 0.908 or 90.8% chance that the findings are real? I explained to him that a P value cannot be interpreted that way. The proper interpretation of the P value is that even if the two drugs really have the same potency (the null hypothesis), there would be a 9.2% chance of observing this large a discrepancy (or larger still) by chance. If I had had a crystal ball, perhaps I could have shown him Chapter 19 of this text!

I took it one step further and computed the CI of the difference. The difference in observed IC_{50}s was −18.5 nM (the order of subtraction was arbitrary, so the difference could have been +18.5 nM; it is important only to be consistent). The 95% CI for the difference was from −41.0 to +4.06 nM. I pointed out that the lower confidence limit is negative (MTX was more potent) and the upper confidence limit is positive (TMQ was more potent), so the 95% CI includes the possibility of no difference in potency (equal IC_{50} values; the null hypothesis). This is consistent with the P value (see Chapter 17). When a P value is greater than 0.05, the 95% CI must include the value specified by the null hypothesis (zero, in this case).

The investigator became enraged. He thought the data in the table would convince any competent pharmacologist that TMQ is, beyond any reasonable doubt, less potent than MTX. Statistics weren't needed, he thought, spouting off half-remembered famous quotes. "When the data speaks for itself, don't interrupt." "There are liars; there are damn liars; and then there are statisticians." "If you need statistics, you've done the wrong experiment."

The investigator sent the manuscript unaltered to another journal, which accepted it.

Now

It is Friday, January 23, 2009. It is a chilly winter day in Buffalo, New York. Barack Obama has just become the president of the United States. There are small, powerful PCs on the desks of virtually all scientists. Powerful statistical PC software is available, at reasonable or no cost, to all scientists. The Internet is a major part of professional and personal life. I am the instructor of an applied biostatistics course. I use *Intuitive Biostatistics* as the main textbook in the course. I just retrieved the published paper from 1975 by Bentham et al. on TMQ and MTX. As I stare at the IC_{50} table reproduced here as Table 46.1, it stares back at me.

The mismatch of statistical reasoning and common sense gnawed at me. I knew the statistical calculations were correct. But I also felt the senior and experienced investigator's scientific intuition and conclusion were also probably correct. Something was wrong, and this chapter is the culmination of decades of angst. I must resolve this 34-year-old quandary. How should have I analyzed these data back in 1975? How could I analyze these data now in 2009?

Before reading on, think about how you would analyze these data.

LOOK BEHIND THE DATA

If I were asked to consult on this project today, I would not begin with Table 46.1. Instead, I would go back to the raw data. Each of the values in Table 46.1 came from analyzing an experiment that measured cell number at one time point in the presence of several different concentrations of drug. The IC_{50} is defined as the concentration of drug that inhibits cell growth to a value halfway between the maximum and minimum values. This raises many questions:

- What are the details of the cell proliferation assay? Which details provide the opportunity for experimental artifacts? Were cells actually counted? Or did they measure some proxy variable (perhaps protein content) that is usually proportional to cell count? Over what period of time was cell growth measured? Has the relationship between cell growth and time been well characterized in previous experiments? Does cell growth slow down, because of cell-to-cell contact inhibition (or depletion of nutrients) as the flasks fill with cells? Are the different drug treatments randomly assigned to the flasks? Is it possible that cell growth depends on where each flask is placed in the incubator?
- How was "100%" cell growth defined? Growth with no drug? What if growth was actually a bit faster in the presence of a tiny concentration of drug? Should the 100% point be defined by averaging the controls? By fitting a curve and letting the curve-fitting program extrapolate to define the top plateau?
- How was 0% cell growth defined? Is "0%" defined to be no cell growth at all? Or cell growth with the largest concentration of drug used? But what if an even larger concentration had been used? Or is 0% defined by a curve-fitting program that extrapolates the curve to infinite drug concentration? The answer to this seemingly simple technical question has a large influence on the estimation of drug potency. The determination of the IC_{50} can be no more accurate than the definitions of 0 and 100.
- How was the IC_{50} determined? By hand with a ruler? By hand with a French curve? By linearizing the raw data and then using linear regression? By fitting the four-parameter concentration-effect model (Chapter 36) to the raw data with nonlinear regression? And if the latter, with what weighting scheme?

Here, we will skip all those questions and assume that the values in Table 46.1 are reliable. But do note that many problems in data analysis actually occur while planning or performing the experiment or while wrangling the data into a form that can be entered into a statistics program.

STATISTICAL SIGNIFICANCE BY CHEATING

One way to solve the problem is to report a one-tail P value, rather than a two-tail P value. And it isn't too hard to justify that decision. All I have to do is state that the experimental hypothesis was to confirm that TMQ is less potent than MTX. The one-tail P value is half the two-tail P value, so it is 0.046. That is less than 0.05, so now the difference is statistically significant. Mission accomplished. That was easy!

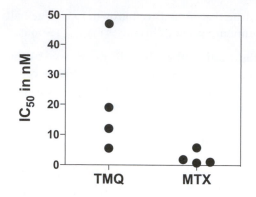

Figure 46.1. The data shown in Table 46.1.

Of course, this is cheating. To justify a one-tail P value, the decision to report a one-tail P value would need to have been made before the data were collected. It wasn't. At that time, it would also be necessary to decide that any data showing that TMQ is more potent than MTX would be attributed to chance and not worth pursuing. In fact, if the results had gone the other way, with MTX being substantially less potent, the investigator would have found an explanation and reported the findings.

USING A t TEST THAT DOESN'T ASSUME EQUAL SDs

One of the assumptions for the unpaired t test—that the data are sampled from populations with equal SDs—seems dubious with these data. Look at Figure 46.1. The TMQ data are way more scattered. This can be quantified by comparing the two SDs. The sample SD for the TMQ data was 18.3 nM, whereas the sample SD for the MTX data was 2.31 nM.

Chapter 30 provides a formal way to assess this discrepancy. If the two populations really have the same SDs, the square of the ratio of the sample SD should follow the F distribution. The ratio is 18.3/2.31 = 7.92, so the square of the ratio is 62.7.

To compute a P value, we first must articulate a null hypothesis. For this particular P value, the null hypothesis is that the two populations have the same standard deviation, and the observed discrepancy is the result of chance. If that were true, then the square of the ratio would be sampled from an F distribution. What is the chance that F would be so high? To answer requires a program that does the calculations (I used the free GraphPad QuickCalcs; see Appendix A) and specifying the df for both the numerator and the denominator of the ratio (both are n-1 or 3). The P value is 0.0033. With such a low P value, it makes sense to reject that null hypothesis.

Now what? A modified t test allows for unequal SDs. With this modified test, the t value is still 2.01, but the P value is now 0.139, with df = 3. The P value

X: DRUG	Y: IC$_{50}$ IN nM
0	5.5
0	12
0	19
0	47
1	0.83
1	1.1
1	1.9
1	5.8

Table 46.2. Data as entered into a regression program.

The X value was defined to be 0 for the drug TMQ and 1 for the drug MTX.

is higher, but perhaps more appropriate, because it does not make an assumption that is probably false. However, according to Moser and Stevens (1992), the decision to use this test should be made as part of the experimental design and should not be based on the results of the F test to compare SDs.

This, perhaps, is a more appropriate way to analyze the data, but it didn't really help. It doesn't bridge the gap between the result that is scientifically obvious and the result computed by formal statistics. In addition, the P value moved in the wrong direction! I know that it is cheating to just run a bunch of rival statistical tests and then pick the one that yields the smallest P value, but the increase in P value with the modified t test surely suggests that something is fundamentally wrong with my thinking!

UNPAIRED t TEST AS LINEAR OR NONLINEAR REGRESSION

Hidden in Chapters 35 and 36 is an intriguing regression approach that might be appropriate for these data. I defined X to equal 0 for the TMQ group and 1 for the MTX group, and defined Y to be the individual IC$_{50}$ values. I then used linear regression to fit a straight line to the data recast as the X,Y pairs shown in Table 46.2. The slope reported by linear regression equals the difference in Y values divided by the difference in X values. The X values for the two drugs differ by 1.0, so the slope quantifies the difference in mean IC$_{50}$'s between TMQ and MTX.

Linear regression calculated that the best-fit slope equals −18.5 nM with a standard error of 9.21. The 95% CI for the true slope (difference in mean IC$_{50}$) was −41.0 to 4.06 nM. The associated P value (testing the null hypothesis that the population slope equals zero) was 0.092. These are exactly the same as results calculated by the simple unpaired t test. I expected this, because Chapter 35 emphasized that the two approaches are equivalent. However, the regression approach is more versatile, because it lets me compensate for nonuniform variance by appropriately weighting the data. Data with more scatter can be given less weight, and data with less scatter can be given more weight. Unfortunately, most linear regression software does not permit this type of weighting! So I switched to nonlinear regression software (which can also fit straight lines).

To apply this weighted regression approach, I fit a straight line to the X,Y data using weighted nonlinear regression (Chapter 36). I assumed that both sets of data were drawn from Gaussian populations, but that the standard deviations of these populations are not equal but instead are proportional to their mean. To fit this model, I asked the regression program to minimize the square of the relative distances of each point from the fitted line (weighting with the reciprocal of the square of the predicted Y). The slope of this line is the difference between IC_{50} values, which is –18.5 nM, with a 95% CI ranging from –42.1 to 5.12 nM. One end of the CI is negative, which corresponds to the IC_{50} of MTX being smaller. But the other end of the CI was positive, which means the IC_{50} of TMQ is smaller. Like before, this method concludes that the data are consistent with no difference in IC_{50}. Because the 95% CI includes zero, the P value must be higher than 0.05. In fact, it was 0.104.

In summary, this alternative logical approach lengthened the CI and increased the P value! I don't seem to be making any real progress.

NONPARAMETRIC MANN–WHITNEY TEST

The t test assumes that the data were sampled from populations with Gaussian distributions. With only four values in each group, it is impossible to seriously assess this assumption. Normality tests (Chapter 24) don't work with such tiny samples.

In fact, I find that normality tests are rarely helpful when used as part of an analysis of a particular experiment, but can be quite useful when characterizing an assay. I prefer to collect many values (dozens to hundreds) while characterizing (developing) an experimental assay. I then examine the distribution of these values (including use of normality tests) to decide how these kind of data should be analyzed. That decision then applies to all experiments that use the assay. In this example, we don't have the large number of measurements we'd need to tell us whether the Gaussian assumption is reasonable for this kind of data.

Rather than assuming the data were sampled from Gaussian populations, we can use the nonparametric Mann–Whitney test instead. With this test, P = 0.057. Although the P value is closer to 0.05, it is still greater than 0.05. Sure, using 0.05 as a threshold for defining statistical significance is arbitrary, but it is widely accepted.

Sure, it is tempting to just erase that last digit and call it 0.05. But that would be cheating. Rounded to two decimal places, the P value is 0.06.

Although you could argue that 0.057 is close enough to "tentatively suggest" that the potencies are different for the two drugs, this is somehow unsatisfying. In my gut, I really know that TMQ is less potent than MTX.

JUST REPORT THE LAST CONFIRMATORY EXPERIMENT?

I considered just presenting the data from the last paired experiment, in which TMQ and MTX were studied simultaneously, with a set of shared control flasks. The individual IC_{50}'s for TMQ and MTX were 19 and 1.9, respectively, with a potency ratio of 10. Perhaps I might consider the first six individual experiments exploratory and the last paired experiment confirmatory.

This last paired experiment's potency ratio is very close to the overall potency ratio of the mean IC_{50}'s of 8.7. Perhaps it would be best to eliminate the table and just list in the text the individual IC_{50}'s for TMQ and MTX and the potency ratio for this last confirmatory experiment and then also state that this experiment was representative of six previous individual exploratory experiments with the two agents.

This seems to be a scientifically ethical approach to the dilemma. However, I like to think of myself as a stubborn, honest, and thorough scientist; I suspect that there is a better solution—one that involves calculating, rather than avoiding, statistics. I want to honestly showcase and analyze all of the experimental work.

Studying TMQ and MTX in paired experiments, with common controls, for the goal of potency ratio assessment, is a good idea. Pairing (Chapter 31) is usually recommended because it reduces variability and so increases power. This example combines data from paired experiments with data from unpaired experiments, and this makes the analysis awkward.

INCREASE SAMPLE SIZE?

Of course, we'd like to get the results we want without collecting more data. But maybe more data are required. Chapter 43 presented an equation to compute the approximate sample size needed to detect a specified difference (w) given an anticipated SD (s) with 80% power and a significance level of 80%.

$$n \approx 16\left(\frac{s}{w}\right)^2 \quad \text{(per group)}$$

To compute a sample size, all we need are values for s and w.

For s, we must enter the anticipated SD. In many situations, we may have lots of prior data to use to estimate this. Here, we have only the data at hand. Our two samples have different standard deviations. The sample SD for the TMQ data was 18.3 nM, whereas the sample SD for MTX was 2.31 nM. One thought might be to average the two and enter s = 10.3. Actually, with the same sample size in both groups, it is better to use the square root of the average of the variances (the square of the SDs). With this procedure, s is approximately 13 nM.

For w, we must enter the smallest difference between mean potencies that we'd find scientifically interesting. It's a bit arbitrary, but to keep the calculations

TMQ	MTX
0.740	−0.081
1.079	0.041
1.279	0.279
1.672	0.763

Table 46.3. The logarithms of the IC_{50} values of TMQ and MTX.

These are the logarithms of the values (in nM) shown in Table 46.1.

easy let's set this to 18 nM, which is a bit smaller than the observed difference of 18.6 nM.

$$n \approx 16\left(\frac{s}{w}\right)^2 \quad \text{(per group)}$$

$$n \approx 16\left(\frac{13}{18}\right)^2 \approx 8 \text{ per group}$$

Each of the eight experiments, per drug, would require 26 flasks of cells measured at multiple time points. This would be an outrageously large amount of work to answer a relatively trivial scientific question for which I am quite sure that I already know the answer.

COMPARING THE LOGARITHMS OF IC_{50} VALUES

Lognormal data

IC_{50} values tend to follow lognormal distributions (Chapter 11) rather than Gaussian distributions. This leads to larger SDs when the mean is larger, as we saw. It can also lead to false identification of outliers (Chapter 25).

Analyzing lognormal data is simple. I first calculated the base 10 (common) logarithms of the 8 IC_{50}'s. The results are shown in Table 46.3 and Figure 46.2. The mean $\log(IC_{50})$ for TMQ is 1.19 and that for MTX is 0.251. The variability of the two sets of $\log(IC_{50})$ values is very similar, with nearly identical sample SDs (0.389 and 0.373). Thus, there is no problem accepting the assumption of the standard two-sample unpaired t test that the two samples come from populations with the same SDs.

Reversing the logarithmic transform (taking the antilog; see Appendix E) converts the values back to their original units. Taking the antilog is the same as taking 10 to that power, and taking the antilog of a mean of logarithms computes the geometric mean (Chapter 11). The corresponding geometric mean for the IC_{50} for TMQ is 15.6 nM and that for MTX is 1.78 nM.

Unpaired t test of log-transformed data

The calculated t ratio is 3.49 and the corresponding P value is 0.013, df = 6. MTX is more potent than TMQ and that discrepancy is statistically significant (with the conventional definition).

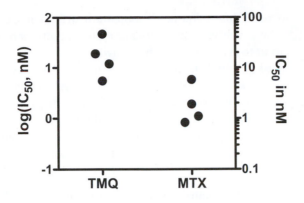

Figure 46.2. The logarithms of the data shown in Figure 46.1.
The left axis shows the logarithms, and the right axis shows the antilogarithms. Comparing the two lets you review the meaning of logarithms. The logarithm of 100 is 2, because $10^2 = 100$. The logarithm of 1.0 is 0.0, because $10^0 = 1.0$. The logarithm of any value between 0 and 1 is negative.

The difference between the $\log(IC_{50})$s is 0.942. Transform this to its antilog to turn it into a potency ratio (the difference in logs is the log of the ratio). The antilog is 10 to that power, or $10^{0.942}$, which equals 8.75. In other words, MTX is almost nine times more potent than TMQ.

95% CI
The 95% CI for the difference in mean $\log(IC_{50})$ ranges from 0.282 to 1.60. Transform each limit to its antilog (10 to that power) to determine the 95% confidence limits of the population potency ratio, 1.91 to 39.8. This interval does not encompass 1.0 (the value of the null hypothesis of equal drug potency), so it is consistent with a P value less than 0.05. With 95% confidence, we can say that MTX is somewhere between twice as potent as TMQ and 40 times as potent. Analyzed this way, the intuition of the investigator is proven to be correct.

Why this is the optimal method
This is probably the best simple way to analyze the data. The t test of the untransformed IC_{50} values is inferior to the t test of the log-transformed IC_{50} values for three important reasons.

- The log transform equalized the two SDs and thus eliminated the assumption violation of unequal variances.
- The log transformation changed the distribution of IC_{50}s from a lognormal distribution to a Gaussian distribution, another assumption of the t test, as suggested in Chapter 11. With only two sets of data, each with only four

values, we really don't know much about the distribution of the population of IC_{50}'s. But extensive past experience with concentration-effect experiments tells us to expect a lognormal distribution.

- The t test asks about differences between means. The t test on log-transformed data essentially asks about ratios. Pharmacologists universally ask about ratios of drug potencies, not differences. Transforming to logarithms helps match the statistical method to the scientific question. The t test of the log-transformed IC_{50} values is a nice statistical translation of the scientific question, "What is the relative potency of TMQ and MTX?".

If I had access to the original raw concentration-effect data, I would likely try to fit a variant of the four-parameter concentration-effect model showcased in Chapter 36, with nonlinear regression, to all of the data at once. I would take into account differences among the experiments run at different times and estimate the overall estimated potency ratio with an accompanying 95% CI. I would take advantage of the true sample size of 203 flasks from eight experiments in my analysis. However, I don't have the original raw data; I just have the eight naked IC_{50}'s in Table 46.1.

SAMPLE SIZE CALCULATIONS REVISITED

Now that we realize the data follow a lognormal distribution, let's go back and redo the sample size calculations. On a log scale, we found that the SD of both groups was 0.38, so we enter into the sample size formula a conservative 0.40 as s. How large a difference in $log(IC_{50})$ are we looking for? Let's say we were looking for an eightfold difference in potency, so the $log(IC_{50})$ values differ by about 0.9. Set $w = 0.9$.

$$n \approx 16 \left(\frac{s}{w} \right)^2 \text{ (per group)}$$

$$n \approx 16 \left(\frac{0.4}{0.9} \right)^2 \text{ (per group)}$$

$$n \approx 3.2 \approx 3 \text{ (per group)}$$

This equation is an approximation that works well with large n. Here, n is tiny and that equation is not accurate. A more complicated equation (by a computer program designed for that purpose) suggests four per group. So the original sample size was indeed sufficient, once the analysis was done properly.

This might be stated in a paper as follows.

A sample size of four in each group was computed to have 80% power to detect as statistically significant ($P < 0.05$) an eightfold difference in potency, assuming that $log(IC_{50})$ values follow a Gaussian distribution with a standard deviation of 0.40.

IS IT OK TO SWITCH ANALYSIS METHODS?

This whole exercise to search for a better statistical analysis than was suggested by the reviewer has left me frustrated.

Data analysis should not be fishing for statistical significance. It is not ethical to conduct multiple statistical procedures on the same data set for the purpose of finding the statistical approach that yields the lowest P value. This whole exercise in analyzing the data this way, then that way, and then another way seems to be scientific fraud.

At the same time, the logarithm method makes scientific sense. As explained in the previous section, this is the optimal method for comparing IC_{50} values. The method matches the scientific context and goals, whereas the other methods do not. Of course, this should have been planned before the data were collected. But it wasn't. Is it OK to switch methods after the fact?

A reality check. This happens all the time in basic research. Many scientists never even think about how to analyze the data until after the experiments are done. But just because it is done commonly doesn't mean it is correct. Chapter 23 pointed out how easy it is to be fooled by multiple analyses. Certainly, clinical trials that will be reviewed by the FDA require that the analysis method be precisely specified in advance.

In this case, I have a strong scientific justification for switching to the proper method. Also, I am responding, albeit indirectly, to comments made by an expert reviewer of the manuscript. Does this rationale make it OK? I think so, but I will let you, the reader, decide for yourself. It certainly would be OK if these were preliminary data, and this whole exercise was done as a way to make decisions about how I will analyze data from future experiments.

THE USEFULNESS OF SIMULATIONS

Analyzing log(IC_{50}) values has more power

For this example, analyzing the log(IC_{50}) values produced a smaller P value than analyzing the IC_{50} values and seems to better match the scientific goals of the study. If the data really do follow a lognormal distribution, how much is lost by analyzing the IC_{50} values rather than the log(IC_{50}) values? Our one example gives a hint of the answer, but only a hint. To find out, I performed Monte Carlo simulations.

Table 46.4 shows the simulated results. The first row in Table 46.4 is the result of 1 million simulated experiments. For each simulated experiment, four values were randomly generated to simulate an experimental measurement of potency for one drug, and four other values were randomly generated to simulate the potency of the other drug. So 8 million values were randomly generated to create the first row of Table 46.4.

The data for one drug were simulated with an IC_{50} of 2 nM, so the logarithm of 2 nM, 0.301, was entered as the mean into the simulation program. The

N PER GROUP	RELATIVE POTENCIES OF TWO DRUGS	DATA ANALYZED	HOW OFTEN IS P < 0.05?
4	Differ by factor of 10	$\log(IC_{50})$	83.6%
4	Differ by factor of 10	IC_{50}	45.6%
7	Differ by factor of 10	$\log(IC_{50})$	99.0%
7	Differ by factor of 10	IC_{50}	79.2%

Table 46.4. Simulations where the drugs have different potencies.

Each row is the result of 1,000,000 simulations. The $\log(IC_{50})$ were simulated using a random number method that generates a Gaussian distribution, and the IC_{50} values were computed by taking the antilog (10 to that power). Therefore, the $\log(IC_{50})$ are sampled from a Gaussian distribution, and the IC_{50} values are sampled from a lognormal distribution. The true population mean IC_{50}s of the two groups in each row differed by a factor of 10 (2 and 20 nM), and the samples included either four or seven IC_{50}s per group. The differences in mean $\log(IC_{50})$ (or IC_{50}) were compared by the unpaired t test, with the assumption of uniform variances.

data for the other drug were simulated using an IC_{50} of 20 nM, so the logarithm of 20 nM, 1.301, was entered into the simulation program. Each $\log(IC_{50})$—all 8 million of them—was chosen using a random number method that simulates sampling from a Gaussian distribution, assuming a mean of 0.301 or 1.301 and a standard deviation of 0.40.

These simulations mimic the example from Chapter 46. The potency of the two drugs differ by a factor of 10, the $\log(IC_{50})$ values vary randomly according to a Gaussian distribution, the SD of the logarithms is 0.4, and n = 4 for each group. The $\log(IC_{50})$ values from each simulated experiment were compared with an unpaired t test, and the P value was tabulated.

The last column of Table 46.4 shows the fraction of the simulated experiments where the P value is less than 0.05, the usual definition of statistical significance. In other words, that last column shows the power of the experimental design (see Chapter 20). For this design, the power was 83.6%. In the remaining simulated experiments (16.4% of them), the P values were greater than 0.05 and so resulted in a not statistically significant conclusion. This happens when the means happen to be close together or the scatter happens to be large among the values in that experiment.

The second row of Table 46.4 shows analyses of IC_{50} values. Each IC_{50} was computed by taking the antilog (10 to that power) of a $\log(IC_{50})$ generated as explained for the first row. The first row simulated sampling $\log(IC_{50})$ values from a Gaussian distribution, and the second row simulated sampling IC_{50} values from a lognormal distribution. The IC_{50} values from each simulated experiment were compared with an unpaired t test, and the P value was tabulated.

In only 45.6% of these experiments was the P value less than 0.05. Because of all three assumption violations that discourage the use of the standard t test on untransformed IC_{50} values (lognormal distribution, unequal variance,

N PER GROUP	RELATIVE POTENCIES OF TWO DRUGS	DATA ANALYZED	HOW OFTEN IS P < 0.05?
4	Equal	log(IC$_{50}$)	5.00%
4	Equal	IC$_{50}$	3.24%
7	Equal	log(IC$_{50}$)	4.99%
7	Equal	IC$_{50}$	3.42%

Table 46.5. Simulations where the null hypothesis is true (drugs have equal potencies).

The simulations were done as explained in Table 46.3, except that these simulations used equal potencies for the two drugs (20 nM, but nearly identical results were obtained when using 2 nM).

differences examined rather than ratios), this approach has much less statistical power (45.6% vs. 83.6%).

Analyzing log(IC$_{50}$) better controls the Type I error rate

Table 46.5 shows simulations identical to those shown in Table 46.4 except that the simulations were done using the same mean IC$_{50}$ for both drugs. In other words, for these simulations the null hypothesis was true—the drugs had equal potency.

The first row shows the analyses of the log(IC$_{50}$) values. These values for both drugs were drawn from the same Gaussian distribution, so the assumptions of a t test are met. If the simulations work as they should, then 5% of these P values should be less than 0.05, and that is precisely what I observed. No surprise here, but this is a good way to check that the simulations worked properly.

The second row shows the analyses of the IC$_{50}$ values. Only 3.23% of these simulated experiments resulted in a P value less than 0.05, although the null hypothesis is true. The data violate one of the assumptions of a t test (Gaussian distribution) and so the definition of statistical significance is off. When P < 0.05 is defined to be statistically significant, you expect that 5% of experiments under the null hypothesis will end up being statistically significant. The Type I error is defined to be 5%. Here, only 3.24% of the experiments under the null hypothesis resulted in a statistically significant result. The Type I error is only 3.24%. Less Type I error might seem to be a good thing, but it is accompanied by a decrease in power, which is definitely not desirable.

Increasing sample size increases power

The third and fourth rows of Table 46.4 show the results of increasing the sample size to seven per group. The power rose to 99.0% for the t test of the log(IC$_{50}$)s. Is this extra effort worth it? It depends on the context of the work, the cost of the experiments (in money and effort), and the consequences of missing a real difference. For this experiment, I think 80% power is plenty and it is not necessary to spend the time and money it would take to increase the sample size to seven experiments.

Increasing the same size to n = 7 increased the power to 79.2% for the t test of the IC_{50}s. This simulation result is similar to our previous sample size calculation with the simple formula.

The third and fourth rows of Table 46.5 show that an increase to n = 7 barely changes the Type I error rates.

Simulating experiments is not hard

These simulations took me an hour or two to set up and less than 20 minutes to compute using a computer purchased in 2008 for about US \$1000. In contrast, it would have taken many hours or even days to complete on many "mainframe" computers in 1975.

Many software packages can perform these simulations (e.g., GraphPad Prism, Minitab, Excel, R, etc.). I used 1,000,000 simulations per experiment to be compulsive. But I would have gotten virtually the same results with 10,000 or even 1,000 simulated experiments. If you plan to design experiments, it is well worth your time to learn how to run these kinds of simulations. You can save a lot of time in the lab using simulations to design your experiments.

OVERALL SUMMARY OF THE PROBLEM

The Case of the Eight Naked IC_{50}'s has been solved. Transforming the IC_{50} values to their logarithms was the critical step, which matched the statistical calculations to the scientific question.

A few final thoughts on this example:

- Lognormal distributions are common in biology. Transforming data to logarithms may seem arcane, but it is actually an important first step for analyzing many kinds of data.
- This Chapter was designed to review as many topics as possible, not to be as realistic as possible. It rambles a bit. But it realistically shows that the search for the best methods for analyzing data can be complicated. Ideally this search should occur before collecting the data or after collecting preliminary data, but before doing the experiments that will be reported. If you analyze final data in many different ways in a quest for statistical significance, you are likely to be misled.
- Statistical methods are all based on assumptions. The Holy Grail of Biostatistics is to find methods that match the scientific problem and where the assumptions are likely to be true (or at least not badly violated). The solution to this problem (using logarithms) was not optimal because it yielded the smallest P value but rather because it melded the statistical analysis to the scientific background and goal. It was a nice translation of the scientific question to a statistical model.

- Simulating data is a powerful tool that can reveal deep insights into data analysis approaches. Learning to simulate data is not hard, and it is a skill well worth acquiring if you plan to design experiments and analyze scientific data.

- Statistical textbooks and software aren't always sufficient to help you analyze data properly. Data analysis is an art form that requires experience as well as courses, textbooks, and software. Until you have that experience, collaborate or consult with others who do. Learning how to analyze data is a journey, not a destination.

CHAPTER 47

Review Problems

I may not have gone where I intended to go, but I think I have ended up where I intended to be.

DOUGLAS ADAMS

*T*hese problems do not cover all the material in the book, but focus *on fundamental areas of statistics that are widely misunderstood. Chapter 48 repeats the questions and includes answers.*

A. PROBLEMS ABOUT CIs OF PROPORTIONS, SURVIVAL CURVES, AND COUNTS

A1. Of the first 100 patients to undergo a new operation, 6 die. Can you calculate the 95% CI for the probability of dying with this procedure? If so, calculate the interval. If not, what information do you need? What assumptions must you make?

A2. A new drug is tested in 100 patients and lowers blood pressure by an average of 6%. Can you calculate the 95% CI for the fractional lowering of blood pressure by this drug? If so, calculate the interval. If not, what information do you need? What is the CI for the fractional lowering of blood pressure? What assumptions must you make?

A3. You use a hemocytometer to determine the viability of cells stained with trypan blue. You count 94 unstained cells (viable) and 6 stained cells (indicating that they are not viable). Can you calculate the 95% CI for the fraction of stained (dead) cells? If so, calculate the interval. If not, what information do you need? What assumptions must you make?

A4. In 1989, 20 of 125 second-year medical students in San Diego failed to pass the biostatistics course (until they came back for an oral exam). Can you calculate the 95% CI for the probability of passing the course? If so, calculate the interval. If not, what information do you need? What assumptions must you make?

A5. Ross Perot won 19% of the vote in the 1992 Presidential Election in the United States. Can you calculate the 95% CI for the fraction of voters who voted for him? If so, calculate the interval. If not, what information do you need? What assumptions must you make?

A6. In your city (population = 1 million) last year a rare disease had an incidence of 25/10,000 population. Can you calculate the 95% CI for the incidence rate? If so, calculate the interval. If not, what information do you need? What assumptions must you make?

A7. Is it possible to calculate the median survival time when some of the subjects are still alive?

A8. Why are survival curves drawn as staircase curves?

A9. A survival curve includes many subjects who were censored because they dropped out of the study because they felt too ill to come to the clinic appointments. Is the survival curve likely to overestimate or underestimate survival of the population?

A10. A study began on January 1, 1991, and ended on December 31, 1994. How will each of these subjects appear on the graph?

   a. Entered March 1, 1991. Died March 31, 1992.
   b. Entered April 1, 1991. Left study March 1, 1992.
   c. Entered January 1, 1991. Still alive when study ended.
   d. Entered January 1, 1992. Still alive when study ended.
   e. Entered January 1, 1993. Still alive when study ended.
   f. Entered January 1, 1994. Died December 30, 1994.
   g. Entered July 1, 1992. Died of car crash March 1, 1993.

A11. A survival study started with 100 subjects. Before the end of the 5th year, no patients had been censored and 25 had died. Five patients were censored in the 6th year, and 5 died in the 7th year. What is the percentage survival at the end of the 7th year? What is the 95% CI for that fraction?

A12. You use a hemocytometer to count white blood cells. When you look in the microscope you see lots of squares and 25 squares enclose 0.1 µL. You count the number of cells in 9 squares and find 50 white blood cells. Can you calculate the 95% CI for the number of cells per microliter? If so, calculate the interval. If not, what information do you need? What assumptions must you make?

A13. In 1988, a paper in *Nature* (Davenas et al., 1988) caused a major stir in the popular and scientific press. The authors claimed that antibodies diluted with even 10^{-120} of the starting concentration stimulated basophils to degranulate. With that much dilution, the probability that even a single molecule of antibody remains in the tube is infinitesimal. The investigators hypothesized that the water somehow "remembered" that it had seen antibody. These results purported to give credence to homeopathy, the theory that extremely low concentrations of drugs are therapeutic.

The assay is simple. Add a test solution to basophils and incubate. Then stain. Count the number of stained cells in a certain volume. Compare the number of cells in control and treated tubes. A low number indicates that many cells had degranulated, because cells that had degranulated won't take up the stain.

The authors present the "mean and standard error of basophil number actually counted in triplicate." In the first experiment, the three control tubes were reported as 81.3 ± 1.2, 81.6 ± 1.4, and 80.0 ± 1.5. A second experiment on another day gave very similar results. The tubes treated with the dilute antibody gave much lower numbers of stained cells, indicating that the dilute antibody had caused degranulation. For this problem, think only about the control tubes.

a. Why are these control values surprising?

b. How could these results have been obtained?

B. PROBLEMS ABOUT SD, SEM, CIs, AND LOGNORMAL DISTRIBUTIONS

B1. Estimate the SD of the age of the students in a typical medical school class (just a rough estimate will suffice).

B2. Estimate the SD of the number of hours slept each night by adults.

B3. The following cholesterol levels were measured in 10 people (mg/dl):

260, 150, 160, 200, 210, 240, 220, 225, 210, 240

Calculate the mean, median, variance, SD, and CV. Make sure you include units.

B4. Add an 11th value (931) to the numbers in Question 3 and recalculate all values.

B5. The level of an enzyme in blood was measured in 20 patients, and the results were reported as 79.6 ± 7.3 units/ml (mean ± SD). No other information is given about the distribution of the results. Estimate what the probability distribution might have looked like.

B6. The level of an enzyme in blood was measured in 20 patients and the results were reported as 9.6 ± 7.3 units/ml (mean ± SD). No other information is given about the distribution of the results. Estimate what the probability distribution might have looked like.

B7. The Weschler IQ scale was created so that the mean is 100 and the standard deviation is 15. What fraction of the population has an IQ greater than 130?

B8. An enzyme level was measured in cultured cells. The experiment was repeated on 3 days; on each day the measurement was made in triplicate. The experimental conditions and cell cultures were identical on each day; the only purpose of the repeated experiments was to determine the value more precisely. The results are shown in Table 47.1 as enzyme activity in units per minute per milligram of membrane protein. Summarize these data as you would for publication. The readers have no interest in the individual results for each day, just in one overall mean with an indication of the scatter. Give the results as mean, error value, and N. Justify your decisions.

	REPLICATE 1	REPLICATE 2	REPLICATE 3
Monday	234	220	229
Tuesday	269	967	275
Wednesday	254	249	246

Table 47.1. Data for Problem 8 of Part C.

B9.   A paper reports that cell membranes have 1,203 ± 64 (mean ± SEM) fmol of receptor per milligram of membrane protein. These data come from nine trials of an experiment.
   a.   Calculate the 95% CI. Explain what it means in plain language.
   b.   Calculate the 90% CI.
   c.   Calculate the CV.

B10. You measure blood pressure in 10 randomly selected subjects and calculate that the mean is 125 and the SD is 7.5 mmHg. Calculate the SEM and 95% CI. Then you measure blood pressure in 100 subjects randomly selected from the same population. What values do you expect to find for the SD and SEM?

B11. Why doesn't it ever make sense to calculate a CI from a population SD (with a denominator of n) as opposed to the sample SD (with a denominator of n–1)?

B12. Data were measured in 16 subjects, and the 95% CI of the mean ranged from 97 to 132. Calculate the 99% CI.

B13. The standard error of the difference between two means is larger than the SE of either mean. Why?

B14. Pullan et al. (1994) investigated the use of transdermal nicotine for treating ulcerative colitis. The plasma nicotine level at baseline was 0.5 ± 1.1 ng/ml (mean ± SD; n = 35). After 6 weeks of treatment, the plasma level was 8.2 ± 7.1 ng/ml (n = 30). Is it more likely that the nicotine levels are sampled from a Gaussian or lognormal distribution?

C. PROBLEMS ABOUT P VALUES AND STATISTICAL SIGNIFICANCE

C1.   You conduct an experiment and calculate that the two-tail P value is 0.08. What is the one-tail P value? What assumptions are you making?

C2.   The FDA requires two-tail statistical tests for Phase III new drug registration trials, defining P<0.05 as statistically significant. What would happen if they required one-tail P values instead, still using the threshold of 0.05 to define significance?

C3.   All members of a class of 111 Pharmacy Practice majors volunteered for a study in which a single blood sample was taken from each student at a single session. All blood samples were analyzed by the same technician for the concentration of a natural human biochemical in plasma, 17β-estradiol. Gender was recorded for each volunteer.

The investigator hypothesized that the 43 males in the class had lower levels of 17β-estradiol than did the 68 females. For the males, the mean level = 17.2 pg/ml; the median level = 15.5 pg/ml. For the females, the mean level = 238 pg/ml; the median level = 146 pg/ml. He then compared the two groups with the Mann–Whitney nonparametric test. The P value was tiny, less than 0.0001. What question is this P value the answer to?

C4. A student wants to determine whether treatment of cells with a particular hormone increases the number of a particular kind of receptors. She and her advisor agree that an increase of less than 100 receptors per cell is too small to care about. Based on the SD of results you have observed in similar studies, she calculates the necessary sample size to have 90% power to detect an increase of 100 receptors per cell. She performs the experiment that number of times, pools the data, and obtains a P value of 0.04.

The student thinks that the experiment makes a lot of sense and thought that the prior probability that her hypothesis was true was 60%. Her advisor is more skeptical and thought that the prior probability was only 5%.

a. Combining the prior probability and the P value, what is the chance that these results are caused by chance? Answer from both the student's perspective and that of the advisor.

b. Explain why two people can interpret the same data differently.

c. How would the advisor's perspective be different if the P value were 0.001 (and the power were still 90%)?

C5. All members of a class of 111 third-year Pharmacy Practice majors volunteered for a study in which a single blood sample was taken from each student. All blood samples were analyzed by the same technician for the concentration of a natural human biochemical in plasma, Compound X, in nanograms per milliliter. No additional patient identifiers or covariates were recorded.

The investigator, after looking over the data from the 111 volunteers (Figure 47.1, left), hypothesized that the subjects came from two distinct populations, one with low values of Compound X and one with high values of Compound X. He divided the data set at the overall median into two groups, a low group (5–44 ng/ml) and a high group (47 – 1,466 ng/ml). There were no values between 44 and 47. For all of the subjects, N = 111; mean = 159; SD = 250; median = 44. For the low group, N = 56; mean = 20.0; SD = 9.45; median = 19.8. For the high group, N = 55; mean = 300; SD = 295; median = 220. The investigator compared the two groups (shown in Figure 47.1, right) using the nonparametric Mann–Whitney test (Chapter 41). The P value was tiny,

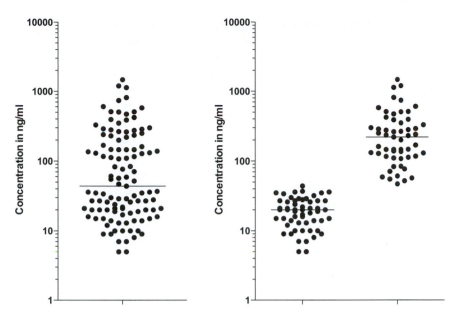

Figure 47.1. Compound X in all students (left panel) and separately for values below and above the median (right panel).

less than 0.0001. Interpret what this P value means and what you can conclude from the study.

C6. Assume that you are reviewing a manuscript prior to publication. The authors have tested many drugs to see whether they increase enzyme activity. All P values were calculated using a paired t test. Each day they also perform a negative control, using just vehicle with no drug. After discussing significant changes caused by some drugs, they state, "In contrast, the vehicle control has consistently given a nonsignificant response (P > 0.05) in each of 250 experiments." Comment on these negative results. Why are they surprising?

C7. The serum level of a hormone (the Y factor) was measured to be 93 ± 1.5 units/ml (mean±SEM) in 100 nonpregnant women and 110 ± 2.3 units/ml in 100 women in the first trimester of pregnancy. The difference between the means is $110-93 = 17$, with a 95% CI extending from 11.6 to 22.4 units/ml.

    a. Interpret that CI.

    b. Estimate the P value.

    d. What assumptions are you making to answer A and B?

    d. Would this be a useful test for diagnosing pregnancy?

C8. Cohen et al. (1993) investigated the use of active cardiopulmonary resuscitation (CPR). In standard CPR, the resuscitator compresses the victim's chest to force the heart to pump blood to the brain (and elsewhere) and then lets go to let the chest expand. Active CPR is done with a suction device. This enables the resuscitator to pull up on the chest to expand it, as well as pressing down to compress it. These investigators randomly assigned cardiac arrest patients to receive either standard or active CPR. Eighteen of 29 patients treated with active CPR were resuscitated. In contrast, 10 of 33 patients treated with standard CPR were resuscitated.

   a. Using Fisher's test, the two-side P value is 0.0207. Explain what this means in plain language.

   b. What would a Type I error mean in this context?

   c. What would a Type II error mean in this context?

C9. Which of the following are inconsistent?

   a. Mean difference = 10. The 95% CI is −20 to 40. P = 0.45.

   b. Mean difference = 10. The 95% CI is −5 to 15. P = 0.02.

   c. Relative risk = 1.56. The 95% CI is 1.23 to 1.89. P = 0.013.

   d. Relative risk = 1.56. The 95% CI is 0.81 to 2.12. P = 0.04.

   e. Relative risk = 2.03. The 95% CI is 1.01 to 3.13. P<0.001.

C10. In response to many case reports of connective tissue diseases after breast implants, the FDA called for a moratorium on breast implants in 1992. Gabriel and investigators (1994) did a prospective study to determine whether there really was an association between breast implants and connective tissue (and other) diseases. They studied 749 women who had received a breast implant and twice that many control subjects. They analyzed their data using survival analysis to account for different times between implant and disease and to correct for differences in age. You can analyze the key findings more simply. They found that 5 of the cases and 10 of the controls developed connective tissue disease.

   a. What null hypothesis would a P value test?

   b. What is that P value (hint: no calculations or computer needed)?

C11. Figure 47.2 shows data from 461 meta-analyses that all showed a statistically significant effect (P < 0.05). A meta-analysis pools data from several (or many) studies to obtain one P value and CI that takes into account all the data. Each symbol in the graph represents one such study. The graph shows that studies with larger samples tend to show a smaller effect size than smaller (presumably less accurate) studies. Ioannidis (2008) presents that as evidence for the winner's curse explained at the end of Chapter 44.

    Figure 47.2 shows Spearman's correlation coefficient and the corresponding P value.

   a. Interpret the meaning of the P value.

   b. The graph is plotted using a logarithmic scale for both axes, but it isn't clear whether the correlation was computed on the raw data or the log-transformed data. Can you tell from the figure? Does it matter? Would the two P values be different or identical?

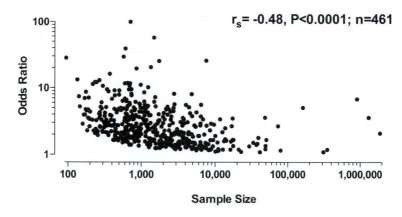

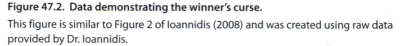

Figure 47.2. Data demonstrating the winner's curse.

This figure is similar to Figure 2 of Ioannidis (2008) and was created using raw data provided by Dr. Ioannidis.

C12. Two gentleman, John and Frank, decided to fly in a hot air balloon from North Carolina, across the Atlantic Ocean, to Europe. After a frightening 5-week journey, the pair finally spotted land. Frank thought that they were now over Ireland. They saw a man in a tweed suit walking along a path. John shouted down to the man, "Where are we?" The man stopped walking, looked up, thought for 5 seconds, and replied, "You're in a balloon." Frank then said to John, "That man must be a statistician." John asked, "How did you know?" What was Frank's answer?

D. PROBLEMS ABOUT SAMPLE SIZE AND POWER

D1. Which will require more subjects, detecting a difference between two proportions where $p_1 = 0.10$ and $p_2 = 0.20$ or between $p_1 = 0.20$ and $p_2 = 0.40$? Assume you are looking for the same difference with the same power and with samples of equal size.

D2. You read the following in a journal: "Before starting the study, we calculated that with a power of 80% and a significance level of 5%, 130 patients would be required in each group to demonstrate a 15-percentage-point reduction in mortality (from the expected rate of 33 down to 18%)." Explain in plain language what this means.

D3. Lymphocytes contain β-adrenergic receptors. Epinephrine binds to these receptors and modulates immune responses. It is possible to count the average number of receptors on human lymphocytes using a small blood sample. You wish to test the hypothesis that people with asthma have fewer receptors. By reading various papers, you learn that there are about 1,000 receptors per cell and that the CV in a normal population is about 25%.

a.   How many asthmatic subjects do you need to determine the receptor number to ± 100 receptors per cell with 95% confidence?

b.   You want to compare a group of normal subjects with a group of asthmatics. How many subjects do you need in each group to have 80% power to detect a mean change of 10% of the receptors using $\alpha = 0.05$ (two-tailed)?

c.   How many subjects do you need in each group to have 95% power to detect a mean difference in receptor number of 5% with $\alpha = 0.01$?

D4.   You are preparing a grant for a study that will test whether a new drug treatment lowers blood pressure substantially. From previous experience, you know that 15 rats in each group is enough and that the SD of measurements in different rats is about 10 mmHg. Prepare a convincing power analysis to justify that sample size.

D5.   The overall incidence of a disease is 1 in 10,000. You think that a risk factor increases the risk. How many subjects do you need if you want to have 80% power to detect a relative risk as small as 1.1 in a prospective study?

E. PROBLEMS ABOUT CORRELATION AND REGRESSION

E1.   Figure 47.3 shows the relationship between the population of countries (or territories) and their area. Each dot is a separate country. All 237 countries are shown. The graph on the left panel shows linear axes. The graph on the right panel shows both axes using a logarithmic axis.

a.   Interpret the P value.

b.   Were the two variables properly assigned to the X-axis and Y-axis?

c.   Would the correlation coefficient or P value be different if the definitions of X and Y were swapped?

d.   What are the advantages of using logarithmic axes?

E2.   Figure 47.4 shows the same data as 47.3, but fit with a linear regression program.

a.   What are the units of the slope? What does it mean?

b.   Interpret the P value.

c.   Imagine that the graph of data remained the same, but the definitions of independent (X) and dependent (Y) variables were switched. Now linear regression is used to find the line that best predicts population (horizontal axis) from area (vertical axis). Would the best-fit line be the same or different?

d.   On logarithmic axes, why is the "line" curved?

e.   On the logarithmic graph, why does the "line" stray so far from many points?

f.   Figure 47.5 was also fit by linear regression. Why is it showing a different line and different R^2?

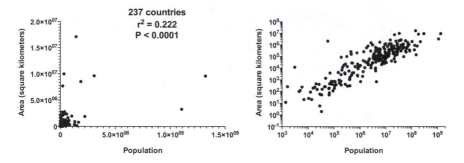

Figure 47.3. Correlation of population versus area of different countries.

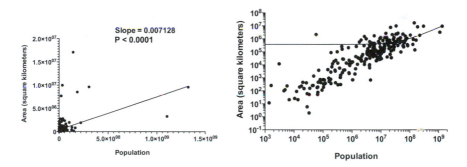

Figure 47.4. Linear regression of population versus area of different countries.

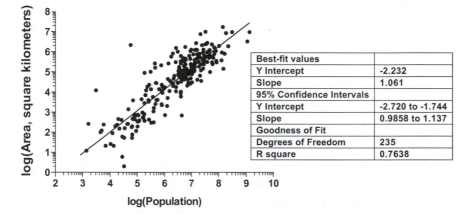

Figure 47.5. Each dot is a different country, with a line fit by linear regression.

E3a. Figure 47.6 (left) shows a log(dose) versus response curve, fit with nonlinear regression. The shaded region shows the 95% CI for the EC_{50} (the dose that provokes a response halfway between the lowest and highest possible responses). Why is this range so wide?

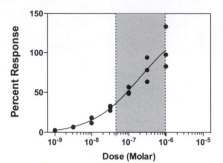
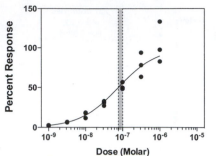

Bottom	-1.587
Top	140.4
LogEC50	-6.684
Hill Slope	0.6616
EC50	2.071e-007
95% Confidence Intervals	
Bottom	-4.519 to 1.345
Top	71.90 to 209.0
LogEC50	-7.349 to -6.019
Hill Slope	0.4425 to 0.8807
EC50	4.476e-008 to 9.577e-007

Bottom	= 0.0
Top	= 100.0
LogEC50	-7.114
Hill Slope	0.8408
EC50	7.699e-008
95% Confidence Intervals	
LogEC50	-7.232 to -6.996
Hill Slope	0.7658 to 0.9157
EC50	5.867e-008 to 1.010e-007

Figure 47.6. Dose–response data fit with nonlinear regression.
Why is the CI for the EC_{50} (shaded) so much narrower on the right?

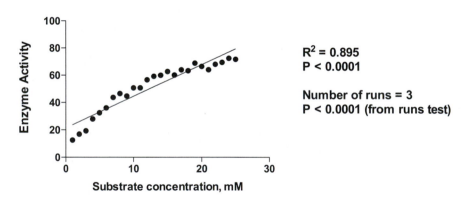

$R^2 = 0.895$
$P < 0.0001$

Number of runs = 3
$P < 0.0001$ (from runs test)

Figure 47.7. Linear regression and runs test.

E3b.   Figure 47.6 (right) shows the same data, also with a log(dose) versus response curve fit by nonlinear regression. Why is the shaded area denoting the 95% CI of the $logEC_{50}$ so much narrower?

E3c.   One of the points has a response greater than 100%. Should it be removed, because that is impossible?

E4a.   Figure 47.7 shows data and a line fit by linear regression. Interpret the R^2 and P value shown on the graph.

E4b.   Figure 47.7 also shows results from a runs test. This is not a test covered in this book. Read about it in other books or on the Web and interpret what the P value means.

VARIABLE	ODDS RATIO	95% CI
Coronary calcium score > 160	14.3	4.9 to 42.3
Age > 55 years old	3.3	1.3 to 8.4
Elevated cholesterol	4.0	1.3 to 12.2
Hypertension	2.6	1.1 to 6.1
Diabetes	4.8	1.6 to 13.9

Table 47.2. Results of logistic regression to predict cardiac events (death, nonfatal myocardial infarction, need for a revascularization procedure).

Data are from a portion of Table 3 from Arad et al. (2000).

E5. Arad and colleagues (2000) performed a large study to see whether measuring calcium in coronary arteries can help predict heart attacks. They studied 1,177 people who were free of cardiac symptoms. They measured calcium in the coronary arteries using a noninvasive method called electron beam computed tomography. The results are reported as a coronary artery calcium score. They followed all these people for 3–4 years and recorded cardiac events (3 people died, 15 had a nonfatal myocardial infarction, and 21 required a revascularization procedure to relieve chest pain). The question is whether the calcium score predicts the occurrence of these cardiac events better than the standard cardiac risk factors (age, high cholesterol, high blood pressure, diabetes). Complete data were available for 787 of the subjects. The data were analyzed by logistic regression, and the results are shown in Table 47.2.

   a. Odds ratios compare the risk in one group with another. When the logistic regression model computes odds ratios, what group is the comparison group?

   b. Which of the five variables make a statistically significant ($P<0.05$) contribution to the model? Which has the highest P value?

   c. Write out the logistic regression model.

   d. What is the predicted odds ratio for someone who is older than 55 who has a coronary artery calcium score greater than 160?

   e. Did this study have enough subjects?

   f. Most of the cardiac events (21 of 39) were people requiring angioplasty or coronary artery surgery to restore blood flow in the coronary arteries. In some cases, the decision to perform these procedures might have been a difficult one. How would the results be affected if the decision to perform the procedures was partially influenced by knowing that the coronary calcium score was high?

   g. Explain in plain language what the odds ratio of 14.3 means.

CHAPTER 48

Answers to Review Problems

*T*he questions from Chapter 47 are all repeated here, along with answers. Reading this chapter can help you review statistics, even if you don't want to actually work the problems.

A. PROBLEMS ABOUT CIs OF PROPORTIONS, SURVIVAL CURVES, AND COUNTS

A1. Of the first 100 patients to undergo a new operation, 6 die. Can you calculate the 95% CI for the probability of dying with this procedure? If so, calculate the interval. If not, what information do you need? What assumptions must you make?

Yes, it is possible to calculate a CI. This is a straightforward calculation of the 95% CI from a proportion. The proportion is 6/100. Chapter 4 explained the modified Wald method for computing the CI. First compute p', the center of the CI.

$$p' \approx \frac{S+2}{n+4} \approx \frac{6+2}{100+4} \approx 0.0769 \approx 7.69\%$$

The margin of error, W, is computed as follows:

$$W \approx 2\sqrt{\frac{.0769(1-0.0769)}{n+4}} \approx 0.0523 = 5.23\%$$

The 95% CI extends from p'-W to p'+W, from 2.46 to 12.92%.

To interpret these results, you must define the population. If these were real data, you'd want to see how the investigators selected the patients. Are they particularly sick? Do they represent all patients with a certain condition or only a small subset? If you can't figure out how the investigators selected their patients, then the data are not very useful. If you can define the population they selected from, you must assume that the 100 patients are representative of these patients and that each was selected independently. If you accept these assumptions, then you can be 95% sure that the overall death rate in the population lies somewhere within the 95% CI.

A2.   A new drug is tested in 100 patients and lowers blood pressure by an average of 6%. Can you calculate the 95% CI for the fractional lowering of blood pressure by this drug? If so, calculate the interval. If not, what information do you need? What is the CI for the fractional lowering of blood pressure? What assumptions must you make?

Although this looks similar to the previous question, it is actually quite different. In the previous question, the percentage was really a proportion. In this question, the percentage is really change in a measured value. The CI cannot be computed without knowing the SD or SEM.

Beware of percentages. Percentages can express a proportion, a relative difference in proportions, a relative difference in a measured value, or many other things. Use the methods of Chapter 4 only with proportions.

A3.   You use a hemocytometer to determine the viability of cells stained with trypan blue. You count 94 unstained cells (viable) and 6 stained cells (indicating that they are not viable). Can you calculate the 95% CI for the fraction of stained (dead) cells? If so, calculate the interval. If not, what information do you need? What assumptions must you make?

This is essentially the same problem as Problem 1 above. The population is the entire tube of cells, and you have assessed the viability of a sample of these cells. Assuming that you mixed the tube well, it is reasonable to assume that your sample is randomly selected from the population. You can calculate a 95% CI for the proportion of viable cells in the entire population. You can say that you are 95% confident that the fraction of stained (dead) cells ranges from 2.5 to 12.9% by the modified Wald method.

A4.   In 1989, 20 of 125 second-year medical students in San Diego failed to pass the biostatistics course (until they came back for an oral exam). Can you calculate the 95% CI for the probability of passing the course? If so, calculate the interval. If not, what information do you need? What assumptions must you make?

It is easy to plug the numbers into a computer program to calculate a CI. But what would it mean? There were only 125 students in 1989, so we don't really have a sample. It would make sense to calculate a CI only if you imagined the 125 students in 1989 to be representative of students in other years (or other cities) and that there is no change in course content, student preparation, exam difficulty, or passing threshold. You would also have to assume that students in future years haven't read this question, because it would give them an incentive to study harder. In fact, the students in 1990 read this question. They got the message that the course required work, and they studied hard. All passed the first time they took the exam.

Because those assumptions are unlikely to be true, I don't think it would be meaningful to calculate a CI. If you are persuaded that the assumptions are met, you can calculate that the 95% CI for passing ranges from 76 to 90%.

A5. Ross Perot won 19% of the vote in the 1992 Presidential Election in the United States. Can you calculate the 95% CI for the fraction of voters who voted for him? If so, calculate the interval. If not, what information do you need? What assumptions must you make?

It wouldn't be meaningful to calculate a CI. We know the exact fraction of voters who voted for each candidate. This is not a poll before the election—these are results from the election. Because we have not sampled from a population, a CI would be pointless and meaningless.

A6. In your city (population = 1 million) last year, a rare disease had an incidence of 25/10,000 population. Can you calculate the 95% CI for the incidence rate? If so, calculate the interval. If not, what information do you need? What assumptions must you make?

First, ask yourself whether it makes sense to calculate a CI. You know the incidence of the disease in the entire population last year, so there is no need for a CI for the incidence of the disease last year. If you assume that the incidence of the disease is not systematically changing from year to year, it may be reasonable to consider last year's population to be a sample from the populations of the next few years. So you can calculate a CI for the overall incidence rate for the next few years.

The problem is stated as number of disease cases per 10,000 population, but 10,000 is not really the denominator, because the data were collected from a population of 1,000,000. So the sample proportion is 2,500 of a population of 1,000,000. Applying the modified Wald method for 95% confidence:

$$p' = \frac{S+2}{n+4} = \frac{2500+2}{1000000+4} = 0.2502$$

$$W \approx 2\sqrt{\frac{p'(1-p')}{n+4}} \approx 2\sqrt{\frac{0.2502(1-0.2502)}{1000000+4}} \approx .0000866 \approx 0.01\%$$

The 95% CI ranges approximately from 0.24 to 0.26%. Assuming that the incidence of the disease is not changing, you can be 95% sure that the true average incidence rate for the next few years will be somewhere within that range.

A7. Is it possible to calculate the median survival time when some of the subjects are still alive?

If you listed all the survival times in order, the median survival time would be the middle survival time. If subjects are still alive, then you don't know their survival time. But you do know that their survival time will be longer than any subject who already died. So you can still find the median time, even if some subjects are still alive, provided that at least half have died. Median survival time is the time at which half the subjects are still alive and half are dead.

A8.   Why are survival curves drawn as staircase curves?

The curves plot the survival of the subjects in your sample. Whenever a subject dies, the percentage survival drops. The percentage survival then remains at a steady plateau until the next patient dies.

You could imagine drawing the curve differently if your goal were to draw your best guess of survival in the population. You might then draw a sloping line from one patient's death to the next. Then the curve would not look like a staircase. But the convention is to draw survival curves showing the survival of your sample, so staircase curves are used.

A9.   A survival curve includes many subjects who were censored because they dropped out of the study because they felt too ill to come to the clinic appointments. Is the survival curve likely to overestimate or underestimate survival of the population?

Because the censored patients are sicker than the average subjects, they tend to die sooner than the noncensored patients. The remaining patients tend to die later than the overall average, and so the data on the remaining patients overestimates the survival of the entire population.

A survival curve can only be interpreted when you assume that the survival of the censored subjects would, on average, equal the survival of the uncensored subjects. If many subjects are censored, this is an important assumption. If the study is large and only a few subjects were censored, then it doesn't matter so much.

A10.   A study began on January 1, 1991, and ended on December 31, 1994. How will each of these subjects appear on the graph?
a.   Entered March 1, 1991. Died March 31, 1992.
b.   Entered April 1, 1991. Left study March 1, 1992.
c.   Entered January 1, 1991. Still alive when study ended.
d.   Entered January 1, 1992. Still alive when study ended.
e.   Entered January 1, 1993. Still alive when study ended.
f.   Entered January 1, 1994. Died December 30, 1994.
g.   Entered July 1, 1992. Died of car crash March 1, 1993.

a.   This subject is shown as a downward step at time = 13 months.
b.   This subject was censored at 11 months. He or she will appear as a blip at time = 11 months.
c.   The subject was alive for the entire 48 months of the study. He or she was censored at time = 48 months. Because the graph ends at 48 months, a blip may or may not be visible.

    d.   This subject was alive for 36 months after starting the trial. He or she was censored at 36 months and will appear as a blip at time = 36 months.

    e.   This subject was alive for 24 months at the time the study ended. He or she appears as a censored subject at time = 24 months.

    f.   This subject died 12 months after starting the trial. He or she will appear as a downward step at time = 12 months.

    g.   This is ambiguous. After 8 months, the subject died of a car crash. This might count as a death or as a censored subject, depending on the decision of the investigator. Ideally, the experimental protocol should have specified how to handle this situation before the data were collected. Some studies only count deaths from the disease being studied, but most studies count deaths from all causes. Some studies analyze the data both ways. Why would you include a death from a car crash in a study of cancer? The problem is that it is impossible to know for sure that a death is really unrelated to the cancer (and its therapy). Maybe the car crash in this example would have been avoided if the study medication hadn't slowed the reaction time or if the cancer hadn't limited peripheral vision.

A11.   A survival study started with 100 subjects. Before the end of the 5th year, no patients had been censored and 25 had died. Five patients were censored in the 6th year, and 5 died in the 7th year. What is the percentage survival at the end of the 7th year? What is the 95% CI for that fraction?

    This book did not give the equations for calculating a survival curve, but it is pretty easy to figure out. At the end of the 5th year, 25 patients had died and 75 are still alive. So the fraction survival is 75%. During the 6th year, 5 subjects are censored. This does not change percentage survival, which remains at 75%. Now 5 subjects die in the next year. At the start of that year, 70 subjects were alive (100−25−5). At the end of the 7th year, 65 subjects are alive. For subjects alive at the start of the 7th year, the probability of surviving that year is 65/70, or 92.86%. The probability of surviving up to the beginning of the 7th year, as we already calculated, is 75%. So the probability of surviving from time zero to the end of the 7th year is the product of those two probabilities, 75% × 92.86% = 69.6%.

    To calculate the CI, compute n as the total number minus those censored before the end of the 7th year. This equals 100−5 = 95. Use the equation in the "How to" section of Chapter 5 with p = 0.696 and n = 95. The margin of error W equals 0.047, so the 95% CI is from 0.696−0.047 to 0.696+0.047, or 0.649 to 0.743, or 64.9 to 74.3%.

A12.   You use a hemocytometer to count white blood cells. When you look in the microscope you see lots of squares and 25 squares enclose 0.1 µL. You count the number of cells in 9 squares and find 50 white blood cells. Can you calculate the 95% CI for the number of cells per microliter? If so, calculate the interval. If not, what information do you need? What assumptions must you make?

You counted 50 cells in 9 squares. To calculate the CI, we must work with the number actually counted, 50. From Table 6.1, you can see that the 95% CI for the average number of cells in 9 squares ranges from 37.1 to 65.9. Because there are 250 squares/µL and 9 were counted, multiply by $(250/9) = 27.77$ to obtain cells per microliter. The 95% CI ranges from 1,030 to 1,830 cells/µL.

A13.   In 1988, a paper in *Nature* (Davenas et al., 1988) caused a major stir in the popular and scientific press. The authors claimed that antibodies diluted with even 10^{-120} of the starting concentration stimulated basophils to degranulate. With that much dilution, the probability that even a single molecule of antibody remains in the tube is infinitesimal. The investigators hypothesized that the water somehow "remembered" that it had seen antibody. These results purported to give credence to homeopathy, the theory that extremely low concentrations of drugs are therapeutic.

The assay is simple. Add a test solution to basophils and incubate. Then stain. Count the number of stained cells in a certain volume. Compare the number of cells in control and treated tubes. A low number indicates that many cells had degranulated, because cells that had degranulated won't take up the stain.

The authors present the "mean and standard error of basophil number actually counted in triplicate." In the first experiment, the three control tubes were reported as 81.3 ± 1.2, 81.6 ± 1.4, and 80.0 ± 1.5. A second experiment on another day gave very similar results. The tubes treated with the dilute antibody gave much lower numbers of stained cells, indicating that the dilute antibody had caused degranulation. For this problem, think only about the control tubes.

a.   Why are these control values surprising?

b.   How could these results have been obtained?

a.   The authors counted only the cells that still had granules. In the results shown, the average number of cells in the volume counted was about 80. If this is true, then the Poisson distribution tells us what we expect to see in different experiments. From Table 6.1, the 95% CI ranges from 63 to 100. If you repeated the experiment many times, you'd expect the number of cells counted to be within this range 95% of the time and outside the range 5% of the time. The results reported by the authors have far less variation than that.

b.   One possibility is that the investigators were lucky and just happened to have so little variation. The chance of having so little variation is very small, so this is quite unlikely. If the cells are well mixed and randomly sampled, the Poisson distribution tells us the distribution of values we expect to see. This is the "best" you can do, assuming perfect experimental technique. Any sloppiness in the experiment will lead to more variability. No matter how carefully you do the experiment, you can't get less scatter than predicted by the Poisson distribution unless you are extremely lucky.

So how then could the results have been obtained? There is no way to be sure, but here is one possibility. It is difficult to count cells in a reliable way. Counting requires some judgment as you ask yourself these kinds of questions: How do you deal with cells on the border? How do you distinguish between real cells and debris? When two cells are stuck together, does that count as one or two? If you know the results you are "supposed" to get, your answers might be swayed to get the count you expect to get.

What do you do when the number of stained cells in a treated sample exceeds the number in the control sample? By chance and assuming the diluted antibodies do nothing, you'd expect half the samples to have more stained cells than the average and half to have less. If the experimenter threw out the data from the samples where the number of stained cells exceeded the control average (because those data seem to be impossible), the data will be biased and give a smaller average. In this case, the results would be impossible to interpret.

For an assay like this one (counting cells manually), it is essential that the person counting the cells not know which tube is which, so he or she can't let the expected results bias the count. Even better, use a machine that counts in an unbiased way. The machines can also count more cells, thus narrowing the CI.

You could also improve the experimental methodology in other ways. Why not count all cells, not just the ones that haven't degranulated? Why not use a more precise assay, such as measuring the amount of histamine releases from the cells instead of the number of cells that have released histamine?

B. PROBLEMS ABOUT SD, SEM, CIs, AND LOGNORMAL DISTRIBUTIONS

B1. Estimate the SD of the age of the students in a typical medical school class (just a rough estimate will suffice).

Without data, you can't determine the SD exactly. But you can estimate it. The mean age of first-year medical students is probably about 23. Lots of students are 1 year older or younger. A few might be a lot younger or a lot older. If you assume that the age distribution is approximately Gaussian, you will include two thirds of the students in a range of ages that extends 1 SD either side of the mean. Therefore, the SD is probably about 1 year. Obviously, it will vary from class to class.

It is likely that the distribution is likely to be skewed (asymmetric) by the presence of a few students much older than the others, which may make the SD a bit larger.

The point of this question is to remind you that the SD is not just a number that falls out of an equation. Rather, the SD describes the scatter of data. If you have a rough idea how the values are scattered, you can estimate the SD without any calculations.

B2. Estimate the SD of the number of hours slept each night by adults.

Without data, you can't know the SD exactly. But you can estimate it. On average, adults sleep about 8 hours. Some sleep more, some less. If you go 1 SD from the mean, you'll include two thirds of the population, assuming that sleep time is roughly Gaussian. I'd estimate that the SD is about 1 hour. If this were true, then about two thirds of adults would sleep between 7 and 9 hours per night, and 95% would sleep between 6 and 10 hours per night.

Again, the point of this question is to remind you that the SD is not just a number that falls out of an equation. Rather, the SD describes the scatter of data. If you have a rough idea how the values are scattered, you can estimate the SD without any calculations.

B3. The following cholesterol levels were measured in 10 people (mg/dl):

260, 150, 160, 200, 210, 240, 220, 225, 210, 240

Calculate the mean, median, variance, SD, and CV. Make sure you include units.

Mean = 211.5 mg/dl
Median = 215 mg/dl
Variance = 1200.28 $(mg/dl)^2$
SD = 34.645 mg/dl
CV = 34.645/211.5 = 16.4%

B4. Add an 11th value (931) to the numbers in Question 3 and recalculate all values.

Mean = 276.9 mg/dl
Median = 220 mg/dl
Variance = 48,142 $(mg/dl)^2$
SD = 219.4 mg/dl
CV = 219.4/276.9 = 79.23%

One value mugh larger than the rest increases the mean, SD, CV, and variance considerably. It has little impact on the median.

B5. The level of an enzyme in blood was measured in 20 patients, and the results were reported as 79.6 ± 7.3 units/ml (means ± SD). No other information is given about the distribution of the results. Estimate what the probability distribution might have looked like.

With no other information to go on, it is reasonable to speculate that the enzyme activity might be roughly Gaussian. If so, then about two thirds of the values should be within 1 SD of the mean, within the range of about 72 to 87, and about 95% of the values should be within 2 SD of the mean (65 to 94).

B6.   The level of an enzyme in blood was measured in 20 patients and the results were reported as 9.6 ± 7.3 units/ml (means $\pm$ SD). No other information is given about the distribution of the results. Estimate what the probability distribution might have looked like.

Again, you might start with the assumption that the distribution is roughly Gaussian. If that were true, then 95% of the population would be within a range defined by the mean ± 2 SD. However this range would include negative numbers, and enzyme activity cannot be negative. Therefore, the distribution cannot possibly be Gaussian with the stated mean and SD. The distribution probably is asymmetrical with a "tail" to the right and may be lognormal. It could also possibly be bimodal.

B7.   The Weschler IQ scale was created so that the mean is 100 and the standard deviation is 15. What fraction of the population has an IQ greater than 130?

The problem asks what fraction of a Gaussian distribution has a value greater than two standard deviations above the mean. Approximately 95% of a Gaussian population is within a range defined by the mean ± 2 SD, so 5% is outside that range. A Gaussian distribution is symmetrical, so 2.5% of a population has a value greater than 2 SD above the mean.

B8.   An enzyme level was measured in cultured cells. The experiment was repeated on 3 days; on each day the measurement was made in triplicate. The experimental conditions and cell cultures were identical on each day; the only purpose of the repeated experiments was to determine the value more precisely. The results are shown in Table 47.1 as enzyme activity in units per minute per milligram of membrane protein. Summarize these data as you would for publication. The readers have no interest in the individual results for each day, just in one overall mean with an indication of the scatter. Give the results as mean, error value, and N. Justify your decisions.

There are two difficulties with this problem. First, you must decide what to do with Tuesday's second replicate. It is wildly out of whack with the others. Deciding what to do with outlying values is a difficult problem, and different scientists have different policies. In this case, I think it is clear that the value can't possibly be correct. Not only is it far, far away from the other two replicates, but it is far, far away from the six replicates measured on other days. Because the experiment was performed with cultured cells, there is no biological variability from day to day. The only contribution to scatter consists of experimental errors. It seems plain to me that the 967 value is clearly incorrect. First, I would look back at the lab notebook and see whether the experimenter noticed anything funny about that tube during the experiment. If there was a known problem with that replicate, then I would feel very comfortable throwing it out. Even otherwise, I would delete it from the analysis, while recording in a lab notebook exactly what I had done. Including that value would throw off the calculations, so the result wouldn't be helpful.

If the rows represented different patients (rather than different experiments on the same cell cultures), then my answer would be different. With different patients, biological variability plays a role. Maybe the large number is correct and the two small numbers are wrong. Maybe the second patient is really different than the first and third. If possible, I'd do the experiment with Patient 2 a second time to find out.

The second problem is how to pool the eight remaining values. It is not really fair to consider these eight independent measurements. The replicates in one day are closer to one another than they are to measurements made on other days. This is expected, because there are more contributions to variability between days than between replicates. So calculating the mean and SD or SEM of all eight values is not valid.

How to compute the CI of a grand mean (often called a consensus mean) is a surprisingly complicated question, with multiple answers, especially since the sample size (after excluding the outlier) is not the same for all three days. A simple approach is to calculate the mean value for each day, then calculate the mean and SEM of the three means, and then calculate a 95% CI. This makes sense if you think of the population as the means of all possible experiments with N = 3. We can be 95% sure that the true mean lies somewhere within the CI.

The three means are 227.7, 272.0, and 249.7. The grand mean is 249.8 with a SEM of 12.8. (n = 3). The 95% CI for the grand mean ranges from 194.7 to 304.9. If you were to repeat a similar experiment many times, the 95% CI would contain the true mean in 95% of experiments. This could be reported as follows:

"The experiment was performed three times in triplicate. After excluding one wildly high value, the mean for each experiment was calculated. The grand mean is 249.8 with a SEM of 12.8 (n = 3). The 95% CI ranges from 194.7 to 304.9."

B9. A paper reports that cell membranes have $1{,}203 \pm 64$ (mean $\pm$ SEM) fmol of receptor per milligram of membrane protein. These data come from nine trials of an experiment.
  a. Calculate the 95% CI. Explain what it means in plain language.
  b. Calculate the 90% CI.
  c. Calculate the CV.

  a. With N = 9, df = 8, and $t^* = 2.3060$ (see Appendix D). So the 95% CI ranges from 1055 to 1351 fmol/mg protein. Assuming that each of the nine experiments was conducted independently, you can be 95% sure that the true mean (if you repeated the experimental trial many times) lies within this range.

b. With df = 8, t* for 90% CI is 1.8595 (see Appendix D). The 90% CI ranges from 1084 to 1322.

c. The coefficient of variation is the SD divided by the mean. The SD equals the SEM times the square root of sample size, 64×3, or 192. So the CV equals 192/1203 or 16.0%. Because the mean and SD have the same units, the CV is a unitless ratio.

B10. You measure blood pressure in 10 randomly selected subjects and calculate that the mean is 125 and the SD is 7.5 mmHg. Calculate the SEM and 95% CI. Then you measure blood pressure in 100 subjects randomly selected from the same population. What values do you expect to find for the SD and SEM?

The SEM is the SD divided by the square root of the sample size, so it equals $7.5/\sqrt{10}$, or 2.37. With n = 10 and df = 9, t* = 2.26. The 95% CI extends 2.26 SEMs on either side of the mean: 119.6 to 130.4 mmHg.

When you increase the sample size, you don't expect the SD to change. The SD measures the scatter of the data, and the scatter doesn't change by sampling more subjects. You'll know the SD more accurately, so the value will probably change. But the SD is just as likely to increase as to decrease when you add more subjects. Your best guess is that the SD will still equal 7.5 mmHg.

The SEM quantifies how well you have determined the population mean. When you increase the sample size, your sample mean will probably be closer to the population mean. So the SEM gets smaller as the sample size gets larger. With n = 100, your best guess for the SEM is $7.5/\sqrt{100}$ or 0.75 mmHg.

Many students mistakenly think that the SD ought to get smaller as the sample size gets larger. Not so. The SD quantifies variability or scatter, and the scatter is real. The values in the population are not all the same. Collecting a larger sample helps you know the SD better, but the size of the SD does not change predictably as the sample size increases. The SD quantifies an attribute of the population, and that attribute (scatter) doesn't change when you sample more subjects.

If you are still confused, think of how the mean will change when you sample more subjects. If you collect a larger sample, you'll know the population mean better and your sample mean from n = 100 won't exactly equal the sample mean from n = 10. But it is just as likely that the mean will increase as decrease. The sample mean quantifies an attribute of the population (its average), and the population doesn't change by sampling more subjects.

The standard error is different. It does not quantify an attribute of the population. It quantifies sampling error, and its value is determined (in part) by the sample size. Collecting bigger samples reduces the value of the standard error of the mean.

B11.   Why doesn't it ever make sense to calculate a CI from a population SD, with a denominator of n, as opposed to the sample SD, with a denominator of n–1?

If you know the population SD, then you must know all the values in the population. If this is true, then you know the population mean exactly, and so there is no point in calculating a CI. CIs are only useful when you are unsure about the true population mean, so you want to calculate a CI to quantify your uncertainty.

B12.   Data were measured in 16 subjects, and the 95% CI of the mean ranged from 97 to 132. Calculate the 99% CI.

Because the CI is symmetrical around the mean, the mean must equal the average of 97 and 132, or 114.5. With 16 subjects, the 95% CI extends in each direction from the mean a distance equal to 2.13 times the SEM. Therefore, the SEM must equal the difference between 132 and 97 divided by twice 2.13. So the SEM is $35/(2 \times 2.13)$, or about 8.22. The SD equals the SEM times the square root of the sample size, which is 4×8.22 or 32.88. To calculate a 99% CI with df=15, $t^* = 2.95$ (see Appendix D). Therefore, the margin of error of the 99% CI equals 2.95 times the SEM, which is 2.95×8.22 or 24.24. The 99% CI extends from 114.5–24.24 to 114.5+24.24: from 90.3 to 138.7. Note that the 99% CI is wider than the 95% CI.

B13.   The standard error of the difference between two means is larger than the SE of either mean. Why?

The SE of a difference quantifies how well you know the difference between two population means. It depends on how well you know each mean as reflected in the two SEMs. Uncertainty in each of the two means contributes to uncertainty in the difference.

B14.   Pullan et al. (1994) investigated the use of transdermal nicotine for treating ulcerative colitis. The plasma nicotine level at baseline was 0.5 ± 1.1 ng/ml (mean±SD; n=35). After 6 weeks of treatment, the plasma level was 8.2 ± 7.1 ng/ml (n=30). Is it more likely that the nicotine levels are sampled from a Gaussian or lognormal distribution?

If the populations were Gaussian, about 95% of the values in the population would be within 2 SDs of the mean and the distribution would be symmetrical around the mean. With the values given in this problem, this would be possible only if nicotine levels could be negative, which is, of course, impossible. Also, the SD is much larger for the group with the larger mean. For these two reasons, the distribution is more likely to be lognormal than Gaussian.

C. PROBLEMS ABOUT P VALUES AND STATISTICAL SIGNIFICANCE

C1.   You conduct an experiment and calculate that the two-tail P value is 0.08. What is the one-tail P value? What assumptions are you making?

You can only calculate a one-tail P value if the direction of the expected change were predicted before the data were collected. If the change occurred in the predicted direction, then the one-tail P value is half the two-tail P value, or 0.04.

If the change occurred in the opposite direction, the situation is more tricky. The one-tail P value answers this question: If the null hypothesis were true, what is the chance of randomly picking subjects such that the difference goes in the direction of the experimental hypothesis with a magnitude as large or larger than that observed? When the result went in the direction opposite to the experimental hypothesis, the one-tail P value equals 1.0 minus half the two-tail value. So the one-tail P value is 0.96.

It really doesn't help to calculate a one-tail P value when the observed difference is opposite in direction to the experimental hypothesis. You should conclude that the P value is very high and the difference was caused by chance.

C2.   The FDA requires two-tail statistical tests for Phase III new drug registration trials, defining $P < 0.05$ as statistically significant. What would happen if they required one-tail P values instead, still using the threshold of 0.05 to define significance?

First, a reality check. When deciding whether to approve a drug, there are many considerations. This problem just considers one—the P value for the difference in treatments for the primary endpoint in the Phase III registration clinical trial. In some cases, this critical P value can have a strong influence on the decision. For this example, we will assume that this one P value is the only information used to decide whether to approve a new drug.

The definition of a 5% significance level (two tailed) is simple. If the new drug really does not work better than whatever it is being compared with (placebo or a standard treatment), there is a 5% chance that random chance will result in a difference large enough to be labeled statistically significant. Half of the time (half of 5%, or 2.5%), this difference will be in the right direction (the new drug worked well) and the drug will be approved. Half of the time, the difference will be in the wrong direction (the new drug worked worse than the standard drug). Although the results are statistically significant, the drug won't be approved because the data show the drug is working significantly *more poorly* than the treatment it is compared with. Effectively, the current policy uses a 2.5% significance level for a one-tail P value to decide on drug approval.

What happens if the policy changes to use a one-tail P value with a 5% threshold for significance? If there is no true underlying superiority of the new treatment, the chance of concluding that a new treatment is statistically significantly better than an older treatment would double from 2.5 to 5%.

By making it easier to declare results statistically significant, this change would also increase power (assuming studies are done with the same sample size). Thus, this alternate policy change would also likely increase the approval rate for drugs that are truly better than the standard. Some of these drugs would have two-tail P values between 0.05 and 0.10. By switching to a one-tail criterion, these P values would be between 0.025 and 0.05, and so the drugs would be approved.

The FDA must find the right balance of approving truly better new drugs, while protecting the public from "me too" and inferior drugs. Switching to a one-tail P value would change this balance, allowing more drugs to be approved. More good drugs would be approved, as would more worthless drugs.

C3.   All members of a class of 111 Pharmacy Practice majors volunteered for a study in which a single blood sample was taken from each student at a single session. All blood samples were analyzed by the same technician for the concentration of a natural human biochemical in plasma, 17β-estradiol. Gender was recorded for each volunteer.

The investigator hypothesized that the 43 males in the class had lower levels of 17β-estradiol than did the 68 females. For the males, the mean level = 17.2 pg/ml; the median level = 15.5 pg/ml. For the females, the mean level = 238 pg/ml; the median level = 146 pg/ml. He then compared the two groups with the Mann–Whitney nonparametric test. The P value was tiny, less than 0.0001. What question is this P value the answer to?

Statistical inference is used to analyze data from a sample to make inferences about a much larger, or infinite, population. The Mann–Whitney test and the t test are statistical procedures for making this kind of generalization or inference from sample to population. In this problem, the investigator seems to be only interested in this particular group of 43 male and 68 female subjects and did not seem to have any more general question in mind. As such, the P value is totally meaningless. It can make sense to summarize the data by stating the medians, as was done in this problem. It might also help to show the minimum and maximum values, or the interquartile range, or the SD. Even better, show a graph of all the values or a graph of their frequency distribution. But P values (and CIs) only make sense when the goal is to extrapolate from sample to population.

PRIOR PROBABILITY = 0.60	RECEPTOR NUMBER REALLY INCREASES BY MORE THAN 100 SITES/CELL	NULL HYPOTHESIS IS TRUE: RECEPTOR NUMBER DOESN'T CHANGE	TOTAL
P < 0.04	540	16	556
P > 0.04	60	384	444
Total	600	400	1,000

Table 48.1. Student's perspective.

C4.   A student wants to determine whether treatment of cells with a particular hormone increases the number of a particular kind of receptor. She and her advisor agree that an increase of less than 100 receptors per cell is too small to care about. Based on the SD of results you have observed in similar studies, she calculates the necessary sample size to have 90% power to detect an increase of 100 receptors per cell. She performs the experiment that number of times, pools the data, and obtains a P value of 0.04.

The student thinks that the experiment makes a lot of sense and thought that the prior probability that her hypothesis was true was 60%. Her advisor is more skeptical and thought that the prior probability was only 5%.

a.   Combining the prior probability and the P value, what is the chance that these results are caused by chance? Answer from both the student's perspective and that of the advisor.

b.   Explain why two people can interpret the same data differently.

c.   How would the advisor's perspective be different if the P value were 0.001 (and the power were still 90%)?

a.   The student's perspective is illustrated in Table 48.1, which shows the results of 1,000 hypothetical experiments.

Of 556 experiments with a P value less than 0.04, receptor number really increases in 540. So the chance that the receptor number really increases is 540/556 = 97.1%, leaving a 2.9% chance that the results are caused by coincidence.

The advisor's perspective is different, as illustrated in Table 48.2.

Of all the hypothetical experiments with P < 0.04, 45/83 = 54.2% occurred when receptor number really increased. The other 45.8% of the low P values were Type I errors, caused by random sampling. So the new evidence is not convincing to the advisor, because she still thinks there is only about a 50% chance that the effect is real.

b.   The results could have been obtained in two ways:

First possibility: The treatment really does not change receptor number, and the change we observed is simply a matter of

PRIOR PROBABILITY = 0.05	RECEPTOR NUMBER REALLY INCREASES BY MORE THAN 100 SITES/CELL	NULL HYPOTHESIS IS TRUE: RECEPTOR NUMBER DOESN'T CHANGE	TOTAL
P < 0.04	45	38	83
P > 0.04	5	912	917
Total	50	950	1,000

Table 48.2. Advisor's perspective.

coincidence. The statistical calculations tell you how unlikely this coincidence would be. For this example, you would see a difference as large or larger than you observed in 4% of experiments, even if the null hypothesis were true.

Second possibility: The hormone really does increase receptor number.

In interpreting the results, you must decide which of these possibilities is more likely. The student in this example thought that the second possibility was probably true even before collecting any data. She is far happier believing this hypothesis is true rather than believing in a coincidence that happens only 1 in every 25 experiments.

The advisor has reasons to think that this experiment shouldn't work. Perhaps she knows that the cells used do not have receptors for the hormone used, so it seems very unlikely that the hormone treatment could alter receptor number. The advisor must choose between believing that an "impossible" experiment worked or believing that a 4% coincidence has occurred. It is a toss up, and the conclusion is not clear.

Interpreting experimental results requires integrating the results from one particular experiment (summarized with a P value) with your prior opinions about the experiment. If different people have different prior opinions, they may reach different conclusions when the P value is only moderately low.

c. Now the advisor must choose between a result that makes no sense to her or a coincidence that happens only 1 time in 1,000. She believes the result, rather than such an unlikely coincidence. See Table 48.3. Although she probably makes this judgment intuitively, you can explain it with Table 48.3. Given the assumptions of this problem, only 1 in 46 results like this would be caused by chance, whereas 45 of 46 reflect a true difference. (To maintain the power with a smaller threshold value of p requires increasing the sample size.)

C5. All members of a class of 111 third-year Pharmacy Practice majors volunteered for a study in which a single blood sample was taken from each student. All blood samples were analyzed by the same technician

PRIOR PROBABILITY = 0.05	RECEPTOR NUMBER REALLY INCREASES BY MORE THAN 100 SITES/CELL	NULL HYPOTHESIS IS TRUE: RECEPTOR NUMBER DOESN'T CHANGE	TOTAL
$P < 0.001$	45	1	46
$P > 0.001$	5	949	954
Total	50	950	1,000

Table 48.3. Advisor's perspective if the P value was 0.001.

for the concentration of a natural human biochemical in plasma, Compound X, in nanograms per milliliter. No additional patient identifiers or covariates were recorded.

The investigator, after looking over the data from the 111 volunteers (Figure 47.1, left), hypothesized that the subjects came from two distinct populations, one with low values of Compound X and one with high values of Compound X. He divided the data set at the overall median into two groups, a low group (5–44 ng/ml) and a high group (47–1,466 ng/ml). There were no values between 44 and 47. For all of the subjects, $n = 111$; mean = 159; SD = 250; median = 44. For the low group, $n = 56$; mean = 20.0; SD = 9.45; median = 19.8. For the high group, $n = 55$; mean = 300; SD = 295; median = 220. The investigator compared the two groups (shown in Figure 47.1, right) using the non-parametric Mann–Whitney test (Chapter 41). The P value was tiny, less than 0.0001. Interpret what this P value means and what you can conclude from the study.

A P value can only be interpreted when you have random samples from populations and you want to make inferences about those populations. Here the investigator created the two groups based on the concentration of Compound X. Of course, the two means and medians are further apart than you'd expect to see by chance. There is zero possibility that chance had anything to do with it. The investigator decided to put the higher values in one group and the lower values in the other. Essentially, this investigator has used statistics to attempt to prove that high numbers are larger than low numbers!

The P value is completely meaningless and provides no help at all in interpreting the data. No conclusion can be reached from these data.

C6. Assume that you are reviewing a manuscript prior to publication. The authors have tested many drugs to see whether they increase enzyme activity. All P values were calculated using a paired t test. Each day, they also perform a negative control, using just vehicle with no drug. After discussing significant changes caused by some drugs, they state, "In contrast, the vehicle control has consistently given a nonsignificant response ($P > 0.05$) in each of 250 experiments." Comment on these negative results. Why are they surprising?

In the negative control experiments, the null hypothesis is true. Therefore, you expect 1 of 20 control experiments to have a P value less than 0.05. In 250 experiments, therefore, you expect to see about $0.05 \times {}^*250 = 12.5$ significant responses. You'd be very surprised to see zero significant responses results among the 250 control experiments.

C7.   The serum level of a hormone (the Y factor) was measured to be 93 ± 1.5 units/ml (mean ± SEM) in 100 nonpregnant women and 110 ± 2.3 units/ml in 100 women in the first trimester of pregnancy. The difference between the means is $110 - 93 = 17$, with a 95% CI extending from 11.6 to 22.4 units/ml.

    a.   Interpret that CI.

    b.   Estimate the P value.

    c.   What assumptions are you making to answer A and B?

    d.   Would this be a useful test for diagnosing pregnancy?

    a.   If we assume that both samples are representative of the overall populations, we can be 95% sure that the mean level of the Y factor in pregnant women is between 11.6 and 22.4 units/ml higher than in nonpregnant women.

    b.   The null hypothesis is that the two means are the same, so the difference between means is zero. Because the 95% CI does not include zero, the P value must be less than 0.05. Because the 95% CI doesn't come near zero, the P value must be a lot less than 0.05.

    c.   We assume that the two samples are representative of the overall populations of pregnant and nonpregnant women of the appropriate age range and that the distribution of Y values is approximately Gaussian. Because the samples are so large, this assumption is not very important so long as the distributions aren't really weird. We do have to assume that the two populations have similar SDs and that the subjects have each been selected independently.

    d.   Don't get trapped by thinking only about the P value and CI. Those results convince us that the difference between the *mean values* is extremely unlikely to be a coincidence. It certainly is not surprising to find that the mean value of the hormone is elevated in pregnant women (it might be surprising to find a hormone whose level does not change in pregnancy!).

But would the test be useful for diagnosing? To answer this question, we need to think beyond means and think about the actual distribution of the values. The problem doesn't present the raw data, but does present the SEM and sample size. It is easy to compute the SDs. This is done by multiplying the SEM by the square root of the sample size. Therefore, the SD of the nonpregnant women is 15; the SD of the pregnant women is 23. You expect about 95% of the values to lie within two SDs either side of the mean. For the nonpregnant women, this interval extends from 63 to 123. For pregnant women, it extends from 64 to 156. The two distributions overlap considerably, so the test would be completely useless as a diagnostic test.

Don't mistake the CI of the mean with the range of the data.

C8.   Cohen et al. (1993) investigated the use of active cardiopulmonary resuscitation (CPR). In standard CPR, the resuscitator compresses the victim's chest to force the heart to pump blood to the brain (and else-where) and then lets go to let the chest expand. Active CPR is done with a suction device. This enables the resuscitator to pull up on the chest to expand it, as well as pressing down to compress it. These investigators randomly assigned cardiac arrest patients to receive either standard or active CPR. Eighteen of 29 patients treated with active CPR were resuscitated. In contrast, 10 of 33 patients treated with standard CPR were resuscitated.

   a.   Using Fisher's test, the two-side P value is 0.0207. Explain what this means in plain language.
   b.   What would a Type I error mean in this context?
   c.   What would a Type II error mean in this context?

   a.   The null hypothesis is that the resuscitation rate is the same for active and standard CPR. If that hypothesis were true, the chance of observing such a large difference (or larger) in a study this size is 2.07%.
   b.   If you set $\alpha = 0.05$, you would conclude that the resuscitation rates are significantly different. You'd be making a Type I error if the resuscitation rates in the overall populations were really identical. You would conclude that there is a real difference, when in fact (but unknown to you) the difference you observed is just a coincidence of sampling.
   c.   If you set $\alpha = 0.01$, you would conclude that the resuscitation rates are not significantly different? If you did this, you'd have made a Type II error if the rates are really different. There is a real difference (but you can't know this), but you conclude that the difference is not statistically significant. The study missed a real difference so make a Type II error.

C9.   Which of the following are inconsistent?
   a.   Mean difference = 10. The 95% CI is –20 to 40. P = 0.45.
   b.   Mean difference = 10. The 95% CI is –5 to 15. P = 0.02.
   c.   Relative risk = 1.56. The 95% CI is 1.23 to 1.89. P = 0.013.
   d.   Relative risk = 1.56. The 95% CI is 0.81 to 2.12. P = 0.04.
   e.   Relative risk = 2.03. The 95% CI is 1.01 to 3.13. P < 0.001.

   a.   Consistent
   b.   Inconsistent. The 95% CI includes 0, so the P value must be greater than 0.05.

    c. Consistent

    d. Inconsistent. The P value is less than 0.05, so the 95% CI for the relative risk cannot include 1.0.

    e. Inconsistent. The P value is way less than 0.05, so the 95% CI must not include 1.0 and shouldn't even come close. But the 95% CI starts at a value just barely greater than 1.00.

C10. In response to many case reports of connective tissue diseases after breast implants, the FDA called for a moratorium on breast implants in 1992. Gabriel and investigators (1994) performed a prospective study to determine whether there really was an association between breast implants and connective tissue (and other) diseases. They studied 749 women who had received a breast implant and twice that many control subjects. They analyzed their data using survival analysis to account for different times between implant and disease and to correct for differences in age. You can analyze the key findings more simply. They found that 5 of the cases and 10 of the controls developed connective tissue disease.

    a. What null hypothesis would a P value test?

    b. What is that P value (hint: no calculations or computer needed)?

    a. The null hypothesis is that there is no association between breast implants and connective tissue diseases. If the null hypothesis is true, the overall incidence of connective tissue diseases among cases ought to equal the incidence among controls.

    b. They used twice as many controls as patients with breast implants, and exactly twice as many controls as cases developed connective tissue disease. This is exactly what you expect under the null hypothesis. The relative risk is exactly 1. The data provide no evidence whatsoever of any association between breast implants and connective tissue disease.

        The P value (two tailed) must be 1.0. The P value answers this question: If the null hypothesis is true, what is the chance of randomly sampling subjects and obtaining such strong evidence (or stronger) that there is an association? Because there was absolutely no evidence of association in this study, 100% of all studies would produce evidence this strong or stronger.

C11. Figure 47.2 shows data from 461 meta-analyses selected because each demonstrated a statistically significant effect ($P < 0.05$). A meta-analysis pools data from several (or many) studies to obtain one P value and CI that takes into account all the data. Each symbol in the graph represents one such study. The graph shows that studies with larger samples tend to show a smaller effect size than smaller (presumably less accurate) studies. Ioannidis (2008) presents that as evidence for the winner's curse explained at the end of Chapter 44.

The figure shows Spearman's correlation coefficient and the corresponding P value.

a. Interpret the meaning of the P value.

b. The graph is plotted using a logarithmic scale for both axes, but it isn't clear whether the correlation was computed on the raw data or the log-transformed data. Can you tell from the figure? Does it matter? Would the two P values be different or identical?

a. Spearman's nonparametric correlation coefficient quantifies the correlation between the rank of the X values (sample size) and the ranks of the Y values (odds ratio). The null hypothesis is that there is no correlation between the two sets of ranks. If that null hypothesis were true, there is less than a 0.01% chance that random chance would lead to a correlation coefficient this far away from zero (or even further).

It only makes sense to interpret the P value if these data are sampled from a larger population. Indeed, it makes sense to think of the meta-analyses summarized here to be representative of other meta-analyses not included here or yet to be published.

b. The nonparametric correlation only analyzes the ranks, not the raw data. The ranks of sample size and odds ratio are the same before and after transforming to logarithms. Thus, the value of r_s will be identical for the raw data and the log-transformed data and so will the corresponding P value.

C12. Two gentleman, John and Frank, decided to fly in a hot air balloon from North Carolina, across the Atlantic Ocean, to Europe. After a frightening 5-week journey, the pair finally spotted land. Frank thought that they were now over Ireland. They saw a man in a tweed suit walking along a path. John shouted down to the man, "Where are we?" The man stopped walking, looked up, thought for 5 seconds, and replied, "You're in a balloon." Frank then said to John, "That man must be a statistician." John asked, "How did you know?" What was Frank's answer?

Frank answered, "He must be a statistician because his answer was 100% correct, but not the answer to the question that you had in mind." I'm not sure of the origin of this joke, but I think it does a good job of illustrating some of the miscommunication and occasional tension between biomedical scientists and statisticians.

D. PROBLEMS ABOUT SAMPLE SIZE AND POWER

D1. Which will require more subjects, detecting a difference between two proportions where $p_1 = 0.10$ and $p_2 = 0.20$ or between $p_1 = 0.20$ and

$p_2 = 0.40$? Assume you are looking for the same difference, with the same power, with samples of equal size.

The equation in Chapter 43 shows that the needed sample size is approximately proportional to $p_{av}(1-p_{av})$, where p_{av} is the average of the two anticipated proportions. For the first scenario, this product is $0.15 \times 0.85 = 0.13$. For the second scenario, the product is $0.30 \times 0.70 = 0.21$. So the second scenario will need more subjects, almost twice as many.

D2. You read the following in a journal: "Before starting the study, we calculated that with a power of 80% and a significance level of 5%, 130 patients would be required in each group to demonstrate a 15-percentage-point reduction in mortality (from the expected rate of 33 down to 18%)." Explain in plain language what this means.

If the null hypothesis were really true (the two treatments are identical in terms of mortality), then there is a 5% chance of obtaining a significant difference by coincidence of random sampling. (The statement that the "significant level is 5%" means that $\alpha = 0.05$.) If the alternative hypothesis is true (that the mortality drops from 33 to 18%), then there is a 80% chance that a study with 130 patients in each group will end up with a statistically significant difference and a 20% chance of ending up with a conclusion of not statistically significant.

D3. Lymphocytes contain β-adrenergic receptors. Epinephrine binds to these receptors and modulates immune responses. It is possible to count the average number of receptors on human lymphocytes using a small blood sample. You wish to test the hypothesis that people with asthma have fewer receptors. By reading various papers, you learn that there are about 1,000 receptors per cell and that the CV in a normal population is about 25%.

a. How many asthmatic subjects do you need to determine the receptor number to plus or minus 100 receptors per cell with 95% confidence?

b. You want to compare a group of normal subjects with a group of asthmatics. How many subjects do you need in each group to have 80% power to detect a mean change of 10% of the receptors using $\alpha = 0.05$ (two tailed)?

c. How many subjects do you need in each group to have 95% power to detect a mean difference in receptor number of 5% with $\alpha = 0.01$?

a. Chapter 43 presented an equation to compute approximate sample size to determine a mean with desired precision. To use this equation, you need to know s, the expected SD of the values. The problem states that the CV is 25%, so s must equal 25% of 1,000 receptors/cell, or 250 receptors/cell. The desired margin of error, w, is stated to be 100 receptors/cell.

$$n \approx 4 \left(\frac{s}{w} \right)^2 \approx 4 \left(\frac{250}{100} \right)^2 \approx 25 \text{ per group}$$

What does this mean? Assume the values distribute according to a Gaussian distribution with a SD of 250 sites/cell and you collect many samples of $n = 25$ and compute the 95% CI of each. You would expect the margin of error of a 95% CI of half of the samples to be smaller than 100 receptors/cell in half of those samples and greater than 100 receptors/cell in the other half.

b. Chapter 43 presented the equation to compute sample size for the difference between two means. The problem states that the margin of error, w, is 10% of the mean receptor number, so $0.10 \times 1,000$, or 100. Use the equation for 80% power to detect a difference with $P < 0.05$.

$$n \approx 16 \left(\frac{s}{w} \right)^2 \approx 16 \left(\frac{250}{100} \right)^2 \approx 100 \quad \text{(per group)}$$

What does this mean? Assume the values distribute according to a Gaussian distribution with a SD of 250 sites/cell and that the two population means differ by 100 receptors per cell. You now perform many experiments with $n = 25$ in each group and compute the 95% CI of the difference between means from each experiment. You would expect to find a statistically significant difference ($P < 0.05$) in 80% (the power) of those experiments and a difference that is not statistically significant in the other 20%.

c. This problem has changed three things from the previous one. The study is looking for a difference that is half as large (5% vs. 10%). This alone would increase the sample size by a factor of 4. You also want more power (95% vs. 80%), which increases the needed sample size. Furthermore, now the definition of statistical significance is stricter, $P < 0.01$ instead of $P < 0.05$. Each of these changes increases the required sample size. All three changes will increase the sample size a lot. How much? This book doesn't give the needed equations or tables, so you'll need to find it in another book or program. GraphPad StatMate computes that 890 subjects are required in each group.

D4. You are preparing a grant for a study that will test whether a new drug treatment lowers blood pressure substantially. From previous experience, you know that 15 rats in each group is enough and that the SD of measurements in different rats is about 10 mmHg. Prepare a convincing power analysis to justify that sample size.

Start with the equation for computing n for comparing two means, plug in the numbers we know, and solve for w:

$$n \approx 16 \left(\frac{s}{w} \right)^2 \quad \text{(per group)}$$

$$15 \approx 16 \left(\frac{10}{w} \right)^2$$

$$w^2 \approx \frac{16}{15} \cdot 100 = 106.7$$

$$w \approx 10.3$$

That equation assumes a standard value of α (0.05) and power (80%). So you could write in a grant: "From previous work, we expected the SD of blood pressure to be 10 mmHg. Setting the significance level to 0.05, we calculated that a study with 15 subjects in each group would have 80% power to detect a mean difference in blood pressures of 10 mmHg."

As this example shows, sample size calculations do not always proceed from the assumptions to the sample size. Sometimes, the sample size is chosen first and then justified. This is OK, so long as the assumptions are reasonable.

D5.   The overall incidence of a disease is 1 in 10,000. You think that a risk factor increases the risk. How many subjects do you need if you want to have 80% power to detect a relative risk as small as 1.1 in a prospective study?

From the problem, p1 equals 0.00010. p2 equals 1.1 times p1 or 0.00011. The margin of error, w, equals the difference between the two proportions. Plug them into the approximate formula:

$$n \approx \frac{16 \cdot p_{av} (1 - p_{av})}{w^2} \quad \text{(in each group)}$$

$$n \approx 16,798,236 \quad \text{(in each group)}.$$

The required sample size is huge! Why such a large sample size? First, the disease is rare, with an incidence of only 1 in 10,000. So it will take a large number of subjects to get a reasonable number with the disease. Because you are looking for a small change in incidence, you will need even larger samples. Detecting small changes in rare diseases is virtually impossible in prospective studies. The required sample size is enormous. That is why case–control studies are so useful.

E. PROBLEMS ABOUT CORRELATION AND REGRESSION

E1.   Figure 47.3 shows the relationship between the population of countries (or territories) and their area. Each dot is a separate country. All

237 countries are shown. The left graph shows linear axes. The right graph shows both axes using a logarithmic axis.
a. Interpret the P value.
b. Where the two variables properly assigned to the X-axis and Y-axis?
c. Would the correlation coefficient or P value be different if the definitions of X and Y were swapped?
d. What are the advantages of using logarithmic axes?

a. P values help you generalize from sample data to make conclusions about the population. They help you extrapolate from your data to a more general situation. These data represent every single country there is. No generalization makes sense, so the P value is entirely without meaning.
b. When cause and effect are clear, the horizontal axis is used to plot the variable that causes the variable plotted in the vertical axis to change. Here, cause and effect are not clear. Do countries with large areas tend to develop large populations? Or do countries with large populations tend to go to war with neighboring countries to increase area? I suspect the former is more common, so I would plot the data the other way, with population on the vertical axis and area on the horizontal axis. But it is not a clear decision.
c. The calculation of the P value and correlation coefficient would be identical if the axes were swapped.
d. The graph on the left uses linear axes. All but a dozen countries are in the lower left corner of the graph, where they cannot be differentiated. A logarithmic scale stretches out lower values and scrunches up larger values. With these data, it is much easier to see the trend.

E2. Figure 47.4 shows the same data as Figure 47.3, but fit with a linear regression program.
a. What are the units of the slope? What does it mean?
b. Interpret the P value.
c. Imagine that the graph of data remained the same, but the definitions of independent (X) and dependent (Y) variables were switched. Now linear regression is used to find the line that best predicts population (horizontal axis) from area (vertical axis). Would the best-fit line be the same or different?
d. On logarithmic axes, why is the "line" curved?
e. On the logarithmic graph, why does the "line" stray so far from many points?
f. Figure 47.5 was also fit by linear regression. Why is it showing a different line and different R^2?

a. The slope quantifies how much Y changes for each unit change in X. So the slope is expressed in units of the Y-axis divided by units of the X-axis, square kilometers per person. Here the slope is 0.007128. So for every increase in population (by 1 person), the area (on average) increases by 0.007128 square kilometers.

b. Normally the P value is easy to interpret from linear regression. The null hypothesis is that the true slope is horizontal (so the slope is 0.0). The P value answers the question: If this null hypothesis is true, what is the chance that randomly sampled data would have a slope as far from 0.0 as did the actual data? But that only makes sense when the data are sampled from a larger population. This graph shows data for every single country that exists. No extrapolation or generalization is needed, so the P value is meaningless.

c. Linear regression minimizes the sum of the square of the discrepancies between actual and predicted Y values. It makes a difference which variable is defined to be X and which is defined to be Y. If you swap the definition of the two variables, a different best-fit line would result. If you keep the axes the same, then linear regression with X and Y defined differently would minimize the sum of the square of the horizontal distances of the points from the line. This is a different line (in almost all cases) than the line that minimizes the sum of the square of the vertical distances of the points from the line. Although the line would be different, R^2 and the P value would be the same.

d. The curve shown on the graph was indeed drawn by linear regression, after fitting the model: area = intercept + slope × population. When drawn on a graph with linear axes, this model appears as a straight line. On a graph with logarithmic axes, the fit of that model appears curved. A linear regression model only appears as a straight line when plotted on ordinary (not logarithmic) axes.

e. The curve on the graph is actually a linear regression line that minimizes the sum of the square of the difference between the actual area and the predicted area. On a linear graph, this method minimizes the sum of squares of the vertical distances between the dots and the line. But the logarithmic scale distorts the scale of the data, so the visible distances of the points from the curve are misleading.

f. Here, the data were transformed to logarithms. The linear regression program was given the log(population) values as X and the log(area) values as Y. The line on the graph fits the model:

$$\log(\text{area}) = \text{intercept} + \text{slope} \times \log(\text{population}).$$

This is a different model than was fit before, so it yields a different best-fit line on the graph and a different R^2 value.

E3a.   Figure 47.6 (left) shows a log(dose) versus response curve, fit with non-linear regression. The shaded region shows the 95% CI for the EC_{50} (the dose that provokes a response halfway between the lowest and highest possible responses). Why is this range so wide?

E3b.   Figure 47.6 (right) shows the same data, also with a log(dose) versus response curve fit by nonlinear regression. Why is the shaded area denoting the 95% CI of the $logEC_{50}$ so much narrower?

E3c.   One of the points has a response greater than 100%. Should it be removed, because that is impossible?

    a.   The results next to the graph show that the nonlinear regression program was asked to find the best-fit values of four parameters. It fit not only the $log(EC_{50})$ and the Hill slope (a measure of how steep the curve is), but also the top and bottom plateaus of the curve. These data simply do not plateau, so the data really give no hint about where the curve will level off. The best-fit value of the top parameter is quite uncertain, with a 95% CI ranging from 72 to 209. This top plateau defines 100%. The EC_{50} can be determined no more accurately than 100% and 0% are defined.

    b.   The Y-axis is labeled "percent response," suggesting that the data have been normalized to some controls. The results on the left were done with constraints so that the nonlinear regression program forces the curve to run from 0 to 100, without fitting the top and bottom plateaus. You can see this because the program does not provide best-fit values, or CI, for the parameters Top or Bottom. With this fit, there is no ambiguity about the top and bottom plateaus of the curve, so there is no ambiguity about the best-fit value of the $log(EC_{50})$. Accordingly, the CI for the EC_{50} is much narrower.

    c.   No! Data points should only be removed when they are clearly in error (and even then some would disagree). The 100% value is the average response with maximum drug. You expect half of the measurements at high drug concentrations to be less than 100% and half to be greater than 100%, so you may have an average greater than 100%. Values greater than 100% are not impossible!

E4a.   Figure 47.7 shows data and a line fit by linear regression. Interpret the R^2 and P value shown on the graph.

E4b.   Figure 47.7 also shows results from a runs test. This is not a test covered in this book. Read about it in other books or on the Web and interpret what the P value means.

    a.   The interpretation of R^2 is straightforward. Of all the variation in enzyme activity, 89.5% is accounted for by a linear relationship between substrate concentration and enzyme activity. That leaves 10.5% that is variation from the linear regression line. This could be caused by random variation or by a systematic trend if the linear regression model was not the best model to explain the data.

b. When you look at Figure 47.7, it seems as though the data points form a curve, not a straight line. If you had an alternative model in mind, you could fit both models and compare as explained in Chapter 35. The runs test is simpler. It just asks whether the data deviate systematically from the line or curve. A run is one or more sequential points on the same side of the line or curve. These data only have three runs: 5 points on the left side that are below the line, 14 points in the middle above the line, and 6 points on the right side below the line. The null hypothesis for the runs test is that each point is randomly and independently above or below the line (or curve). The P value answers this question: What is the chance that random sampling would result in as few runs as observed or fewer? Here the P value is tiny. From this, you can conclude that the curvature of the data is statistically significant and that the straight line model is probably not the best model for these data.

E5. Arad and colleagues (2000) performed a large study to see whether measuring calcium in coronary arteries can help predict heart attacks. They studied 1,177 people who were free of cardiac symptoms. They measured calcium in the coronary arteries using a noninvasive method called electron beam computed tomography. The results are reported as a coronary artery calcium score. They followed all these people for 3–4 years and recorded cardiac events (3 people died, 15 had a nonfatal myocardial infarction, and 21 required a revascularization procedure to relieve chest pain). The question is whether the calcium score predicts the occurrence of these cardiac events better than the standard cardiac risk factors (age, high cholesterol, high blood pressure, diabetes). Complete data were available for 787 of the subjects. The data were analyzed by logistic regression, and the results are shown in Table 47.3.

a. Odds ratios compare the risk in one group with another. When the logistic regression model computes odds ratios, what group is the comparison group?

b. Which of the five variables make a statistically significant ($P < 0.05$) contribution to the model? Which has the highest P value?

c. Write out the logistic regression model.

d. What is the predicted odds ratio for someone who is older than 55 and has a coronary artery calcium score greater than 160?

e. Did this study have enough subjects?

f. Most of the cardiac events (21 of 39) were people requiring angioplasty or coronary artery surgery to restore blood flow in the coronary arteries. In some cases, the decision to perform these procedures might have been a difficult one. How would the results be affected if the decision to perform the procedures was partially influenced by knowing that the coronary calcium score was high?

g. Explain in plain language what the odds ratio of 14.3 means.

IF	THEN SET	OTHERWISE
Coronary calcium score > 160	$X_1 = 1$	$X_1 = 0$
Age > 55 years old	$X_2 = 1$	$X_2 = 0$
Elevated cholesterol	$X_3 = 1$	$X_3 = 0$
Hypertension	$X_4 = 1$	$X_4 = 0$
Diabetes	$X_5 = 1$	$X_5 = 0$

Table 48.4. Definitions of the independent variables for multiple regression.

a. The comparison group is the one defined by setting all independent variables to zero. With this model, the comparison group is people who have a coronary artery calcium score less than 160, who are less than 55 years old, and who do not have elevated cholesterol, hypertension, or diabetes.

b. None of the five CIs includes an odds ratio of 1.0 (the null hypothesis), so all five P values must be less than 0.05. The odds ratio for hypertension is closest to 1.0, so it will have the highest P value.

c. The model is

$$\ln(OR) = X_1 \ln(14.3) + X_2 \ln(3.3) + X_3 \ln(4.0) + X_4 \ln(2.6) + X_5 \ln(4.8).$$

The five X variables are defined in Table 48.4.

d. Using the definitions of Table 48.4, X_1 and X_2 are equal to 1.0 and the rest of the X variables are equal to 0. So,

$$\ln(OR) = \ln(14.3) + \ln(3.3) = 2.67 + 1.19 = 3.85$$

$$OR = e^{3.85} = 47.2.$$

If you assume that coronary events are rare, this can be interpreted as a relative risk. Compared with people younger than 55 with low coronary artery calcium scores, people older than 55 with high coronary artery calcium score have about 47 times the risk of having a myocardial infarction or requiring coronary artery surgery or angioplasty.

e. Chapter 43 discussed sample size for studies to be analyzed with multiple logistic regression. There are no firm rules, but Chapter 43 gives several guidelines. The number of subjects needed is based on the number of independent variables included in the regression model (m) and the number of events (n). In this study, there were 39 events (3 people died, 15 had a nonfatal myocardial infarction, and 21 required a revascularization procedure to relieve chest pain), so n = 39. The model has five independent variables, so m = 5 (actually, they included and then rejected a few other variables, but we won't discuss those here). So there were about eight events per variable (n = 7.8 m). The sample size was a bit lower than the lowest recommended. Of course, when planning a study, the investigators rarely can choose the number of events. Instead, they choose the number of subjects and must predict the number of events.

f.   The whole point of the study is to ask whether the high coronary artery calcium score is associated with more cardiac events. More than half of the events tracked by this study were procedures (angioplasty or coronary artery surgery) to increase flow through blocked coronary arteries. If the decision to perform these procedures was based on the high coronary calcium levels, then the study would be meaningless. It would show that high calcium levels in coronary arteries are associated with procedures performed because the calcium level is high. Testing that kind of tautology is not helpful.

The authors recognized this problem and tried to avoid it. They did not count procedures performed on patients without acute symptoms and did not count procedures performed because of the high calcium levels. But it seems that the people deciding whether to perform the angioplasty or coronary artery bypass knew the calcium score and could have used that score as part of their decision-making process. If this happened, the results would be impossible to interpret.

g.   It is easiest to think of an odds ratio as an approximation of a relative risk. The odds ratio reported by logistic regression for having a coronary artery calcium score greater than 160 equals 14.3. Logistic regression is used when the outcome is binary. Here, the outcome is having a coronary event (death, heart attack, or need for angioplasty or coronary artery surgery) within 3–4 years.

Someone with a calcium score greater than 160 has 14.3 times the risk of having a coronary event than someone who has a calcium score less than 160 but is in the same age group (greater or less than 55) and is matched for the other three variables (presence or absence of elevated cholesterol, elevated blood pressure, or diabetes).

Of course, this odds ratio is meaningful only within the population these investigators studied. They decided not to include anyone who already had a heart attack, so this study cannot compute the odds ratio for having a second heart attack. The study excluded anyone who had chest pains, so the results cannot be used to predict future coronary events in someone with chest pain.

Appendices

APPENDIX A

___

Statistics With GraphPad

WHAT IS GRAPHPAD PRISM?

All the figures in this book were created with GraphPad Prism, and most of the analyses mentioned in this book can be performed with Prism (but not multiple and logistic regression).

GraphPad Prism, available for both Windows and Macintosh computers, combines scientific graphing, curve fitting, and basic biostatistics. It differs from other statistics programs in many ways:

- Statistical guidance. Prism helps you make the right choices and make sense of the results. If you like the style of this book, then you'll appreciate the help built in to Prism.
- Analysis checklists. After completing any analysis in Prism, click the clipboard icon to see an analysis checklist. Prism shows you a list of questions to ask yourself to make sure you've picked an appropriate analysis.
- Nonlinear regression. Some statistics programs can't fit curves with nonlinear regression and others provide only the basics. Nonlinear regression is one of Prism's strengths, and it provides many options (remove outliers, compare models, compare curves, interpolate standard curves, etc.).
- Automatic updating. Prism remembers the links between data, analysis choices, results, and graphs. When you edit or replace the data, Prism automatically updates the results and graphs.
- Analysis choices can be reviewed and changed at any time.
- Error bars. You don't have to decide in advance. Enter raw data and then choose whether to graph each value or the mean with SD, SEM, or CI. Try different ways to present the data.

WHAT YOU NEED TO KNOW BEFORE LEARNING
GRAPHPAD PRISM

Prism is designed so you can just plunge in and use it without reading instructions. But avoid the temptation to sail past the Welcome dialog so you can go straight to the analyses. Instead, spend a few moments understanding the choices on the Welcome dialog (Figure A1). This is where you start a new data table and graph, open a Prism file, or clone a graph from one you've made before.

The key to using Prism effectively is to choose the right kind of table for your data, because Prism's data tables are arranged differently than those used by most statistics programs. For example, if you want to compare three means with one-way ANOVA, you enter the three sets of data into three different columns in a data table formatted for entry of column data. With some other programs, you'd enter all the data into one column and also enter a grouping variable into

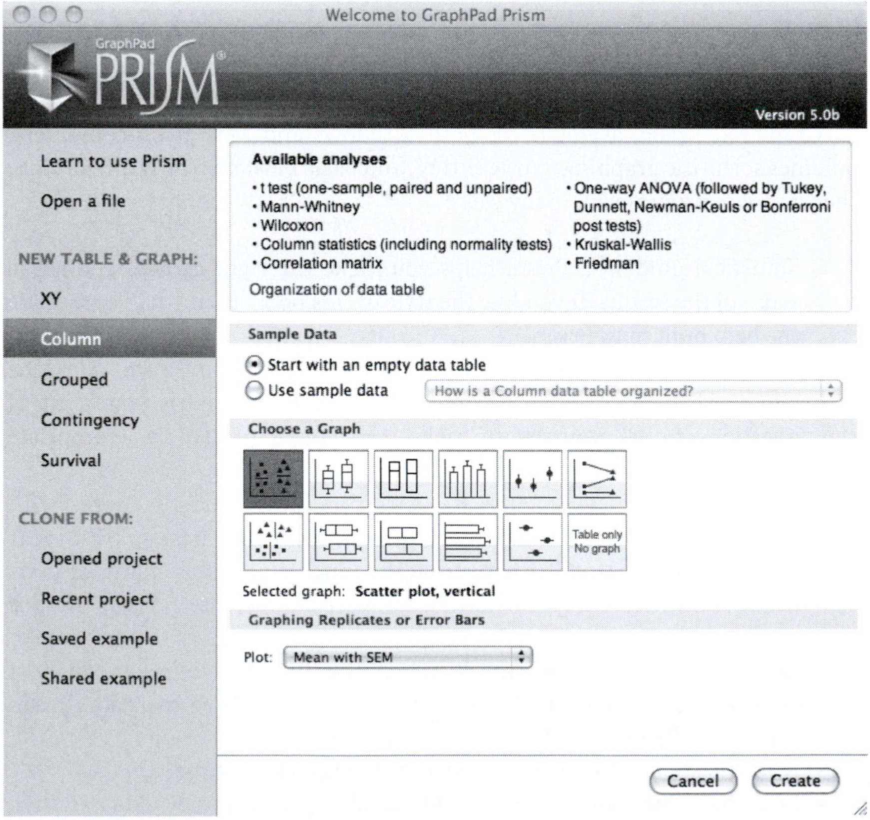

Figure A1. The Welcome dialog of GraphPad Prism.
Before entering data, you must choose which kind of data table is appropriate for your data. You can also choose sample data sets, complete with instructions.

another column to define which group each value belongs to. Prism does not use grouping variables.

To understand how the various tables are organized, start by choosing some of the sample data sets built in to Prism. These sample data sets come with explanations about how the data are organized and how to perform the analysis you want. After experimenting with several sample data sets, you'll be ready to analyze your own data.

You can download a free demo from www.graphpad.com. The demo is fully functional for 30 days (and can be extended for 15 more days).

ABOUT GRAPHPAD SOFTWARE

History

I wrote the first GraphPad program in 1984 and founded GraphPad Software, Inc., in 1989. The statistics programs available then were wonderful tools for statisticians, but were overkill for scientists and researchers with limited statistical backgrounds. I created GraphPad Software to provide data analysis software designed for students and scientists, with plenty of statistical guidance built in. Today, a dozen full-time programmers develop GraphPad programs. More than a hundred thousand scientists and students around the world use Prism, and thousands use our free Web QuickCalcs every day.

GraphPad StatMate

GraphPad StatMate helps you decide how many data points you'll need for an experiment (Figure A2). The concepts of power and sample size were explained in Chapter 43.

Some programs ask how much statistical power you desire and how large an effect you are looking for and then tell you what sample size you should use. The problem with this approach is most people find those questions impossible to answer. You want to design a study with very high power to detect very small effects and with a very strict definition of statistical significance. But doing so requires a huge number of subjects, more than you can afford.

StatMate uses a unique approach. First, you define the experimental system. If you are comparing two means, you must estimate the SD (from previous data). StatMate then shows you a table of the size of the effect (difference between means) that can be detected as a function of power (various values shown) and sample size. This table shows you the tradeoffs among power, sample size, and detectable effect.

StatMate also helps you interpret experiments where the effect is not statistically significant. This doesn't prove that a treatment had zero effect (see Chapter 19), only that the observed effect is not greater than you'd often see by chance. StatMate shows you the power of your completed experiment to detect various hypothetical differences.

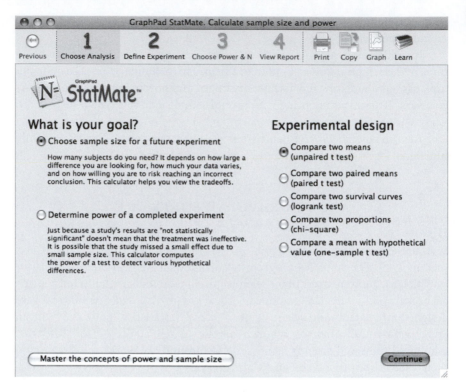

Figure A2. The opening screen of GraphPad StatMate.

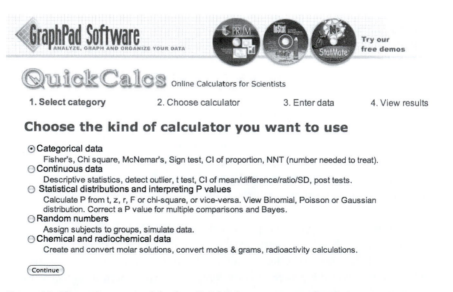

Figure A3. The main screen of the free QuickCalcs at www.graphpad.com.

GraphPad InStat

GraphPad InStat makes it really simple to do basic statistical calculations. Unlike Prism, it doesn't make customizable graphs, doesn't fit curves with nonlinear regression, doesn't analyze survival data, and cannot do two-way ANOVA. The advantage of InStat is that it guides you through every step, so there is no learning curve at all.

Free GraphPad Web QuickCalcs

QuickCalcs are free calculators on www.graphpad.com. We call them calculators because you enter data and instantly get back results, without saving or opening files.

The QuickCalcs system offers a diverse array of calculations (Figure A3). The most popular calculators include t test, outlier detection, chi-square, CI of a proportion or count, and calculating a P value from a statistical ratio (i.e., t or F). All of the calculators are either self-explanatory or link to longer explanations.

Statistics With Excel

THE PROS AND CONS OF USING EXCEL FOR STATISTICAL CALCULATIONS

Microsoft Excel is widely used and is a great program for managing and wrangling data sets. Excel has some statistical capabilities, and many also use it to do some statistical calculations.

The use of Excel for statistics is somewhat controversial, and some recommend that Excel not be used for statistics. One problem is that Excel is far from a complete statistics program. It lacks nonparametric tests, multiple comparison tests following ANOVA, and many others tests. Another problem is that Excel reports statistical results without all the supporting details other programs provide.

More seriously, Excel uses some poor algorithms for computing statistics, which can lead to incorrect results (Knusel, 2005; McCullough & Wilson, 2005). Microsoft responded to these criticisms and fixed many issues in Excel 2003 (Microsoft, 2006). Don't use earlier versions of Excel for statistical work.

Unfortunately, some errors remain in Excel 2007 for Windows and Excel 2008 for Mac. McCullough and Hellser (2008) pointed out many erroneous results produced by Excel 2007 (especially its Solver) and concluded, "Microsoft has repeatedly proved itself incapable of providing reliable statistical functionality." Yalta (2008) reached a similar conclusion, that "the accuracy of various statistical functions in Excel 2007 range from unacceptably bad to acceptable but inferior." In contrast, Pace (2008) concludes that Microsoft has fixed the important bugs, leaving only statistical bugs that are trivial or obscure. He concludes that Excel 2007 is a reasonable choice for analyzing the kinds of data most academics and professionals collect.

Given these problems, you should use another program to check important calculations, especially if your data seem unusual or include missing values.

WHAT YOU NEED TO KNOW BEFORE USING EXCEL FOR STATISTICS

- If you want to compute the mean of a range of numbers, there is no MEAN() function. Use the AVERAGE() function.
- Excel has no function to compute the SEM. You'll need to compute from the SD and n using this equation:

   STDEV (range)/SQRT (COUNT (range))

- To compute most CIs, you must know the critical value of t (called t* in this book) for specified number of df and confidence (C, in percent, usually 95). Do not use Excel's Confidence() function, which is based on the z (normal) distribution, rather than the t distribution, and so has limited utility. Use this syntax:

   TINV (1–0.01 * C, df)

- The Help within Excel does not always provide useful information about statistical functions. Google for other sources of information.
- Excel provides an Analysis ToolPak, which can perform some statistical tests. You need to use the Add-in manager to install it before you can use it. Unlike Excel equations, the results of the ToolPak are not linked to the data. If you edit the data, the results remain fixed until you run the analysis again.
- Beware of Excel's RANK() function. Nonparametric tests give all tied values the average of the ranks they tie for. Excel's RANK() function gives all tied values the lowest of the ranks they tie for, and the other ranks are not used.
- Beware of the NORMDIST(z) function (Gaussian distribution). It looks like it ought to be similar to the TDIST(t) function (Student t distribution), but the two work very differently. Experiment with sample data before using that function.
- The excellent book by Pace (2008) gives many details about using Excel to do statistical calculations. It can be purchased as either a printed book or as a pdf download.

Statistics With R

Some things in R are incredibly easy to do; other tasks are bizarrely difficult. Such an environment can be strange and perplexing at first.

Matt Briggs (2008)

WHAT IS R?

R is a popular software environment (for Windows, Macintosh, and Unix computers) for manipulating, analyzing, and graphing data. Two short introductions are a short article by Burns (2005) and a longer one by Robinson (2008). Learn about R, and download it, from: www.r-project.org.

WHAT YOU NEED TO KNOW BEFORE LEARNING R

- R is free and widely available.
- R is a programming environment. You write commands and get back answers. This gives it great power, but also makes it hard to get started.
- You don't interact with R via dialogs and menus and buttons like most Windows and Mac software. Instead, using R feels like having an instant message session with the computer.
- Almost every statistical and bioinformatics analysis has been implemented in R. It is comprehensive.
- Running some analyses require that you first install add-on software (called a package), as well as R.
- When you run an analysis, the results are stored in an object and R presents only a few key results. You can then enter new commands to query that object to get more details.
- The R language is case sensitive. If you accidentally enter an uppercase letter ("A") when R expects a lowercase letter ("a"), the command won't work.

- You can save R commands in files and then run those R programs. This means you can share R files.
- R is related to S. If you read about a statistical method implemented in S (or S-plus), it will almost certainly also work in R.
- R comes with only a rudimentary spreadsheet-like data editor. You can type values into its session or ask it to read text files. Extensions provide table editors and let it access databases or files created by other statistics programs.
- R includes lots of online help to explain its syntax, but this online help generally assumes you already understand the tests you are using and the results they produce.

APPENDIX D

Values of the t Distribution Needed to Compute CIs

df	DESIRED CONFIDENCE LEVEL				df	DESIRED CONFIDENCE LEVEL			
	80%	90%	95%	99%		80%	90%	95%	99%
1	3.0777	6.3138	12.7062	63.6567	27	1.3137	1.7033	2.0518	2.7707
2	1.8856	2.9200	4.3027	9.9248	28	1.3125	1.7011	2.0484	2.7633
3	1.6377	2.3534	3.1824	5.8409	29	1.3114	1.6991	2.0452	2.7564
4	1.5332	2.1318	2.7764	4.6041	30	1.3104	1.6973	2.0423	2.7500
5	1.4759	2.0150	2.5706	4.0321	35	1.3062	1.6896	2.0301	2.7238
6	1.4398	1.9432	2.4469	3.7074	40	1.3031	1.6839	2.0211	2.7045
7	1.4149	1.8946	2.3646	3.4995	45	1.3006	1.6794	2.0141	2.6896
8	1.3968	1.8595	2.3060	3.3554	50	1.2987	1.6759	2.0086	2.6778
9	1.3830	1.8331	2.2622	3.2498	55	1.2971	1.6730	2.0040	2.6682
10	1.3722	1.8125	2.2281	3.1693	60	1.2958	1.6706	2.0003	2.6603
11	1.3634	1.7959	2.2010	3.1058	65	1.2947	1.6686	1.9971	2.6536
12	1.3562	1.7823	2.1788	3.0545	70	1.2938	1.6669	1.9944	2.6479
13	1.3502	1.7709	2.1604	3.0123	75	1.2929	1.6654	1.9921	2.6430
14	1.3450	1.7613	2.1448	2.9768	80	1.2922	1.6641	1.9901	2.6387
15	1.3406	1.7531	2.1314	2.9467	85	1.2916	1.6630	1.9883	2.6349
16	1.3368	1.7459	2.1199	2.9208	90	1.2910	1.6620	1.9867	2.6316
17	1.3334	1.7396	2.1098	2.8982	95	1.2905	1.6611	1.9853	2.6286
18	1.3304	1.7341	2.1009	2.8784	100	1.2901	1.6602	1.9840	2.6259
19	1.3277	1.7291	2.0930	2.8609	150	1.2872	1.6551	1.9759	2.6090
20	1.3253	1.7247	2.0860	2.8453	200	1.2858	1.6525	1.9719	2.6006
21	1.3232	1.7207	2.0796	2.8314	250	1.2849	1.6510	1.9695	2.5956
22	1.3212	1.7171	2.0739	2.8188	300	1.2844	1.6499	1.9679	2.5923
23	1.3195	1.7139	2.0687	2.8073	350	1.2840	1.6492	1.9668	2.5899
24	1.3178	1.7109	2.0639	2.7969	400	1.2837	1.6487	1.9659	2.5882
25	1.3163	1.7081	2.0595	2.7874	450	1.2834	1.6482	1.9652	2.5868
26	1.3150	1.7056	2.0555	2.7787	500	1.2832	1.6479	1.9647	2.5857

The margin of error of many CIs equals the standard error times a critical value of the t distribution tabulated above. Its value depends on the desired confidence level and the number of df, which equals n minus the number of parameters estimated.

Excel can compute the values tabulated above. Don't use Excel's Confidence() function, which is based on the z (normal) distribution, rather than the t distribution, and so has limited utility. Use this formula for a specified number of df and confidence (C, in percent, usually 95):

TINV (1–0.01*C, df)

APPENDIX E

A Review of Logarithms

COMMON (BASE 10) LOGARITHMS

The best way to understand logarithms is through an example. If you take 10 to the third power (10×10×10), the result is 1,000. The logarithm is the inverse of that power function. The logarithm (base 10) of 1,000 is the power of 10 that gives the answer 1,000. So the logarithm of 1,000 is 3. If you multiply 10 by itself 3 times, you get 1,000.

You can take 10 to a negative power. For example, taking 10 to the −3 power is the same as taking the reciprocal of 10^3. So 10^{-3} equals $1/10^3$, or 0.001. The logarithm of 0.001 is the power of 10 that equals 0.001, which is −3.

You can take 10 to a fractional power. Ten to the ½ power equals the square root of 10, which is 3.163. So the logarithm of 3.163 is 0.5.

Ten to the zero power equals 1, so the logarithm of 1.0 is 0.0.

You can take the logarithm of any positive number. The logarithms of values between zero and 1 are negative; the logarithms of values greater than 1 are positive. The logarithms of zero and all negative numbers are undefined; there is no power of 10 that gives a negative number or zero.

OTHER BASES

The logarithms shown in the previous section are called base 10 logarithms, because the computations take 10 to some power. These are also called common logarithms.

You can compute logarithms for any power. Mathematicians prefer natural logarithms, using base e (2.7183...). By convention, natural logarithms are used in logistic and proportional hazards regression (Chapter 37).

Biologists sometimes use base 2 logarithms, often without realizing it. The base 2 logarithm is the number of doublings it takes to reach a value. So the log base 2 of 16 is 4 because if you start with 1 and double it four times (2, 4, 8, and

16), the result is 16. Immunologists often serially dilute antibodies by factors of 2, so they often graph data on a log2 scale. Cell biologists use base 2 logarithms to convert cell counts to number of doublings.

Logarithms using different bases are proportional to each other. So converting from natural logs to common logs is sort of like changing units. Divide a natural logarithm by 2.303 to compute the common log of the same value. Multiply a common log by 2.303 to obtain the corresponding natural log.

NOTATION

Unfortunately, the notation is used inconsistently.

The notation "log(x)" usually means the common (base 10) logarithm, but some computer languages use it to mean the natural logarithm.

The notation "ln(x)" always means natural logarithm.

The notation "$\log_{10}(x)$" clearly shows that the logarithm uses base 10.

LOGARITHMS CONVERT MULTIPLICATION INTO ADDITION

Logarithms are popular because of this equation:

$$\log (A \cdot B) = \log(A) + \log(B)$$

Similarly, as shown in Chapter 11, logarithms transform a lognormal distribution into a Gaussian distribution.

ANTILOGARITHMS

The antilogarithm (also called an antilog) is the inverse of the logarithm transform. Because the logarithm (base 10) of 1,000 equals 3, the antilogarithm of 3 is 1,000. To compute the antilogarithm of a base 10 logarithm, take 10 to that power.

To compute the antilogarithm of a natural logarithm, take e to that power. The natural logarithm of 1,000 is 6.980. So the antilogarithm of 6.908 is $e^{6.908}$, which is 1,000. Spreadsheets and computer languages use the notation exp(6.908).

REFERENCES

Agresti, A., & Coull, B. A. (1998). Approximate is better than exact for interval estimation of binomial proportions. *American Journal of Statistics, 52*, 119–126.

Allen, M. C., Donohue, P. K., & Dusman, A. E. (1993). The limit of viability—Neonatal outcome of infants born at 22 to 25 weeks' gestation. *The New England Journal of Medicine, 329*, 1597–1601.

Altman, D. G. (1990). *Practical statistics for medical research.* London: Chapman & Hall/CRC.

Altman, D. G., & Bland, J. M. (1995). Absence of evidence is not evidence of absence. *BMJ (Clinical Research Ed.), 311*, 485.

Altman, D. G., & Bland, J. M. (1998). Time to event (survival) data. *BMJ (Clinical Research Ed.), 317*, 468–469.

Anscombe, F. J. (1973). Graphs in statistical analysis. *The American Statistician, 27*, 17–21.

Arad, Y., Spadaro, L. A., Goodman, K., Newstein, D., & Guerci, A. D. (2000). Prediction of coronary events with electron beam computed tomography. *Journal of the American College of Cardiology, 36*, 1253–1260.

Arden, R., Gottfredson, L. S., Miller, G., & Pierce, A. (2008). Intelligence and semen quality are positively correlated. *Intelligence, 37*, 277–282.

Austin, P. C., & Goldwasser, M. A. (2008). Pisces did not have increased heart failure: Data-driven comparisons of binary proportions between levels of a categorical variable can result in incorrect statistical significance levels. *Journal of Clinical Epidemiology, 61*, 295–300.

Austin, P. C., Mamdani, M. M., Juurlink, D. N., & Hux, J. E. (2006). Testing multiple statistical hypotheses resulted in spurious associations: A study of astrological signs and health. *Journal of Clinical Epidemiology, 59*, 964–969.

Babyak, M. A. (2004). What you see may not be what you get: A brief, nontechnical introduction to overfitting in regression-type models. *Psychosomatic Medicine, 66*, 411–421.

Bakhshi, E., Eshraghian, M. R., Mohammad, K., & Seifi, B. (2008). A comparison of two methods for estimating odds ratios: Results from the National Health Survey. *BMC Medical Research Methodology, 8*, 78.

Barnett, V., & Lewis, T. (1994). *Outliers in statistical data* (3rd ed.). Chichester, UK: Wiley. ISBN=0471930946.

Barter, P. J., Caulfield, M., Eriksson, M., Grundy, S. M., Kastelein, J. J., Komajda, M., Lopez-Sendon, J., et al. (2007). Effects of torcetrapib in patients at high risk for coronary events. *The New England Journal of Medicine, 357,* 2109–2122.

Bausell, R. B. (2007). *Snake oil science: The truth about complementary and alternative medicine.* Oxford, UK: Oxford University Press. ISBN=0195313682.

Benjamini, Y., & Hochberg, Y. (1995). Controlling the false discovery rate: A practical and powerful approach to multiple testing. *Journal of Royal Statistical Society, B, 57,* 290–300.

Bickel, P. J., Hammel, E. A., & O'Connell, J. W. (1975). Sex bias in graduate admissions: Data from Berkeley. *Science, 187,* 398–404.

Blumberg, M. S. (2004). *Body heat: Temperature and life on earth.* Cambridge, MA: Harvard University Press. ISBN=0674013697.

Borkman, M., Storlien, L. H., Pan, D. A., Jenkins, A. B., Chisholm, D. J., & Campbell, L. V. (1993). The relation between insulin sensitivity and the fatty-acid composition of skeletal-muscle phospholipids. *The New England Journal of Medicine, 328,* 238–244.

Briggs, W. M. (2008). *Breaking the law of averages: Real-life probability and statistics in plain english.* ISBN=0557019907. Raleigh, NC: Lulu, ISBN 0557019907

Briggs, W. M. (2008) *Do not calculate correlations after smoothing data.* Retrieved June 21, 2009 25, 2008, from http://wmbriggs.com/blog/?p=86/

Briggs, W. M. (2008) *On the difference between mathematical ability between boys and girls.* Retrieved June 21, 2009, from http://wmbriggs.com/blog/?p=163/

Brown, L. D., Cai, T. T., & DasGupta, A. (2001). Interval estimation for a binomial proportion. *Statistical Science, 16,* 101–133.

Brownstein, C. A., & Brownstein, J. S. (2008). Estimating excess mortality in post-invasion Iraq. *New England Journal of Medicine, 358,* 445–448.

Burnham, K., & Anderson, D. (2003). *Model selection and multi-model inference* (2nd ed.). New York, Springer. ISBN=0387953647.

Burns, P. (2005) *A guide for the unwilling S user.* Retrieved January 26, 2009, from http://www.burns-stat.com/pages/Tutor/unwilling_S.pdf.

Campbell, M. J. (2006). *Statistics at square two* (2nd ed.). London: Blackwell. ISBN= 1-4051-3409-9.

Cantor, W. J., Fitchett, Dl, Borgundyagg, B., Ducas, J. Heffernam, M., et al. (2009) Routine early angioplasty after fibrinolysis for acute myocardial infarction, *The New England Journal of Medicine, 360,* 2705–2718.

Chan, A. W., Hrobjartsson, A., Haahr, M. T., Gotzsche, P. C., & Altman, D. G. (2004). Empirical evidence for selective reporting of outcomes in randomized trials: Comparison of protocols to published articles. *Journal of the American Medical Association, 291,* 2457–2465.

Clopper, C. J., & Pearson, E. S. (1934). The use of confidence or fiducial limits illustrated in the case of the binomial. *Biometrika, 26,* 404–413.

Cohen, J. (1988). *Statistical power analysis for the behavioral sciences* (2nd ed.). Hillsdale, NJ: Erlbaum. ISBN=0805802835.

Cohen, T. J., Goldner, B. G., Maccaro, P. C., Ardito, A. P., Trazzera, S., Cohen, M. B., et al. (1993). A comparison of active compression–decompression cardiopulmonary resuscitation with standard cardiopulmonary resuscitation for cardiac arrests occurring in the hospital. *The New England Journal of Medicine, 329,* 1918–1921.

Cooper, D. A., Gatell, J. M., Kroon, S., Clumeck, N., Millard, J., Goebel, F. D., et al. (1993). Zidovudine in persons with asymptomatic HIV infection and CD4+ cell counts greater than 400 per cubic millimeter. The European–Australian Collaborative Group. *The New England Journal of Medicine, 329*, 297–303.

Cramer, H. (1999). *Mathematical methods of statistics.* Princeton, NJ: Princeton University Press. ISBN=0691005478.

Crichton, M. (2003). *Environmentalism as religion.* Retrieved November 9, 2008, from http://www.michaelcrichton.net/speech-environmentalismaseligion.html

Crichton, M. (2005). *The case for skepticism on global warming.* Retrieved November 9, 2008, from http://www.michaelcrichton.net/speech-ourenvironmentalfuture.html

Cumming, G., Fidler, F., & Vaux, D. L. (2007). Error bars in experimental biology. *The Journal of Cell Biology, 177*, 7–11.

Darwin, C. (1876). *The effects of cross and self fertilisation in the vegetable kingdom.* London: Murray.

Davenas, E., Beauvais, F., Amara, J., Oberbaum, M., Robinzon, B., Miadonna, A., et al. (1988). Human basophil degranulation triggered by very dilute antiserum against IgE. *Nature, 333*, 816–818.

Denes-Raj, V., & Epstein, S. (1994). Conflict between intuitive and rational processing: When people behave against their better judgment. *Journal of Personality and Social Psychology, 66*, 819–829.

Ellsberg, D. (1961). Risk, ambiguity, and the savage axioms. *Quarterly Journal of Economics, 75*, 643–669.

Ewigman, B. G., Crane, J. P., Frigoletto, F. D., LeFevre, M. L., Bain, R. P., & McNellis, D. (1993). Effect of prenatal ultrasound screening on perinatal outcome. RADIUS Study Group. *The New England Journal of Medicine, 329*, 821–827.

Feinstein, A. R., Sosin, D. M., & Wells, C. K. (1985). The Will Rogers phenomenon. Stage migration and new diagnostic techniques as a source of misleading statistics for survival in cancer. *The New England Journal of Medicine, 312*, 1604–1608.

Fisher, R. A. (1935). *The design of experiments.* Hafner: Oxford University Press. ISBN =0198522290.

Fisher, R. A. (1936). Has Mendel's work been rediscovered? *Annals of Science, 1*, 115–137.

Fleming, T. R. (2006). Standard versus adaptive monitoring procedures: A commentary. *Statistics in Medicine, 25*, 3305–3512; discussion 3313–3314, 3326–3347.

Frazier, E. P., Schneider, T., & Michel, M. C. (2006). Effects of gender, age and hypertension on beta-adrenergic receptor function in rat urinary bladder. *Naunyn-Schmiedeberg's Archives of Pharmacology, 373*, 300–309.

Freedman, D. (1983). A note on screening regression equations. *The American Statistician, 37*, 152–155.

Freedman, D. (2007). *Statistics* (4th ed.). New York: Norton.

Gabriel, S. E., O'Fallon, W. M., Kurland, L. T., Beard, C. M., Woods, J. E., & Melton, L. J.,3rd. (1994). Risk of connective-tissue diseases and other disorders after breast implantation. *The New England Journal of Medicine, 330*, 1697–1702.

Gelman, A., & Hill, J. (2007). *Data analysis using regression and multilevel/hierarchical models.* New York: Cambridge press. ISBN=978-0-521-68689-1.

Gilovich, T. (1985). The hot hand in basketball: On the misperception of random sequences. *Cognitive Psychology, 17*, 295–314.

Gilovich, T. (1991). *How we know what isn't so.* New York: Free Press. ISBN=0029117062.

Glantz, S. A., & Slinker, B. K. (2000). *Primer of applied regression and analysis of variance* (2nd ed.). New York: McGraw–Hill. ISBN=0071360867.

Goddard, S. (2008). *Is the earth getting warmer, or cooler?* Retrieved June 13, 2008, from http://www.theregister.co.uk/2008/05/02/a_tale_of_two_thermometers/

Good, P. I., & Hardin, J. W. (2006). *Common errors in statistics (and how to avoid them)*. Hoboken, NJ: Wiley. ISBN=0471794317.

Gotzsche, P. C. (2006). Believability of relative risks and odds ratios in abstracts: Cross sectional study. *BMJ (Clinical Research Ed.), 333,* 231–234.

Gould, S. J. (1997). *Full house: The spread of excellence from Plato to Darwin.* New York: Three Rivers Press. ISBN=0609801406.

Greco, W. R. (1989). Importance of the structural component of generalized nonlinear models for joint drug action. *Proceedings of the American Statistics Association, Biopharmaceutics Section,* 183–189.

Green, S. (1991). How many subjects does it take to do a regression analysis? *Multivariate Behavioral Research, 26,* 499–510.

Guyatt, G. H., Keller, J. L., Jaeschke, R., Rosenbloom, D., Adachi, J. D., & Newhouse, M. T. (1990). The n-of-1 randomized controlled trial: clinical usefulness. Our three-year experience. *Annals of Internal Medicine, 112,* 293–299.

Hand, D. J., Daly, F., McConway, K., Lunn, D., & Ostrowski, E. (1993). *A handbook of small data sets.* London: Chapman & Hall/CRC. ISBN=0412399202.

Hanley, J. A., & Lippman-Hand, A. (1983). If nothing goes wrong, is everything alright? *Journal of the American Medical Association, 259,* 1743–1745.

Harter, H. L. (1984). Another look at plotting positions. *Communications in Statistics— Theory and Methods, 13,* 1613–1633.

Hartung, J. (2005). Statistics: When to suspect a false negative inference. In *American Society of Anesthesiology 56th Annual Meeting Refresher Course Lectures* (Lecture 377, pp. 1–7). Philadelphia: Lippincott.

Heal, C. F., Buettner, P. G., Cruickshank, R., & Graham, D. (2009). Does single application of topical chloramphenicol to high risk sutured wounds reduce incidence of wound infection after minor surgery? Prospective randomised placebo controlled double blind trial. *British Medical Journal, 338,* 211–214.

Hetland, M. L., Haarbo, J., Christiansen, C., & Larsen, T. (1993). Running induces menstrual disturbances but bone mass is unaffected, except in amenorrheic women. *The American Journal of Medicine, 95,* 53–60.

Hoenig, J. M., & Heisey, D. M. (2001). The abuse of power: The pervasive fallacy of power. Calculations for data analysis. *American Statistician, 55,* 1–6.

Hollis, S., & Campbell, F. (1999). What is meant by intention to treat analysis? Survey of published randomised controlled trials. *BMJ (Clinical Research Ed.), 319,* 670–674.

Hsu, J. (1996). *Multiple comparisons: Theory and methods.* Boca Raton, FL: Chapman & Hall/CRC. ISBN=0412982811.

Hsu, M., Bhatt, M., Adolphs, R., Tranel, D., & Camerer, C. F. (2005). Neural systems responding to degrees of uncertainty in human decision-making. *Science, 310,* 1680–1683.

Huber, P. J. (2003). *Robust statistics.* Hoboken, NJ: Wiley–Interscience. ISBN=0471650722.

Hunter, D. J., Manson, J. E., Colditz, G. A., Stampfer, M. J., Rosner, B., Hennekens, C., et al. (1993). A prospective study of the intake of vitamins C, E, and A and the risk of breast cancer. *New England Journal of Medicine, 329,* 234–240.

Hyde, J. S., Lindberg, S. M., Linn, M. C., Ellis, A. B., & Williams, C. C. (2008). Diversity. Gender similarities characterize math performance. *Science, 321*, 494–495.

Ioannidis, J. P. (2005). Why most published research findings are false. *PLoS Medicine, 2*, e124.

Ioannidis, J. P. (2008). Why most discovered true associations are inflated. *Epidemiology, 19*, 640–648.

Kales, S. N., Soteriades, E. S., Christophi, C. A., & Christiani, D. C. (2007). Emergency duties and deaths from heart disease among firefighters in the United States. *The New England Journal of Medicine, 356*, 1207–1215.

Katz, M. H. (2006). *Multivariable analysis: A practical guide for clinicians.* Cambridge, UK: Cambridge University Press. ISBN=052154985x.

Kaul, A., & Diamond, G. (2006). Good enough: A primer on the analysis and interpretation of noninferiority trials. *Annals of Internal Medicine, 145*, 62–69.

Kirk, A. P., Jain, S., Pocock, S., Thomas, H. C., & Sherlock, S. (1980). Late results of the Royal Free Hospital prospective controlled trial of prednisolone therapy in hepatitis B surface antigen negative chronic active hepatitis. *Gut, 21*, 78–83.

Knusel, L. (2005). On the accuracy of statistical distributions in Microsoft Excel 2003. *Computational Statistics and Data Analysis, 48*, 445–449.

Kuehn, B. (2006). Industry, FDA warm to "adaptive" trials. *Journal of the American Medical Association, 296*, 1955–1957.

Lanzante, J. R. (2005). A cautionary note on the use of error bars. *Journal of Climate, 18*, 3699–3703.

Laupacis, A., Sackett, D. L., & Roberts, R. S. (1988). An assessment of clinically useful measures of the consequences of treatment. *The New England Journal of Medicine, 318*, 1728–1733.

Lee, K. L., McNeer, J. F., Starmer, C. F., Harris, P. J., & Rosati, R. A. (1980). Clinical judgment and statistics. Lessons from a simulated randomized trial in coronary artery disease. *Circulation, 61*, 508–515.

Lehman, E. (2007). *Nonparametrics: Statistical methods based on ranks.* New York: Springer. ISBN=0387352120.

Lenth, R. V. (2001). Some practical guidelines for effective sample size determination. *The American Statistician, 55*, 187–193.

Levine, M., & Ensom, M. H. (2001). Post hoc power analysis: An idea whose time has passed? *Pharmacotherapy, 21*, 405–409.

Levins, R. (1966). The strategy of model building in population biology. *American Scientist, 54*, 421–431.

Lewin, T. (2008). *Math scores show no gap for girls, study finds.* Retrieved July 26, 2008, from http://www.nytimes.com/2008/07/25/education/25math.html

Limpert, E., Stahel, W. A., & Abbt, M. (2001). Log-normal distributions across the sciences: Keys and clues. *Biosciences, 51*, 341–352.

Lucas, M. E. S., Deen, J. L., von Seidlein, L., Wang, X., Ampuero, J., Puri, M., et al. (2005). Effectiveness of mass oral cholera vaccination in Beira, Mozambique. *The New England Journal of Medicine, 352*, 757–767.

Ludbrook, L., & Lew, M. J. (2009). Estimating the risk of rare complications: Is the "rule of three" good enough? *Australian and New Zealand Journal of Surgery, 79*, 565–570.

Machin, D., Cheung, Y. B., & Parmar, M. (2006). *Survival analysis: A practical approach* (2nd ed.). Chichester, UK: Wiley. ISBN=0470870400.

Mackowiak, P. A., Wasserman, S. S., & Levine, M. M. (1992). A critical appraisal of 98.6 degrees F, the upper limit of the normal body temperature, and other legacies of Carl Reinhold August Wunderlich. *Journal of the American Medical Association, 268*, 1578–1580.

Manly, B. F. J. (2006). *Randomization, bootstrap and Monte Carlo methods in biology* (3rd ed.). London: Chapman & Hall/CRC. ISBN=1584885416.

Maxwell, S. E., & Delaney, H. D. (2004). *Designing experiments and analyzing data.* Mahwah, NJ: Erlbaum. ISBN=0805837183.

McCullough, B. D., & Hellser, D. A. (2008). On the accuracy of statistical procedures in Microsoft Excel 2007. *Computational Statistics and Data Analysis, 52*, 4570–4578.

McCullough, B. D., & Wilson, B. (2005). On the accuracy of statistical procedures in Microsoft Excel 2003. *Computational Statistics and Data Analysis, 49*, 1244.

Meyers, M. A. (2007). *Happy accidents: Serendipity in modern medical breakthroughs.* New York: Arcade. ISBN=1559708190.

Micceri, T. (1989). The unicorn, the normal curve, and other improbable creatures. *Psychological Bulletin, 105*, 156–166.

Microsoft. (2006). *Description of improvements in the statistical functions in Excel 2003 and in Excel 2004 for Mac.* Retrieved December 16, 2008, from http://support.microsoft.com/kb/828888

Mills, J. L. (1993). Data torturing. *New England Journal of Medicine, 329*, 1196.

Montori, V. M., Kleinbart, J., Newman, T. B., Keitz, S., Wyer, P. C., Moyer, V., et al. (2004). Tips for learners of evidence-based medicine: 2. Measures of precision (confidence intervals). *Canadian Medical Association Journal ,171*, 611–615.

Moser, B. K., & Stevens, G. R. (1992). Homogeneity of variance in the two-sample means test. *The American Statistician, 46*, 19–21.

Motulsky, H. J., & Brown, R. E. (2006). Detecting outliers when fitting data with non-linear regression—A new method based on robust nonlinear regression and the false discovery rate. *BMC Bioinformatics, 7*, 123.

Motulsky, H., & Christopoulos, A. (2004). *Fitting models to biological data using linear and nonlinear regression: A practical guide to curve fitting.* New York: Oxford University Press.

Motulsky, H. J., O'Connor, D. T., & Insel, P. A. (1983). Platelet alpha 2-adrenergic receptors in treated and untreated essential hypertension. *Clinical Science, 64*, 265–272.

New Scientist. (2007, November 10). *NASA blows millions on flawed airline safety survey.* Retrieved May 25, 2008, from http://www.newscientist.com/channel/opinion/mg19626293.900-nasa-blows-millions-on-flawed-airline-safety-survey.html

Nikles, C. J., Yelland, M., Glasziou, P. P., & Del Mar, C. (2005). Do individualized medication effectiveness tests (n-of-1 trials) change clinical decisions about which drugs to use for osteoarthritis and chronic pain? *American Journal of Therapeutics, 12*, 92–97.

Pace, L. A. (2008). *The Excel 2007 data & statistics cookbook* (2nd ed.). Anderson, SC: TwoPaces. ISBN=978-0-9799775-2-7.

Parker, R. A., & Berman, N. G. (2003). Sample size: More than calculations. *The American Statistician, 57*, 166–170.

Paulos, J. A. (2007). *Irreligion: A mathematician explains why the arguments for god just don't add up.* New York: Hill and Wang. ISBN=0809059193.

Payton, M. E., Greenstone, M. H., & Schenker, N. (2003). Overlapping confidence intervals or standard error intervals: What do they mean in terms of statistical significance? *Journal of Insect Science, 3*, 34–40.

Pielke, R. (2008). *Prometheus: Forecast verification for climate science, part 3.* Retrieved April 20, 2008, from http://sciencepolicy.colorado.edu/prometheus/archives/climate_change/001315forecast_verificatio.html

Pullan, R.D., Rhodes, J., Gatesh, S. et al. Transdermal nicotine for active ulcerative colitis. *New England Journal of Medicine, 330: 811–815.*

Ridker, P. M., Danielson, E., Fonseca, F. A. H., Genest, J., Gotto, A. M., Jr., Kastelein, J. J. P., et al. (2008). Rosuvastatin to prevent vascular events in men and women with elevated C-reactive protein. *The New England Journal of Medicine, 359,* 2195–2207.

Roberts, S. (2004). Self-experimentation as a source of new ideas: Ten examples about sleep, mood, health, and weight. *The Behavioral and Brain Sciences, 27,* 227–262; discussion 262–287.

Robinson, A. (2008) *icebreakeR.* Retrieved January 26, 2009, from http://cran.r-project.org/doc/contrib/Robinson-icebreaker.pdf

Rosman, N. P., Colton, T., Labazzo, J., Gilbert, P. L., Gardella, N. B., Kaye, E. M., et al. (1993). A controlled trial of diazepam administered during febrile illnesses to prevent recurrence of febrile seizures. *The New England Journal of Medicine, 329,* 79–84.

Rothman, K. J. (1990). No adjustments are needed for multiple comparisons. *Epidemiology,* 1, 43–46.

Russo, J. E., & Schoemaker, P. J. H. (1989). *Decision traps. The ten barriers to brilliant decision-asking and how to overcome them.* New York: Simon & Schuster. ISBN=0671726099.

Sawilowsky, S. S. (2005). Misconceptions leading to choosing the t test over the Wilcoxon Mann–Whitney test for shift in location parameter. *Journal of Modern Applied Statistical Methods, 4,* 598–600.

Schoemaker, A. L. (1996). What's normal?—Temperature, gender, and heart rate. *Journal of Statistics Education, 4:2.* Retrieved May 5, 2007 from http://www.amstat.org/publications/jse/v4n2/datasets.shoemaker.html

Seaman, M. A., Levin, J. R., & Serlin, R. C. (1991). New developments in pairwise multiple comparisons: Some powerful and practicable procedures. *Psychological Bulletin, 110,* 577–586.

Sheskin, D. J. (2007). *Handbook of Parametric and Nonparametric Statistical Procedures: Fourth Edition.* New York, NY: Chapman & Hall/CRC. ISBN=1584888148.

Simon, S. (2005, May 16). *Stats: Standard deviation versus standard error.* Retrieved March 5, 2008, from http://www.childrens-mercy.org/stats/weblog2005/standarderror.asp

Snapinn, S. M. (2000). Noninferiority trials. *Current Control Trials in Cardiovascular Medicine, 1,* 19–21.

Sparling, B. (2001). *Ozone history.* Retrieved June 13, 2008, from http://www.nas.nasa.gov/About/Education/Ozone/history.html

Spector, R., Vesell, E.S. (2006a). The heart of drug discovery and development: rational target selection. *Pharmacology, 77:* 85–92.

Spector R., Vesell, E.S. (2006b). Pharmacology and statistics: recommendations to strengthen a productive partnership. *Pharmacology,* 78:113–122.

Staessen, J. A., Lauwerys, R. R., Buchet, J. P., Bulpitt, C. J., Rondia, D., Vanrenterghem, Y., et al. (1992). Impairment of renal function with increasing blood lead concentrations in the general population. The Cadmibel Study Group. *The New England Journal of Medicine, 327,* 151–156.

Taubes, G. (1995). Epidemiology faces its limits. *Science, 269,* 164–169.

Thun, M. J., & Sinks, T. (2004). Understanding cancer clusters. *CA: A Cancer Journal for Clinicians, 54,* 273–280.

Tierney, J. (2008) *A spot check of global warming*. Retrieved April 20, 2008, from http://tierneylab.blogs.nytimes.com/2008/01/10/a-spot-check-of-global-warming/

Turner, E. H., Matthews, A. M., Linardatos, E., Tell, R. A., & Rosenthal, R. (2008). Selective publication of antidepressant trials and its influence on apparent efficacy. *The New England Journal of Medicine, 358*, 252–260.

van Belle, G. (2008). *Statistical rules of thumb* (2nd ed.). New York: Wiley–Interscience. ISBN=0470144483.

Velleman, P. F., & Wilkinson, L. (1993). Nominal, ordinal, interval, and ratio typologies are misleading. *The American Statistician, 47*, 65–72.

Vickers, A. J. (2006a). Michael Jordan won't accept the null hypothesis: Notes on interpreting high P values. *Medscape Business of Medicine, 7:1*. Retrieved May 23, 2008, from http://www.medscape.com/viewarticle/531928_print.

Vickers, A. J. (2006b). Shoot first and ask questions later: How to approach statistics like a real clinician. *Medscape Business of Medicine, 7:2*. Retrieved June 19, 2009, from http://www.medscape.com/viewarticle/540898

Vittinghoff, E., Glidden, D. V., Shiboski, S. C., & McCulloch, C. E. (2007). *Regression methods in biostatistics: Linear, logistic, survival, and repeated measures models (statistics for biology and health)*. New York: Springer. ISBN=0387202757.

Vos Savant, M. (1997). *The power of logical thinking: Easy lessons in the art of reasoning…and hard facts about its absence in our lives*. New York: St. Martin's Griffin. ISBN=0312156278.

Welch, A. (1998). *If he's explaining beauty, he's just doing his job*. Retrieved February 17, 2009, from http://www.fsu.edu/~fstime/FS-Times/Volume4/aug98web/14aug98.html

Wellek, S. (2002). *Testing statistical hypotheses of equivalence*. Boca Raton, FL: Chapman & Hall/CRC. ISBN=1584881607.

Westfall, P., Tobias, R., Rom, D., Wolfinger, R., & Hochberg,Y. (1999) *Multiple comparisons and multiple tests using the SAS system*. Cary, NC: SAS Publishing. ISBN=1580253970.

Wilcox, R. R. (2001). *Fundamentals of modern statistical methods: Substantially improving power and accuracy*. New York: Springer-Verlag. ISBN=0387951571.

Wolff, A. (2002, Jan. 21). *That old black magic*. Retrieved May 25, 2008, from http://sportsillustrated.cnn.com/2003/magazine/08/27/jinx/

Xu, F., & Garcia, V. (2008). Intuitive statistics by 8-month-old infants. *Proceedings of the National Academy of Sciences of the United States of America, 105*, 5012–5015.

Yalta, A. T. (2008). The accuracy of statistical distributions in Microsoft Excel 2007. *Computational Statistics and Data Analysis, 52*, 4579–4586.

Yamagishi, K. (1997). When a 12.86% mortality is more dangerous than 24.14%: Implications for risk communication. *Applied Cognitive Psychology, 11*, 495–506.

Zhang, J. H., Chung, T. D., & Oldenburg, K. R. (1999). A simple statistical parameter for use in evaluation and validation of high throughput screening assays. *Journal of Biomolecular Screening, 4*, 67–73.

Ziliak, S., & McCloskey, D. N. (2008). *The cult of statistical significance: How the standard error costs us jobs, justice, and lives*. Ann Arbor, MI: University of Michigan Press. ISBN=0472050079.

Zollner, S., & Pritchard, J. K. (2007). Overcoming the winner's curse: Estimating penetrance parameters from case–control data. *American Journal of Human Genetics, 80*, 605–615.

INDEX